HELE

Baillière's
CLINICAL ENDOCRINOLOGY AND METABOLISM

INTERNATIONAL PRACTICE AND RESEARCH

Baillière's

CLINICAL ENDOCRINOLOGY AND METABOLISM

INTERNATIONAL PRACTICE AND RESEARCH

Volume 1/Number 1
February 1987

Reproductive Endocrinology

H. G. BURGER MD, FRACP
Guest Editor

Baillière Tindall London Philadelphia Toronto
Mexico City Sydney Tokyo Hong Kong

Baillière Tindall   33 The Avenue
W.B. Saunders   Eastbourne, East Sussex BN21 3UN, UK

West Washington Square
Philadelphia, PA 19105, USA

1 Goldthorne Avenue
Toronto, Ontario M8Z 5T9, Canada

Apartado 26370—Cedro 512
Mexico 4, DF Mexico

9 Waltham Street
Artarmon, NSW 2064, Australia

10/fl, Inter-Continental Plaza, 94 Granville Road
Tsim Sha Tsui East, Kowloon, Hong Kong

Exclusive Agent in Japan:
Maruzen Co. Ltd. (Journals Division)
3–10 Nihonbashi 2-chome, Chuo-ku, Tokyo 103, Japan

ISSN 0950–351X

ISBN 0–7020–1206–8 (single copy)

Baillière's Clinical Endocrinology and Metabolism is published four times each year by Baillière Tindall. Annual subscription prices are:

TERRITORY	ANNUAL SUBSCRIPTION	SINGLE ISSUE
1. UK & Republic of Ireland	£35.00 post free	£15.00 post free
2. USA & Canada	US\$60.00 post free	US\$25.00 post free
3. All other countries	£45.00 post free	£18.50 post free

The editor of this publication is Nicholas Dunton, Baillière Tindall,
33 The Avenue, Eastbourne, East Sussex BN21 3UN, England.

Baillière's Clinical Endocrinology and Metabolism was published from 1972 to 1986 as *Clinics in Endocrinology and Metabolism*.

Typeset by Phoenix Photosetting, Chatham.
Printed and bound in Great Britain by Mackays of Chatham Ltd.

Contributors to this issue

JUDY ADAMS SRN, SRCN, DMU, Senior Ultrasonographer, Department of X-Ray and Imaging, The Middlesex Hospital, Mortimer Street, London W1N 8AA, UK.

DAVID T. BAIRD DSc, MB, ChB, FRCP, FRCOG, Clinical Research Professor, Medical Research Council, Centre for Reproductive Biology, 37 Chalmers Street, Edinburgh EH3 9EW, UK.

ETIENNE EMILE BAULIEU MD, PhD, Professor of Biochemistry, Medical School, Université Paris Sud; Director of Research, U 33 INSERM, Hôpital Bicêtre, 78 rue du Gal Leclerc, 94270 Bicêtre, France.

MANDY BESANKO BSc (Honours), Monash University, Department of Obstetrics and Gynaecology, Queen Victoria Medical Centre, 172 Lonsdale Street, Melbourne, Australia 3000.

WILLIAM J. BREMNER MD, PhD, Associate Professor of Medicine, University of Washington School of Medicine; Chief, Endocrine Section, Veterans Administration Medical Centre (182B), 1660 Columbian Way, Seattle, Washington 98108, USA.

C. G. D. BROOK MA, MD, FRCP, DCH, Consultant Paediatric Endocrinologist, The Middlesex Hospital, Mortimer Street, London W1N 8AA, UK.

H. G. BURGER MD, FRACP, Director, Medical Research Centre and Department of Endocrinology, Prince Henry's Hospital, St Kilda Road, Melbourne, Australia 3004; Professor of Medicine, Monash University, Melbourne, Australia.

IAIN J. CLARKE BAgricSci, MAgricSci, PhD, Senior Research Officer, Medical Research Centre, Prince Henry's Hospital, St Kilda Road, Melbourne, Australia 3004.

JAMES T. CUMMINS MBBS, FRCS, FRACS, Neurosurgeon, St Vincent's Hospital, Melbourne; Senior Research Fellow, Institute of Medical Research, St Vincent's Hospital, Melbourne; Honorary Research Associate, Prince Henry's Hospital, St Kilda Road, Melbourne, Australia 3004.

D. M. de KRETSER MD, FRACP, Professor of Anatomy, Monash University, Melbourne, Australia; Physician, Reproductive Medicine Clinic, Prince Henry's Hospital, St Kilda Road, Melbourne, Australia 3004.

MARIA L. DUFAU MD, PhD, Head, Molecular Endocrinology Section, Endocrinology & Reproduction Research Branch, National Institute of Child Health and Human Development, National Institutes of Health, Building 10, Room 8C-407, 9000 Rockville Pike, Bethesda, Maryland 20892, USA.

J. K. FINDLAY BAgSc (Hons), PhD, Associate Director, Medical Research Centre, Prince Henry's Hospital, St Kilda Road, Melbourne, Victoria, Australia 3004.

HAMISH M. FRASER PhD, Senior Scientist, Medical Research Council, Centre for Reproductive Biology, 37 Chalmers Street, Edinburgh EH3 9EW, UK.

R. E. GARFIELD MD, McMaster University, Health Sciences Center, Departments of Neurosciences and Obstetrics & Gynecology, Hamilton, Ontario L8S 48L, Canada.

DAVID L. HEALY BMed Sci, MBBS, PhD, FRACOG, Wellcome Trust Senior Clinical Research Fellow, Medical Research Centre, Prince Henry's Hospital & Monash University, Department of Obstetrics & Gynaecology, Queen Victoria Medical Centre, 172 Lonsdale Street, Melbourne, Australia 3000.

PETER HINDMARSH BSc, MB, MRCP, Paediatric Research Registrar, The Middlesex Hospital, Mortimer Street, London W1N 8AA, UK.

HOWARD SAUL JACOBS MD, FRCP, Professor of Reproductive Endocrinology, The Middlesex Hospital Medical School, Mortimer Street, London W1N 8AA, UK.

MAXWELL JONES BSc, Monash University, Department of Obstetrics & Gynaecology, Queen Victoria Medical Centre, 172 Lonsdale Street, Melbourne, Australia 3000.

HOWARD L. JUDD MD, Professor, Department of Obstetrics & Gynecology; Chief, Division of Reproductive Endocrinology, University of California, Los Angeles, School of Medicine, 22-177 Center for Health Sciences, Los Angeles, California 90024, USA.

ULRICH A. KNUTH Dr med Max-Planck-Clinical Research Unit for Reproductive Medicine, Steinfurter Strasse 107, D-4400 Münster, FRG.

F. MARTINEZ MD, Monash University, Department of Obstetrics & Gynaecology, Queen Victoria Medical Centre, 172 Lonsdale Street, Melbourne, Australia 3000.

ALVIN M. MATSUMOTO MD, Assistant Professor of Medicine, University of Washington School of Medicine; Staff Physician, Geriatrics Research, Education, and Clinical Center, Division of Gerontology and Geriatric Medicine, Veterans Administration Medical Center, 1660 South Columbian Way, Seattle, Washington 98108, USA.

R. I. McLACHLAN MBBS, FRACP, Research Fellow, Medical Research Centre, Prince Henry's Hospital; Physician, Reproductive Medicine and Endocrine Clinics, Prince Henry's Hospital, St Kilda Road, Melbourne, Australia 3004.

VIVIEN McLACHLAN BSc, Monash University, Department of Obstetrics & Gynaecology, Queen Victoria Medical Centre, 172 Lonsdale Street, Melbourne, Australia 3000.

LYNN MORROW BSc, Monash University, Department of Obstetrics & Gynaecology, Queen Victoria Medical Centre, 172 Lonsdale Street, Melbourne, Australia 3000.

EBERHARD NIESCHLAG Prof Dr Med, Max-Planck-Clinical Research Unit for Reproductive Medicine, Department of Experimental Endocrinology, University Women's Hospital, Steinfurter Strasse 107, D-4400 Münster, FRG.

SUMIHIDE OKAMATO MD, Monash University, Department of Obstetrics & Gynaecology, Queen Victoria Medical Centre, 172 Lonsdale Street, Melbourne, Australia 3000.

GAIL P. RISBRIDGER BSc (Hons), Dip Ed, PhD, Senior Research Officer, Department of Anatomy, Monash University, Clayton, Victoria, Australia 3168.

D. M. ROBERTSON MSc, Fil Dr (Karolinska Institute), Senior Research Fellow, Department of Anatomy, Monash University, Clayton, Victoria, Australia 3168.

PETER ROGERS BSc, PhD, Monash University, Department of Obstetrics & Gynaecology Queen Victoria Medical Centre, 172 Lonsdale Street, Melbourne, Australia 3000.

RICHARD STANHOPE BSc, MB, MRCP, Clinical Lecturer in Growth and Development, The Institute of Child Health, London WC1; Honorary Senior Registrar in Paediatric Endocrinology, The Middlesex Hospital, Mortimer Street, London W1N 8AA, UK.

ALEX THOMAS BSc, Monash University, Department of Obstetrics & Gynaecology, Queen Victoria Medical Centre, 172 Lonsdale Street, Melbourne, Australia 3000.

JOHANNES VELDHUIS MD, Professor of Medicine, Division of Endocrinology & Metabolism, University of Virginia School of Medicine, Box 202, Charlottesville, Virginia 22908, USA.

Table of contents

Foreword/H. G. BURGER   ix

1   Pulsatility of reproductive hormones: physiological basis and clinical implications   1
I. J. CLARKE & J. T. CUMMINS

2   Pulsatility of reproductive hormones: applications to the understanding of puberty and to the treatment of infertility   23
C. G. D. BROOK, H. S. JACOBS, R. STANHOPE, J. ADAMS & P. HINDMARSH

3   Clinical applications of LHRH analogues   43
M. FRASER & D. T. BAIRD

4   Endocrinology of the hypothalamic–pituitary–testicular axis with particular reference to the hormonal control of spermatogenesis   71
A. M. MATSUMOTO & W. J. BREMNER

5   Inhibin—a non-steroidal regulator of pituitary follicle stimulating hormone   89
R. I. McLACHLAN, D. M. ROBERTSON, D. de KRETSER & H. G. BURGER

6   Endocrine approaches to male fertility control   113
U. A. KNUTH & E. NIESCHLAG

7   Contributions of in vitro fertilization to knowledge of the reproductive endocrinology of the menstrual cycle   133
D. L. HEALY, S. OKAMATO, L. MORROW, A. THOMAS, M. JONES, V. McLACHLAN, M. BESANKO, F. MARTINEZ & P. A. W. ROGERS

8   Pathophysiological relationships between the biological and immunological activities of luteinizing hormone   153
M. L. DUFAU & J. D. VELDHUIS

9   Oestrogen replacement therapy: physiological considerations and new applications   177
H. L. JUDD

10   The antiprogesterone steroid RU486: a short pharmacological and clinical review, with emphasis on the interruption of pregnancy   207
R. E. GARFIELD & E. E. BAULIEU

11   Intragonadal control mechanisms   223
J. K. FINDLAY & G. P. RISBRIDGER

Index   244

FORTHCOMING ISSUES

Baillière's Clinical Endocrinology and Metabolism
INTERNATIONAL PRACTICE AND RESEARCH

May 1987
Neuroendocrinology of Stress
A. GROSSMAN

August 1987
Lipoprotein Metabolism
J. SHEPHERD

November 1987
Techniques for Metabolic Measurement in Man
K. G. M. M. ALBERTI, P. D. HOME & R. TAYLOR

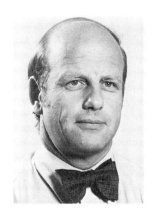

Foreword

To select a series of topics representative of recent advances in reproductive endocrinology was an exciting challenge—and the invited contributors have more than done justice to their briefs. It was logical to begin with gonadotrophin releasing hormone (luteinizing hormone releasing hormone, LHRH), which is central to the control of reproductive function. Clarke and Cummins were pioneers in the demonstration that LHRH secretion into hypophyseal portal blood was indeed pulsatile; they have provided a clear conceptual basis for the following chapter in which Jacobs, Brook and their colleagues report their elegant demonstrations that the processes of puberty and ovulation can be restored in a physiological manner by appropriate pulsatile LHRH administration to patients deficient in the hormone. The paradoxically suppressive effect of continuous LHRH administration (achieved with long-acting agonist analogues) can be exploited in a variety of clinical disorders in which a medical 'gonadotrophin withdrawal' is desirable, as described comprehensively by Fraser and Baird.

Although much remains to be learned about the precise roles of follicle stimulating hormone (FSH) and luteinizing hormone (LH) in the control of human spermatogenesis, the clinical investigations of Bremner and Matsumoto have provided important new insights which they clearly summarize. Inhibin has been a shadowy concept for many years but its recent isolation, structural characterization and assay have now given it full endocrine authenticity, well described by McLachlan and colleagues in a review which points to a number of possible clinical applications. The Editor makes no apology for the inclusion of an extensive chapter on this topic!!

Nieschlag's contributions to the development of endocrine approaches to male fertility regulation have been of fundamental importance in the search for an effective and safe male contraceptive and the state of the art is reviewed in the chapter from his group.

The Monash University In Vitro Fertilization (IVF) Programme has achieved widespread recognition for its pioneering efforts in the field and Healy and his colleagues describe the contribution of IVF to our knowledge of the hormonal events of the normal cycle and its derangements.

There is a growing awareness of the need for caution in the interpretation of radioimmunoassay data for the gonadotrophins, elegantly highlighted by Veldhuis and Dufau in their substantial studies of the relationships between biological and immunological LH activity.

The endocrinology of the menopause has advanced greatly and Judd's scholarly contribution provides a highly readable account of the basis for oestrogen replacement and the various avenues by which this can be achieved.

Another interesting development in the area of gonadal steroids has been the characterization of antiprogestational steroids—their physiological and clinical applications are summarized in a provocative chapter by Baulieu and Garfield.

Finally, an area of extremely rapid recent progress has been in the identification of a variety of intragonadal regulatory mechanisms, clearly and comprehensively described by Findlay and Risbridger.

I am indeed grateful to all the contributors to this outstanding volume of Clinics—the more so as many of them have had associations with our research team in Melbourne (including Clarke, Cummins, Baird, Bremner, McLachlan and his colleagues, Healy and his colleagues, Judd, Findlay and Risbridger).

H. G. BURGER

1

Pulsatility of reproductive hormones: physiological basis and clinical implications

I. J. CLARKE
J. T. CUMMINS

It is now well accepted that the release of hormones from the anterior pituitary is variably pulsatile in nature. This chapter is concerned with the mechanisms underlying the pulse patterns for the gonadotrophins and pro-lactin. On the one hand there is indisputable evidence that neural mechanisms are involved in pulsatile gonadotrophin secretion with luteinizing hormone releasing hormone (LHRH) serving as the conduit between the hypothalamus and the pituitary. In this circumstance, the reason for the existence of pulsatility may be that neural systems are inherently episodic and that translation from neural to endocrine mechanisms necessitates pulsatile rather than continuous signalling. On the other hand there is evidence that basal pulsatile secretion of prolactin from the pituitary gland does not require hypothalamic inputs.

We will briefly consider the patterns of gonadotrophin and sex steroid pulsatility that are seen in the blood and relate this to the patterns of LHRH secretion. The way in which gonadal steroids regulate pulsatile LHRH secretion will be reviewed and then the neural systems that generate or modulate pulsatility will be addressed. With regard to prolactin secretion, we will consider the evidence for the inherent pulsatility of the lactotrophs.

PULSATILITY OF GONADOTROPHINS AND SEX STEROIDS

After the establishment of radioimmunoassays and the adoption of repeti-tive sampling techniques at suitably short time intervals it became apparent that the secretion of the gonadotrophins was pulsatile in men (Nankin and Troen, 1971; Naftolin et al, 1972) and in women (Midgley and Jaffe, 1971). The coincidence of luteinizing hormone (LH) and follicle stimulating hormone (FSH) pulses is relatively high; in normal men it was found that 85% of FSH pulses were associated with LH pulses (Matsumoto and Bremner, 1984) and in women the figure was 70% (Backstrom et al, 1982).

In ovariectomized (OVX) rats Lumpkin et al (1984) found that 83% of FSH pulses were associated with LH pulses. On the other hand 37% of LH pulses occurred in the absence of FSH pulses. This, coupled with a difference in pulse frequency for the two gonadotrophins led these authors to speculate that two separate mechanisms are involved in releasing LH and FSH. In a later study, Culler and Negro-Vilar (1986) have found that pulsatile FSH secretion continues but LH secretion does not in OVX rats given LHRH antiserum. This could be due to a separate releasing factor for FSH or an inherent pulsatility of the FSH-secreting gonadotrophs. In cows studied during the luteal phase, 90–100% of LH pulses were accompanied by FSH pulses (Walters et al, 1984).

Temporal relationships between LH pulses and testosterone pulses have been observed in males of various species, including sheep (Lincoln, 1976), but this pattern is more difficult to discern in men (Baker et al, 1975; Burger and Lee, 1983). In the ram, LH pulses produce testosterone pulses, but FSH pulses are not distinct (Lincoln and Fraser, 1979), perhaps because of the long biological half-life in this species.

In a study of women during the follicular phase, up to 80% of LH pulses were followed by oestrogen pulses (Backstrom et al, 1982). The relationship between LH pulses and oestrogen pulses is found to be much more explicit when ovarian venous blood is sampled in sheep that have an ovary transplanted to the neck (Baird, 1978). In the mid- and late-luteal phase of the human menstrual cycle large LH pulses also stimulate the production of progesterone pulses from the corpus luteum (Filicori et al, 1984); this has not been seen in sheep although an infusion of LHRH, causing LH release, does increase plasma progesterone levels in ewes during the luteal phase of the oestrous cycle (Martin, 1984).

Recently there has been some indication that LH pulses can be classified as 'large' or 'small'. The question arises as to whether or not the 'small' pulses are real and, if so, whether they are physiologically meaningful? Veldhuis et al (1984) found that intensified rates of venous blood sampling in men could 'unmask' a significant number of LH pulses that were not previously seen; as the frequency of sampling increased the mean amplitude of pulses decreased indicating the detection of more 'small' pulses. In women who were sampled at 10 min intervals, Filicori et al (1984) also identified large (>5 mIU/ml) and small (<5 mIU/ml) LH pulses. There was no significant correlation between the overall LH interpulse interval and mean oestrogen or progesterone levels in the luteal phase but progesterone levels were significantly correlated with the number of small pulses. The emergence of smaller pulses as the luteal phase progressed was taken as evidence that the steroids acted on the pituitary to dampen LH pulse amplitude. This is supported by a study in cows which showed that the amplitude of LH pulses, but not FSH pulses, was lower in the mid-luteal phase compared to the early luteal phase (Walters et al, 1984). In the light of these observations, it would appear that small pulses may be of some physiological importance.

PULSATILITY OF LHRH

There is overwhelming evidence that pulses of LH from the pituitary gland are the direct result of LHRH pulses secreted from the median eminence into the hypophyseal portal blood. This was amply demonstrated by the sampling of LHRH in the portal blood and LH in the peripheral blood of conscious OVX ewes which showed a one-to-one relationship between large LHRH and LH pulses (Clarke and Cummins 1982) (Figure 1). The use of the portal access model (Clarke and Cummins, 1982) and the push–pull perfusion technique (Levine et al, 1982) has also raised the issue of 'small' pulses of LHRH that are not accompanied by pulses of LH. There is some question of the reality of these small pulses which may arise from spurious artefacts in the LHRH assays. Possible measurement errors are very difficult to identify because the baseline levels of LHRH in portal blood are close to the limit of detection. Also, it is often difficult to reassay portal samples because of the small volumes collected. Notwithstanding these problems,

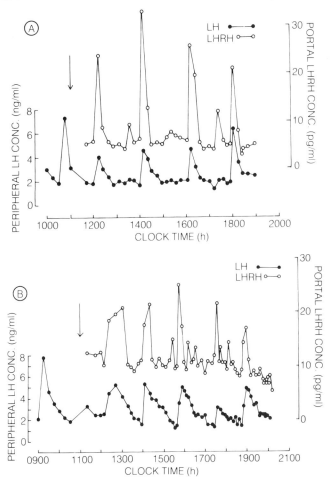

Figure 1. Hypophyseal portal LHRH concentrations and jugular venous LH concentrations in OVX ewes. The arrow indicates the time at which portal blood vessels were lesioned. From Clarke and Cummins (1982), with permission.

there is a clear difference in the patterns of LH secretion in the two sheep shown in Figure 1 which may help to convince us that 'small' pulses are indeed real. In the case where more small LHRH pulses were seen (Figure 1B) there appeared to be an attenuation of the decay of the LH pulses. In fact, the 'small' LH pulses observed in men and women (see above) may result from small LHRH pulses.

PATTERNS OF PULSATILITY

In men there is very little consistency in the pulse pattern of LH and FSH either between or within subjects (Krieger et al, 1972; Yen et al, 1972a). This makes it extremely difficult to define the reproductive status of an individual, especially with regard to LH secretion, without repetitive sampling (Judd, 1979; Burger and Lee, 1983). The day to day pattern of LH and testosterone secretion is much more repeatable in rams (Schanbacher and Ford, 1976).

In females the LH pulse pattern is dependent upon the stage of the oestrous/menstrual cycle. During the luteal stage of the cycle the pulse frequency is relatively low in women (Yen et al, 1972a; Santen and Bardin, 1973) and in sheep (Baird, 1978; Hauger et al, 1977). In more recent studies of women, Backstrom et al (1982) found that the frequency of pulses was greater during the late luteal phase than in the early–mid-luteal phase yet Filicori et al (1984) found a gradual slowing of pulse frequency across this time of the cycle. This discrepancy is not yet resolved. Both studies showed that LH pulse amplitude was progressively reduced during the luteal phase. In the follicular phase of the cycle there is a marked increase in LH pulse frequency in women (Backstrom et al, 1982) and in sheep (Baird, 1978). This is associated with an increase in the secretion of oestrogen from the developing ovarian follicle(s) and leads to the preovulatory LH surge by the positive feedback effect. At the time of the surge there is a large increase in the frequency and the amplitude of LH pulses in rats (Gallo, 1981), monkeys (Marut et al, 1981), sheep (Baird, 1978; Karsch et al, 1983), cows (Rahe et al, 1980) and women (Djahanbakhch et al, 1984).

GONADAL FEEDBACK AND LHRH/LH PULSATILITY

The low frequency of LH pulses during the luteal phase of the oestrous/ menstrual cycle suggests that progesterone has a negative feedback effect to limit LHRH pulsatility at this time. This effect could be the result of synergism with oestrogen or other ovarian steroids. There is good evidence from experimental models that this is indeed the case. For example, Martin et al (1983) found that the LH pulse frequency in ovariectomized ewes studied during the breeding season could be markedly reduced by a combined oestrogen and progesterone treatment; given individually at the same dosages neither steroid had any effect. Because of the direct relationship between LHRH and LH, these data suggest that the steroid combination acts at a central level, rather than on the pituitary gland. Definitive evidence that oestrogen and progesterone can act to limit LHRH secretion has recently been obtained using the portal access model (Clarke et al, 1985). In another series of experiments in OVX ewes, Goodman and Karsch (1980) found that progesterone reduced pulse frequency whilst oestrogen reduced pulse amplitude, the latter being an effect on the pituitary gland (Goodman et al, 1981). The reason that Goodman and Karsch (1980) found an effect of progesterone alone whereas Martin et al (1983) did not may have been the higher doses used in the former study; breed differences in the sheep may also have been a significant factor. Since both oestrogen and progesterone are secreted during the luteal phase of the oestrous/menstrual cycle it seems more reasonable to consider the feedback effects of the combination rather than of the individual steroids.

During the oestrogen-dominant follicular phase of the female cycle the LH pulse frequency approximates or exceeds that seen in hypergonado-trophic, hypogonadal individuals, where no gonadal feedback occurs (Djahanbakhch et al, 1984). Thus, it is hardly surprising that physiological oestrogen treatment does not limit the frequency of LH pulses in OVX animals (Goodman and Karsch, 1980; Martin et al, 1983). If anything, oestrogen may increase pulse frequency at this time (Karsch et al, 1983). This may explain the progressive increase in pulse frequency that is seen across the human follicular phase (see above).

A fundamental question that has been much pondered is the mechanism of the positive feedback effect that generates the preovulatory LH surge. Is this due to an increase in the frequency and/or amplitude of LHRH pulses, or is it due to an enhancement of pituitary responsiveness of LHRH? There is no doubt that oestrogen enhances pituitary gland responsiveness to LHRH (Van Dieten et al, 1974; Yen et al, 1974; Coppings and Malven, 1976) and increases the 'self-priming' effect of LHRH (Aiyer et al, 1974). This heightened responsiveness is seen during the preovulatory period in all species so far studied (Reeves et al, 1971; Cooper et al, 1973; Yen and Lein, 1976) and there can be little doubt that this is a major contributory factor in the generation of the LH surge. Since LH pulses are more frequent at the time of the LH surge than at any other time (see above), it also seems reasonable to expect that LHRH pulse frequency is enhanced at this time. Data from rats (Sarkar et al, 1976), monkeys (Neill et al, 1977) and women (Miyake et al, 1980; Elkind-Hirsch et al, 1982) show that there is a rise in LHRH secretion in portal blood in the preovulatory period, but these studies did not indicate whether this was due to a change in frequency and/or amplitude of LHRH pulses. More recently this aspect has been studied in OVX ewes and monkeys given oestrogen injections. With the portal access model, Clarke and Cummins (1985) found that there was an increase in LHRH pulse frequency at the time of the LH surge. Using the push–pull perfusion technique, Schillo et al (1985) found variable patterns of LHRH secretion in oestrogen-treated OVX ewes. A particular feature of this study was the large-amplitude LHRH pulse seen at the start of the LH surge in two sheep. In oestrogen-treated OVX monkeys, Levine et al (1985) also found variable LHRH profiles; some animals showed bursts of LHRH secretion whereas others showed a consistent pattern of high pulse frequency and amplitude. At this stage it seems that more than one pattern of LHRH secretion may be able to facilitate an LH surge, but additional studies are needed to clarify this point.

The chronically OVX animal may not be the most appropriate model for the study of LHRH secretion during oestrogen-induced surges because of the long-term deprivation of steroids and the inherently high pulse frequency. A much better model may be the anoestrous ewe in which both of these problems are overcome and in which an LH surge may be induced by oestrogen (Goding et al, 1969).

In cycling ewes the pattern of LHRH secretion is extremely difficult to ascertain because of the very low levels in portal blood. In spite of this, recent findings (Clarke et al, 1986a) indicate that the patterns of LHRH secretion at the time of the surge may vary between animals. In some cases there was a sustained elevation in LHRH secretion during the LH surge whereas in others this was not apparent. Also, we sometimes saw a large LHRH pulse at the start of the LH surge, reminiscent of the patterns observed in oestrogen-treated OVX ewes by Schillo et al (1985).

In males the issue of feedback effects on LHRH/LH pulsatility appears more straightforward than in females. Since LH surges do not occur, only negative feedback effects are relevant and the question is quite simply whether or not testosterone and/or its metabolites affect pulse frequency. In castrated rams, testosterone and either its androgenic or oestrogenic metabolites reduced LH pulse frequency (D'Occhio et al, 1983), although the doses of oestrogen and 5α-dihydrotestosterone (5α-DHT) that were used exceeded the physiological range. In a further study (Schanbacher, 1984), physiological doses of oestradiol were found to reduce LH pulse frequency. In men the infusion of 5α-DHT reduced LH pulse frequency whereas infusions of oestrogen reduced pulse amplitude but did not affect frequency (Santen, 1975). Since oestrogen blunted the pituitary response to LHRH, it was concluded that the reduction in pulse amplitude by this steroid was due to pituitary action. On the other hand, testosterone or 5α-DHT probably has an effect on the neural mechanisms regulating LHRH/LH pulse frequency.

NEURAL MECHANISMS INVOLVED IN PULSE GENERATION

Recordings of multi-unit activity within the mediobasal hypothalamus have shown that neural activity can be correlated with pulsatile discharges of LH (Thiery and Pelletier, 1981; Kawakami et al, 1982; Wilson et al, 1984). These studies demonstrate the existence of a neural pacemaker that governs the activity of LHRH neurons but indicate neither the nature nor the site of this centre.

Early studies by Sawyer (1952, 1963) indicated that central α-adrenergic systems were involved in ovulatory mechanisms. More recently, α-adrenergic blocking agents—but not β-blockers—have been shown to inhibit LH pulsatility in monkeys (Bhattacharya et al, 1972) and sheep (Jackson, 1977). Kaufman et al (1985) showed that α_1- and dopamine-blockers—but not an α_2-blocker—could inhibit the multi-unit activity in the mediobasal hypothalamus that correlates with LH pulses. A number of recent reviews have considered the large body of evidence that shows how central catecholaminergic pathways may control the function of LHRH neurons (Barraclough and Wise, 1982; Kalra and Kalra, 1982, 1983, 1984a,b; Kalra, 1986; Kalra and Leadem, 1984; Ramirez et al, 1984). We will not replough this ground here but, instead, will cover salient and recent issues.

To consider the relevant neuronal systems that may regulate the LHRH neurons it is necessary to briefly consider the neuroanatomical arrangement of the latter. Extensive neuroanatomical studies of LHRH neuronal systems have now been performed in a number of species (see Hoffman, 1983, for review). The ubiquitous finding is that the most dense bed of LHRH-containing perikarya is found in the preoptic/septal region of the brain. Some positive cells may also be found in the mediobasal hypothalamus, being present in relatively larger numbers in some species, e.g. baboons (Marshall and Goldsmith, 1980) and monkeys (Silverman et al, 1982) than in others, e.g. sheep (Lehman et al, 1986). These LHRH neurons project fascicles of axons into the external zone of the median eminence where LHRH is stored in neuronal terminals prior to release.

Afferent projections into the preoptic area or the mediobasal hypothalamus, from any part of the brain, may be relevant to the function of LHRH neurons. In particular, these regions receive noradrenergic innervation from the A_1–A_3 and A_5–A_7 cell groups of the brain stem (Lindvall and Bjorklund, 1974; Day et al, 1980; Berk and Finkelstein, 1981), and electron-microscopic studies show that catecholaminergic neurons make synaptic contact with LHRH-containing neurons in the preoptic area (Nakai et al, 1985). Given that the aminergic inputs to the hypothalamus are fundamentally involved in the function of LHRH neurons, it becomes possible to identify brain centres from which pulse patterns might originate. In the present discussion we will consider two possibilities: that the pulse generator resides within the hypothalamus or that it is extrinsic.

Studies in which the Halasz knife has been used to isolate or deafferentate the hypothalamus suggest the existence of a pulse generator within the mediobasal hypothalamus. In the rhesus monkey the creation of mediobasal hypothalamic 'islands' did not eliminate LH pulsatility (Krey et al, 1975). In rats, Blake and Sawyer (1974) also found that LH pulses persisted after complete hypothalamic deafferentation. In a later experiment, Arendash and Gallo (1978) found that if the knife cuts were made caudal to the suprachiasmatic nucleus then pulsatility was eliminated. Deafferentation which left the ventromedial, paraventricular, dorsal–medial hypothalamic and suprachiasmatic nuclei and mammillary bodies intact did not inhibit pulsatility, whereas smaller islands, in which the rostral extent of the cut passed through the anterior region of the arcuate nucleus, eliminated pulsatility (Soper and Weick, 1980). Neither anterior hypothalamic cuts nor anterior arcuate nucleus lesions had an effect individually, but in combination these two insults prevented pulsatility. It was thus concluded that either an extrahypothalamic pathway or the arcuate nucleus could generate pulses and perhaps one system may function in the absence of the other. Anterior hypothalamic deafferentation in the sheep has also been found to prevent pulsatility only when the cuts were made through the anterior part of the arcuate nucleus (Jackson et al, 1978; Thiery et al, 1978).

Although the above experiments suggest that the pulse generator resides within the hypothalamus, they do not rule out the possibility that, in normal circumstances, afferent inputs are involved. Furthermore, these experiments were performed with OVX animals, in which the system is 'free running' without steroidal regulation. The positive feedback effect of oestrogen to elicit an LH surge is eliminated by anterior hypothalamic deafferentation in sheep (Jackson et al, 1978; Thiery et al, 1978) and in rats (Halasz and Pupp, 1965). In these species therefore, the rostrally located LHRH neurons are vital for this feedback function. This is not the case in the monkey (Krey et al, 1975) and suggests that the rostrally located LHRH neurons are of less importance in this species. The long-term negative feedback action of oestrogen appears to be exerted at the hypothalamic level since oestrogen treatment increased the mediobasal content of LHRH in anterior hypothalamic deafferentated rats (Kalra, 1976) but further studies are required to examine this function more thoroughly and identify the hypothalamic centre(s) involved.

What, then, is the role of the extrahypothalamic centres in regard to LHRH/LH pulsatility? An attempt to answer this question was made by Clifton and Sawyer (1969) who transected the ascending noradrenergic pathways in the rat and effected an 83% depletion of hypothalamic noradrenaline. In spite of some short-term perturbations, this procedure had no effect on cyclicity. Further treatment with diethyldithiocarbamate (a noradrenaline synthesis inhibitor) caused anovulation in some, but not all, animals. It was concluded that noradrenergic inputs may play some role, perhaps modulatory rather than mandatory. Other studies (e.g. Kawakami and Arita, 1980) showed that transection through the ventromedial part of the midbrain could block ovulation. Franci and Antunes-Rodrigues (1985) have shown that lesions in the locus coeruleus blocked the pro-oestrous LH surge in rats and caused oestrous cycles to become erratic and irregular. The lesions also affected tonic LH release in castrated rats suggesting that A_6 noradrenergic afferents are involved in tonic, as well as surge, release of gonadotrophins.

As mentioned above, extrahypothalamic inputs are of crucial importance in the generation of the preovulatory LH surge, particularly in non-primate species, and are probably important in steroidal modulation of the pulse generator. Steroidal feedback could be effected by direct action on hypothalamic centres but may also be conducted via the afferent inputs. Taking into account the brain centres that contain steroid receptors and the centres thought to play some role in reproductive function, Stumpf and Jennes (1984) have presented an hypothesis of anatomical and functional interrelationships. They have considered the allocortex–brain stem–core circuit in terms of steroid sites of action and peptidergic and aminergic systems and point out that the three components are inextricably intertwined. With the realization that peptidergic neurotransmitters are of major importance as well as the amines, the picture has become, as one might expect, increasingly more complex. It is interesting to note that oestrogen does not concentrate in LHRH neurons but does so in some of the β-endorphin- and dynorphin-containing cells of the mediobasal hypothalamus (Morrell et al, 1985), the latter being implicated in steroidal feedback mechanisms.

NEUROPEPTIDERGIC INVOLVEMENT IN PULSATILITY

Opioid peptides

A wide range of neuropeptides have now been found to influence LHRH/LH pulsatility. Most notable are the opioid peptides (β-endorphin, met-enkephalin, dynorphin) which may regulate gonadotrophin and prolactin secretion. This has been adequately demonstrated by the administration of opiate antagonists to a variety of species. Treatment with compounds such as naloxone or naltrexone leads to increases in LH secretion in men (Ellingboe et al, 1982), women (Quigley and Yen, 1980; Ropert et al, 1981), female monkeys (Van Vugt et al, 1983), male and female rats (Bruni et al, 1977; Cicero et al, 1980) and sheep (Ebling and Lincoln, 1985; Brooks et al, 1986). The effect is variously manifested by an increase in LH pulse frequency and, in some cases, pulse amplitude. Direct measurements of LHRH secretion have not yet been made in a way that allows us to determine whether LHRH pulse frequency and/or amplitude are increased. One aspect of the responses to naloxone that has not been adequately explained is the variability of incidence and pattern that is seen between or within studies. For example, Van Vugt et al (1983) found that only 60% of monkeys responded to naloxone during the luteal phase and 40% during the follicular phase of the menstrual cycle. Another feature that has attracted only minimal attention is that the effects of naloxone can be quite transitory (Ebling and Lincoln, 1985). Whereas some studies have shown that morphine inhibits LH secretion (Cicero et al, 1980; Ebling and Lincoln, 1985), others (Piva et al, 1986) have shown the reverse effect. These factors are of some concern when it is generally considered that opioids exert an inhibitory influence and hypotheses regarding steroidal feedback are based on this (Ferin et al, 1984).

Opiate agonist and antagonist effects appear dependent upon gonadal steroids, and in females, naloxone responsiveness is more pronounced during the progesterone dominant luteal phase (Quigley and Yen, 1980; Van Vugt et al, 1983; Brooks et al, 1986). Nevertheless, effects have been seen in the oestrogen-dominant follicular phase (Quigley and Yen, 1980; Blank and Roberts, 1982; Brooks et al, 1986). In males, castration eliminates the naloxone response but steroidal replacement reinstates it (Bhanot and Wilkinson, 1983, 1984; Petraglia et al, 1984). In female rats, castration may not eliminate the naloxone effect (Sylvester et al, 1982) suggesting that, in this sex, there may not be an absolute requirement for steroidal background. However, in the same study it was found that naloxone could restore pulsatile LH secretion that had been blocked by steroid treatment, suggesting involvement of opioid pathways in the negative feedback mechanism. The opioid systems also appear to be involved in the positive feedback effect as demonstrated by morphine blockade (Kalra and Kalra, 1983).

Regarding the site of endogenous opioid action and the neural circuitry involved, this has been reviewed recently by Kalra (1986). It seems that opioid inputs can modulate the aminergic inputs to the LHRH system either at the level of the LHRH cell bodies or the LHRH neuronal terminals in the median eminence. Although there is a high density of opiate receptors in the locus coeruleus (Pert et al, 1976), the implantation of naloxone at this level had no effect (Kalra, 1981). Intrahypothalamic implantations were effective and the probable site of action was the opiate receptor containing, and LHRH cell-body rich, preoptic area. It appears that the median eminence contains very few opiate receptors so modulation at this level is probably minimal.

The evidence that opioid pathways are involved in the feedback effects of steroids on LHRH secretion is quite compelling. However, a major question that needs to be addressed is whether the opioid inputs are totally obligatory or, as the results of long-term treatments suggest (Ebling and Lincoln, 1985), feedback systems can operate without these mechanisms.

Other neuropeptides

As more peptides have been found in the central nervous system, the number that have been found to affect gonadotrophin secretion has also grown. Thus, significant roles have been invoked for substance P (SP), neuropeptide Y (NPY) and vasoactive intestinal peptide (VIP).

SP networks are found in most hypothalamic nuclei (Ljungdahl et al, 1978). Studies in monkeys (Eckstein et al, 1980) failed to show any effect of SP on gonadotrophin secretion, but evidence from rats does indicate a possible role in LHRH/LH secretion. For example, the intracerebroventricular (ICV) injection of SP abolished LH surges in one study and injection of SP antiserum raised gonadotrophin levels (Kerdelhue et al, 1982). In contrast, others (Dees et al, 1985) have found that ICV injections of SP antiserum or SP antagonist reduced plasma LH levels. Although the data are conflicting with regard to SP, it appears as though this neuropeptide may be involved in controlling LH secretion and more work needs to be done to clarify its role.

NPY-like immunoreactive perikarya and fibres have been localized in brain regions that overlap the LHRH system (O'Donahue et al, 1985; Sawchenko et al, 1985). ICV injections of NPY decreased LH secretion in OVX rats but increased secretion in steroid-primed rats (Kalra and Crowley, 1984). Also temporal changes in NPY and LHRH levels in the median eminence run parallel in steroid-treated OVX rats (Crowley et al, 1985). Since NPY appears to coexist with catecholamines (Everitt et al, 1984), there is a strong chance that both may act together on LHRH neurons.

As with SP and NPY, the VIP-containing regions of the hypothalamus overlap the LHRH system. Bolus ICV injections elevated plasma LH levels in rats (Vijayan et al, 1979) whereas infusions reduced LH pulse frequency (Alexander et al, 1985). Again, it is too early to say whether or not VIP may act as a neuromodulator and more definitive studies are required.

In conclusion, there is evidence that at least four neuropeptides may be involved in regulating the LHRH system. An attractive hypothesis is that LHRH neurons possess inherent pulsatility that is regulated by aminergic systems and that the peptidergic systems may act in concert with the amines, e.g. NPY, or as neuromodulators of the aminergic inputs, e.g. opioids. Very elaborate experimental designs will be required to unravel the interrelationships that presumably exist between these various neuronal systems.

THE FUNCTIONAL SIGNIFICANCE OF LHRH PULSES

LHRH provides a link between the central nervous system and the pituitary gland. Since secretion is controlled by neural mechanisms and these are, of necessity, dependent upon cyclic rather than continuous transmission, it comes as no surprise that LHRH secretion is pulsatile. In functional terms, the pituitary secretion of LH and FSH can be achieved only by a pulsatile mode of LHRH stimulation and not by a continuous mode (Belchetz et al, 1978). LH pulsatility is a strict reflection of LHRH pulsatility, but FSH secretion per se does not depend upon LHRH pulses. In circumstances where LHRH inputs are removed (Clarke et al, 1986b; Culler and Negro-Vilar, 1986), LH secretion ceases but FSH secretion may continue for weeks at an ever-diminishing rate. One possible explanation of these results is that FSH secretion is a function of pituitary stores of FSH, the latter being maintained by LHRH; thus deprivation of LHRH leads to gradual depletion of pituitary stores of FSH and a concomitant decline in secretion.

Although LH and, in man and rats, FSH levels in plasma reflect episodic secretion, this pulsatility may not be necessary for gonadal function. Thus, the gonads of both sexes may respond to unphysiological treatment with exogenous gonadotrophins with very long half-lives (e.g. pregnant mare serum gonadotrophin or human chorionic gonadotrophin).

PULSATILE PROLACTIN SECRETION

In contrast to the well defined hypothalamic control of gonadotrophin secretion by LHRH, the neural factors relevant to the control of prolactin (PRL) release are poorly defined. The profusion of putative control systems is hardly surprising given the variety of physiological situations which influence plasma PRL levels, such as sleep (Weitzman et al, 1975), reproductive status (Tyson et al., 1972b), suckling or stress (Frantz et al, 1972), feeding (Quigley et al, 1981) and exercise (Shangold et al, 1981). The lengthening list of neuropeptides adds to the complexity of the situation since many of these have been found to either stimulate or inhibit PRL release.

There is good evidence that the secretion of PRL is pulsatile in humans, rats, cows, goats and sheep (for refs see Lamming et al, 1974). From studies of transplanted pituitary glands (Shin and Reifel, 1981), pituitary stalk-sectioned monkeys (Pavasuthipaisit et al, 1981) and sheep with isolated pituitary glands (Thomas et al, 1986) it seems that the lactotrophs possess an inherent capacity to secrete PRL in a pulsatile fashion. Also, when monkey hemipituitaries were perfused in vitro (Stewart et al, 1985) or when pituitary cells were superfused in cell culture (Denef and Andries, 1983), pulsatile PRL release was observed. The frequency of prolactin pulses was similar in sheep before and after hypothalamopituitary disconnection (HPD), suggesting that this is not determined by a central pulse generator. Since the rise in plasma PRL after HPD was associated with an increased pulse amplitude it seems possible that amplitude, not frequency, is the parameter that is under direct hypothalamic inhibition.

Further support for the assertion that changes in plasma PRL levels mainly result from changes in amplitude is given by the effects of oestrogen, which increases the amplitude of episodic PRL release in man (Vetekemans and Robyns, 1975), monkey (Frawley and Neill, 1980) and rats (Meites et al, 1972), and glucocorticoids which inhibit the basal and induced PRL responses in man (Copinschi et al, 1975) and rats (Euker et al, 1975).

It is most unlikely that the lactrotroph pulsatility would be the result of random activity such that apparent pulses occur when the spontaneous secretory activity of a number of cells occurs in unison. The inherent pulsatility may involve some form of intercellular communication. Denef has championed the viewpoint that lactotrophs are profoundly influenced by paracrine effects perhaps involving the gonadotrophs (see Denef et al, 1986, for review). There is strong evidence from cell aggregate studies that LHRH 'is capable of stimulating PRL release not by a direct action on the lactrotrophs but through a stimulus transfer from the gonadotrophs to the lactrotrophs'. These observations are supported by the in vivo studies of Tan et al (1986) who have shown that the synchrony between the LH and PRL in both phases of the human menstrual cycle is due to activation of both the gonadotroph and the lactotroph by endogenous LHRH. On the other hand, in studies of the isolated ovine pituitary gland (Thomas et al, 1986) and in lactotroph-enriched, gonadotroph-poor rat pituitary cell cultures (Denef and Andries, 1983) there was no pulsatile LHRH stimulus, so that the release of PRL in a pulsatile manner must have been intrinsic and not the result of a signal via the gonadotrophs.

In contrast to the intrinsic pulsatility during basal secretion, the almost instantaneous rises in plasma PRL levels that occur following the initiation of suckling or stress provide good evidence for central releasing mechanisms. The neural systems involved in controlling PRL secretion will not be detailed but excellent reviews have recently been provided by Neill (1980), Yen (1982), Leong et al (1983), McCann et al (1984), and Ben-Jonathan (1985). Many putative plasma releasing factors have been identified including thyrotrophin releasing hormone (TRH), VIP, porcine intestinal peptide, angiotensin II, neurotensin and SP.

TRH can liberate PRL in a variety of circumstances but there is still disagreement on its role as a physiological PRL releasing hormone particularly as TSH and PRL are not released in parallel. There is no elevation of TSH during suckling despite the marked elevation of PRL (Gautvik et al, 1973) and TRH-immunized ewes show a marked reduction in TSH levels without any major influences on PRL levels in various physiological situations (Fraser and McNeilly, 1982). Stress, which produces a rise in plasma PRL, has even been reported to cause a rapid decline in circulating TSH levels (Ducommun et al, 1966) further suggesting that the prolactin response to stress is not TRH dependent. In the late stages of nursing (21–56 days) there were only small PRL responses to suckling, but TRH administered after a bout of suckling was able to cause PRL release (Tyson et al, 1972a).

Recent studies in the rat have strongly indicated a role for VIP as a PRL releasing factor. Antiserum to VIP blunts the PRL secretion induced by cerebroventricular administration of 5-hydroxytryptamine (serotonin) (Kato et al, 1984), delays the PRL response to suckling and abolishes the PRL response to ether stress (Abe et al, 1985). Also VIP is present in high concentrations in the rat hypophyseal portal blood (Said and Porter, 1979; Shimatsu et al, 1983) and may be localized on lactotrophs (Morel et al, 1982). VIP causes release of PRL in vitro (Enjalbert et al, 1980) and in vivo (Kato et al, 1978). Whereas this presents a convincing story for the rat, the same may not be true for other species. For example, recent studies in the sheep have failed to demonstrate VIP in hypophyseal portal blood (I. J. Clarke, J. T. Cummins, G. B. Thomas and S. R. Bloom, unpublished data 1986).

It is a well held belief that hypothalamic dopamine is a PRL inhibiting factor, maintaining a constant negative input via the portal blood. Indeed, dopamine levels in the portal blood of rats are substantially higher than peripheral levels (Reymond et al, 1983) and dopamine infusions are able to inhibit PRL secretion in a wide range of species (see Ben-Jonathan, 1985, for references). In order to investigate whether alterations in dopamine input could account for the pulsatile secretory pattern of prolactin that occur, for example, after suckling, Frawley and Neill (1984) conducted the following experiment in stalk-sectioned monkeys. Dopamine infusions were given with brief intermissions and when the infusion rate was decreased it was found that PRL pulses occurred. These authors suggested that a diminution of hypothalamic dopamine secretion could be a pulse-generating mechanism. It remains possible that the inherent pulsatility of the lactotroph is tonically suppressed by an inhibitory factor, possibly dopamine, and further efforts are needed to identify mechanisms of PRL inhibition and release.

SUMMARY

The secretion of LHRH from the median eminence, into hypophyseal portal blood provides a signal whereby the central nervous system interfaces with the endocrine system. The pulsatile nature of this system originates from phasic neural signals and, except in extreme cases where pulses are eliminated by the pituitary action of steroids, pulse frequency is determined by LHRH secretion. Steroidal feedback and other extrinsic influences that affect pulse frequency act via neural afferents to the LHRH neurons. Amplitude regulation may be by way of steroidal influence at the level of the pituitary gland, or indirectly via changes in LHRH pulse frequency. In this chapter, we have attempted to outline our current knowledge of factors regulating LHRH pulsatility and how this is transmitted into pulsatile gonadotrophin secretion.

Regarding PRL secretion, we have outlined evidence that pulsatility is inherent in the lactotrophs, requiring no hypothalamic input. The possible roles of PRL releasing factors in circumstances like suckling and stress and of PRL inhibiting factors have been discussed with reference to the pulsatile nature of PRL secretion.

REFERENCES

Abe H, Engler D, Molitch M, Bollinger-Gruber J & Reichlen S (1985) Vasoactive intestinal peptide is a physiological mediator in the rat. *Endocrinology* **116:** 1383–1390.

Aiyer MS, Chiappa SA & Fink G (1974) A priming effect of luteinizing hormone releasing factor on the pituitary gland in the female rat. *Journal of Endocrinology* **62:** 573–588.

Alexander MJ, Clifton DK & Steiner RA (1985) Vasoactive intestinal polypeptide effects a central inhibition of pulsatile luteinizing hormone secretion in ovariectomized rats. *Endocrinology* **117:** 2134–2139.

Arendash GW & Gallo RV (1978) Apomorphine-induced inhibition of episodic LH release in ovariectomized rats with complete hypothalamic deafferentation. *Proceedings of the Society for Experimental Biology and Medicine* **159:** 121–125.

Backstrom CT, McNeilly AS, Leask RM & Baird DT (1982) Pulsatile secretion of LH, FSH, prolactin, oestradiol and progesterone during the human menstrual cycle. *Clinical Endocrinology* **17:** 29–42.

Baird DT (1978) Pulsatile secretion of LH and ovarian estradiol during the follicular phase of the sheep estrous cycle. *Biology of Reproduction* **18:** 359–364.

Baird DT, Swanston IA & McNeilly AS (1981) Relationship between LH, FSH and prolactin concentration and the secretion of androgens and estrogens by the preovulatory follicle in the ewe. *Biology of Reproduction* **24:** 1013–1025.

Baker HWG, Santen RJ, Burger HG et al (1975) Rhythms in the secretion of gonadotropins and gonadal steroids. *Journal of Steroid Biochemistry* **6:** 793–801.

Barraclough CA & Wise PM (1982) The role of catecholamines in the regulation of pituitary luteinizing hormone and follicle-stimulating hormone secretion. *Endocrine Reviews* **3:** 91–119.

Belchetz PE, Plant TM, Nakai Y, Keogh EJ & Knobil E (1978) Hypophysial responses to continuous and intermittent delivery of hypothalamic gonadotropin-releasing hormone. *Science* **202:** 631–633.

Ben-Jonathan N (1985) Dopamine: a prolactin-inhibiting hormone. *Endocrine Reviews* **6:** 564–589.

Berk ML & Finkelstein JA (1981) Afferent projections to the preoptic area and hypothalamic regions in the rat brain. *Neuroscience* **6:** 1601–1624.

Bhanot R & Wilkinson M (1983) Opiatergic control of LH secretion is eliminated by gonadectomy. *Endocrinology* **112:** 399–401.

Bhattacharya AN, Dierschke DJ, Yamaji T & Knobil E (1972) The pharmacological blockade of the circhoral mode of LH secretion in the ovariectomized rhesus monkey. *Endocrinology* **90:** 778–786.

Blake CA & Sawyer CH (1974) Effects of hypothalamic deafferentation on the pulsatile rhythm in plasma concentrations of luteinizing hormone in ovariectomized rats. *Endocrinology* **94:** 780–786.

Blank MS & Roberts DL (1982) Antagonist of gonadotropin-releasing hormone blocks naloxone-induced elevations in serum luteinizing hormone. *Neuroendocrinology* **35:** 309–312.

Brooks AN, Lamming GE, Lees PD & Haynes NH (1986) Opioid modulation of LH secretion in the ewe. *Journal of Reproduction and Fertility* **76:** 693–708.

Bruni JF, Van Vugt D, Marshall S & Meites J (1977) Effects of naloxone, morphine, and methionine enkephalin on serum prolactin, luteinizing hormone, follicle stimulating hormone, thyroid stimulating hormone and growth hormone. *Life Sciences* **21:** 461–466.

Burger HG & Lee VWK (1983) Patterns of secretion and metabolism of the gonadotrophic hormones. *Monographs on Endocrinology* **25:** 1–11.

Cicero TJ, Badger TM, Wilcox RD, Meyer B & Meyer E (1980) Morphine decreases luteinizing hormone by an action on the hypothalamic pituitary axis. *Journal of Pharmacology and Experimental Therapeutics* **203:** 548–555.

Clarke IJ & Cummins JT (1982) The temporal relationship between gonadotropin releasing hormone (GnRH) and luteinizing hormone (LH) secretion in ovariectomized ewes. *Endocrinology* **111:** 1737–1739.

Clarke IJ & Cummins JT (1985) Increased GnRH pulse frequency associated with estrogen-induced LH surges in ovariectomized ewes. *Endocrinology* **116:** 2376–2383.

Clarke IJ, Karsch FJ & Cummins JT (1985) Oestrogen and progesterone stop GnRH pulses in ovariectomized anoestrous ewes. *Proceedings of the Australian Society for Reproductive Biology, 17th Annual Conference.* Abstract 28.

Clarke IJ, Thomas GB, Doughton BW et al (1986a) Gonadotropin-releasing hormone secretion during the ovine estrous cycle. *Proceedings of the 68th Meeting of the Endocrine Society*, Anaheim, USA. Abstract 468.

Clarke IJ, Burman KR, Doughton BW & Cummins JT (1986b) Effects of constant infusion of gonadotrophin-releasing hormone (GnRH) in ovariectomized ewes with hypothalamo-pituitary disconnection: further evidence for differential control of LH and FSH secretion and the lack of a priming effect. *Journal of Endocrinology* **111:** 43–49.

Clifton DK & Sawyer CH (1979) LH release and ovulation in the rat following depletion of hypothalamic norepinephrine: chronic vs acute effects. *Neuroendocrinology* **28:** 442–449.

Cooper KJ, Fawcett CP & McCann SM (1973) Variations in pituitary responsiveness to luteinizing hormone releasing factor during the rat oestrous cycle. *Journal of Endocrinology* **57:** 187–188.

Copinschi G, L'Hermitte M, Leclerq R et al (1975) Effects of glucocorticoids on pituitary hormonal response to hypoglycaemia inhibition of prolactin. *Journal of Clinical Endocrinology and Metabolism* **40:** 442–449.

Coppings RJ & Malven PV (1976) Biphasic effect of estradiol on mechanisms regulating LH release in ovariectomized sheep. *Neuroendocrinology* **21:** 146–156.

Crowley WR, Tessel RE, O'Donahue TL, Adler BA & Kalra SP (1985) Effects of ovarian hormones on the concentrations of immunoreactive neuropeptide Y in discrete brain regions of the female rat: correlation with serum luteinizing hormone (LH) and median eminence LH-releasing hormone. *Endocrinology* **117:** 1151–1155.

Culler MD & Negro-Vilar A (1986) Evidence that pulsatile follicle-stimulating hormone secretion is independent of endogenous luteinizing hormone-releasing hormone. *Endocrinology* **118:** 609–612.

Day TA, Blessing W & Willoughby JO (1980) Noradrenergic and dopaminergic projections to the medial preoptic area of the rat. A combined horseradish peroxidase/catecholamine fluorescence study. *Brain Research* **193:** 543–548.

Dees WL, Skelley CW & Kozlowski GP (1985) Central effects of an antagonist and an antiserum to substance P on serum gonadotropin and prolactin secretion. *Life Sciences* **37:** 1627–1631.

Denef C & Andries M (1983) Evidence for paracrine interaction between gonadotrophs and lactotrophs in pituitary cell aggregates. *Endocrinology* **112:** 813–822.

Denef C, Baes M & Schramme C (1986) Paracrine interactions in the anterior pituitary gland: role in the regulation of prolactin and growth hormone secretion. In Ganong WF & Martini L (eds) *Frontiers in Neuroendocrinology*, vol. 9, pp 115–148. New York: Raven Press.

Djahanbakhch O, Warner P, McNeilly AS & Baird DT (1984) Pulsatile release of LH and oestradiol during the periovulatory period in women. *Clinical Endocrinology* **20:** 579–589.

D'Occhio MJ, Schanbacher BD & Kinder JE (1983) Androgenic and oestrogenic steroid participation in feedback control of luteinizing hormone secretion in male sheep. *Acta Endocrinologica* **102**: 499–504.

Ducommun P, Sakiz E & Guillemin R (1966) Lability of plasma TSH levels in the rat in response to non-specific exteroceptive stimuli. *Proceedings of the Society for Experimental Biology and Medicine* **121**: 921–923.

Ebling FJP & Lincoln GA (1985) Endogenous opioids and the control of seasonal LH secretion in Soay rams. *Journal of Endocrinology* **107**: 341–353.

Eckstein N, Wehrenberg WB, Louis K et al (1980) Effects of substance P on anterior pituitary secretion in the female rhesus monkey. *Neuroendocrinology* **31**: 338–342.

Elkind-Hirsch K, Ravnikar U, Schiff I, Tulchinsky D & Ryan KJ (1982) Determinations of endogenous immunoreactive luteinizing hormone-releasing hormone in human plasma. *Journal of Clinical Endocrinology and Metabolism* **54**: 602–607.

Ellingboe J, Veldhuis JD, Mendelson JH, Kuehnle JC & Mello NK (1982) Effect of endogenous opioid blockage on the amplitude and frequency of pulsatile luteinizing hormone secretion in normal men. *Journal of Clinical Endocrinology and Metabolism* **54**: 854–857.

Enjalbert A, Arancibia S, Ruberg M et al (1980) Stimulation of in vitro prolactin release by vasoactive intestinal peptide. *Neuroendocrinology* **31**: 200–204.

Euker JS, Meites J & Riegle GD (1975) Effects of acute stress on serum LH and prolactin in intact, castrate and dexamethasone-treated male rats. *Endocrinology* **96**: 85–92.

Everitt BJ, Hokfelt L, Terenius K, Mutt U & Goldstein M (1984) Differential co-existence of neuropeptide Y (NPY)-like immunoreactivity with catecholamines in the central nervous system in the rat. *Neuroscience* **11**: 443–462.

Ferin M, Van Vugt D & Wardlaw S (1984) The hypothalamic control of the menstrual cycle and the role of endogenous opioid peptides. *Recent Progress in Hormone Research* **40**: 441–485.

Filicori M, Butler JP & Crowley WF (1984) Neuroendocrine regulation of the corpus luteum in the human. Evidence for pulsatile progesterone secretion. *Journal of Clinical Investigation* **73**: 1638–1647.

Franci JAA & Antunes-Rodrigues J (1985) Effect of locus ceruleus lesion on luteinizing hormone secretion under different experimental conditions. *Neuroendocrinology* **41**: 44–51.

Frantz AG, Kleinberg DL & Noel GL (1972) Studies on prolactin in man. *Recent Progress in Hormone Research* **28**: 527–590.

Fraser HM & McNeilly AS (1982) Effect of chronic immunoneutralization of thyrotropin-releasing hormone on the hypothalamic–pituitary–thyroid axis, prolactin, and reproductive function in the ewe. *Endocrinology* **111**: 1964–1973.

Frawley LS & Neill JD (1980) Effect of estrogen on serum prolactin levels in rhesus monkeys after hypophyseal stalk transection. *Biology of Reproduction* **22**: 1089–1093.

Frawley LS & Neill JD (1984) Brief decreases in dopamine result in surges of prolactin secretion in monkeys. *American Journal of Physiology* **247**: E778–E780.

Gallo RV (1981) Pulsatile LH release during the ovulatory LH surge on proestrus in the rat. *Biology of Reproduction* **24**: 100–104.

Gautvik KM, Weintraub BD, Graeber CT et al (1973) Serum prolactin and TSH: Effects of nursing and pyroGlu-His-Pro-NH$_2$ administration in post partum women. *Journal of Clinical Endocrinology and Metabolism* **37**: 135–139.

Goding JR, Catt KJ, Brown JM et al (1969) Radioimmunoassay for ovine luteinizing hormone. Secretion of luteinizing hormone during estrus and following estrogen administration in the sheep. *Endocrinology* **85**: 133–142.

Goodman RL & Karsch FJ (1980) Pulsatile secretion of luteinizing hormone: differential suppression by ovarian steroids. *Endocrinology* **107**: 1286–1290.

Goodman RL, Bittman EL, Foster DL & Karsch FJ (1981) The endocrine basis of the synergistic suppression of luteinizing hormone by estradiol and progesterone. *Endocrinology* **109**: 1414–1417.

Halasz B & Pupp L (1965) Hormone secretion of the anterior pituitary gland after physical interruption of all nervous pathways to the hypophysiotrophic area. *Endocrinology* **77**: 553–562.

Hauger RL, Karsch FJ & Foster DL (1977) A new concept for the control of the estrous cycle of the ewe based on the temporal relationships between luteinizing hormone, estradiol and progesterone in peripheral serum and evidence that progesterone inhibits tonic LH secretion. *Endocrinology* **101**: 807–817.

Hoffman GE (1983) LHRH neurons and their projections. In Sano Y, Ibata Y, Zimmerman EA (eds) *Structure and Function of Peptidergic and Aminergic Neurons*, pp 183–202. Tokyo: Japan Scientific Societies Press.

Jackson GL (1977) Effect of adrenergic blocking drugs on secretion of luteinizing hormone in the ovariectomized ewe. *Biology of Reproduction* **16**: 543–548.

Jackson GL, Kuehl D, McDowell K & Zaleski A (1978) Effect of hypothalamic deafferentation on secretion of luteinizing hormone in the ewe. *Biology of Reproduction* **17**: 808–819.

Judd HL (1979) Biorhythms of gonadotropins and testicular hormone secretion. In Krieger DT (ed.) *Endocrine Rhythms*, pp 299–324. New York: Raven Press.

Kalra SP (1976) Tissue levels of luteinizing hormone-releasing hormone in the pre-optic area and hypothalamus, and serum concentrations of gonadotropins following anterior hypothalamic deafferentation and estrogen treatment of the female rat. *Endocrinology* **99**: 101–107.

Kalra SP (1981) Neural loci involved in naxolone-induced luteinizing hormone release: effects of a norepinephrine synthesis inhibitor. *Endocrinology* **109**: 1805–1810.

Kalra SP (1986) Neural circuitry involved in the control of LHRH secretion: a model for preovulatory LH release. In Ganong WF & Martini L (eds) *Frontiers in Neuroendocrinology*, vol. 9, pp 31–76. New York: Raven Press.

Kalra SP & Crowley WR (1984) Norepinephrine-like effects of neuropeptide Y on LH release in the rat. *Life Sciences* **35**: 1173–1176.

Kalra SP & Kalra PS (1982) Stimulatory role of gonadal steroids on luteinizing hormone releasing hormone secretion. In Motta M, Zanisi M & Piva F (eds) *Pituitary Hormones and Related Peptides*, pp 157–170. New York: Academic Press.

Kalra SP & Kalra PS (1983) Neural regulation of luteinizing hormone secretion in the rat. *Endocrine Reviews* **4**: 311–351.

Kalra SP & Kalra PS (1984a) Opioid–adrenergic–steroid connection in regulation of luteinizing hormone secretion in the rat. *Neuroendocrinology* **38**: 418–426.

Kalra SP & Kalra PS (1984b) Intrahypothalamic environment controlling LHRH secretion. In McKerns K (ed.) *Regulation of Target Cell Responsiveness*, pp 127–184. New York: Plenum.

Kalra SP & Leadem CA (1984) Control of luteinizing hormone secretion by endogenous opioid peptides. In Delitala G, Motta M & Serio M (eds) *Opioid modulation of endocrine function*, pp 171–184. New York: Raven Press.

Karsch FJ, Foster DL, Bittman EL & Goodman RL (1983) A role of estradiol in enhancing luteinizing hormone pulse frequency during the follicular phase of the estrous cycle of sheep. *Endocrinology* **113**: 1333–1339.

Kato Y, Iwasaki Y, Iwasaki J et al (1978) Prolactin release by vasoactive intestinal polypeptide in rats. *Endocrinology* **103**: 554–558.

Kato Y, Shimatsu A, Matsushita N et al (1984) Regulation of pituitary hormone secretion by VIP and related peptides. In Labrie F & Proulx L (eds) *Endocrinology*, pp 175–179. Amsterdam: Elsevier Science Publishers.

Kaufman JM, Kesner JS, Wilson RC & Knobil E (1985) Electrophysiological manifestation of luteinizing hormone-releasing hormone pulse generator activity in the rhesus monkey: influence of α-adrenergic and dopaminergic blocking agents. *Endocrinology* **116**: 1327–1333.

Kawakami M & Arita J (1980) Involvement of the ventromedial part of the midbrain in the control of proestrous surge of gonadotropins and prolactin in the rat. *Neuroendocrinology* **30**: 337–343.

Kawakami M, Vemura T & Hayashi R (1982) Electrophysiological correlates of pulsatile gonadotrophin release in rats. *Neuroendocrinology* **35**: 63–67.

Kerdelhue B, Lenoir V, Pasqualini C, El Abed A & Millar RP (1982) Rôle modulateur de la substance P, un undecapeptide, dans l'excrétion des gonadotrophins hypophysaires induite par le GnRH. *Les Colloques del'INSERM* **110**: 221–240.

Krey LC, Butler WR & Knobil E (1975) Surgical disconnection of the medial basal hypothalamus and pituitary function in the rhesus monkey. 1. Gonadotropin secretion. *Endocrinology* **96**: 1073–1087.

Krieger DT, Ossowski R, Fogel M & Allen W (1972) Lack of circadian periodicity of serum FSH and LH levels. *Journal of Clinical Endocrinology and Metabolism* **35**: 619–623.

Lamming GE, Moseley SR & McNeilly JR (1974) Prolactin release in the sheep. *Journal of Reproduction and Fertility* **40**: 151–168.

Lehman MN, Robinson JE, Karsch FJ & Silverman AJ (1986) Immunocytochemical localization of luteinizing hormone-releasing hormone (LHRH) pathways of the sheep brain during anestrus and the mid-luteal phase of the estrus cycle. *Journal of Comparative Neurology* **244**: 19–35.

Leong DA, Frawley LS & Neill JD (1983) Neuroendocrine control of prolactin secretion. *Annual Review of Physiology* **45**: 109–127.

Levine JE, Pau K-Y, Ramirez VD & Jackson GL (1982) Simultaneous measurement of luteinizing hormone-releasing hormone and luteinizing hormone release in unanaesthetized, ovariectomized sheep. *Endocrinology* **111**: 1449–1455.

Levine JE, Norman RL, Gliessman PM et al (1985) In vivo gonadotropin-releasing hormone release and serum luteinizing hormone measurements in ovariectomized, estrogen-treated rhesus monkeys. *Endocrinology* **117**: 711–721.

Lincoln GA (1976) Seasonal variation in the episodic secretion of luteinizing hormone and testosterone in the ram. *Journal of Endocrinology* **69**: 213–226.

Lincoln GA & Fraser HM (1979) Blockade of episodic secretion of luteinizing hormone in the ram by the administration of antibodies to luteinizing hormone releasing hormone. *Biology of Reproduction* **21**: 1239–1245.

Lindvall O & Bjorklund A (1974) The organisation of the ascending CA neuron system in the rat brain as revealed by the glycoxylic acid fluorescence method. *Acta Physiologica Scandinavica Supplement* **412**: 1–48.

Ljungdahl A, Hokfelt T & Nillson G (1978) Distribution of substance P-like immunoreactivity in the central nervous system of the rat. *Neuroscience* **3**: 861–886.

Lumpkin MD, De Paolo LV and Negro-Vilar A (1984) Pulsatile release of follicle-stimulating hormone in ovariectomized rats is inhibited by porcine follicular fluid (inhibin). *Endocrinology* **114**: 201–206.

Marshall PE & Goldsmith PC (1980) Neuroregulatory and neuroendocrine GnRH pathways in the hypothalamus and forebrain of the baboon. *Brain Research* **193**: 353–372.

Martin GB (1984) Factors affecting the secretion of luteinizing hormone in the ewe. *Biological Reviews* **59**: 1–87.

Martin GB, Scaramuzzi RJ & Henstridge JD (1983) Effects of oestradiol, progesterone and androstenedione on the pulsatile secretion of luteinizing hormone in ovariectomized ewes during spring and autumn. *Journal of Endocrinology* **96**: 181–193.

Marut EL, Williams RF, Cowan BD et al (1981) Pulsatile pituitary gonadotropin secretion during maturation of the dominant follicle in monkeys: estrogen positive feedback enhances the biological activity of LH. *Endocrinology* **109**: 2270–2272.

Matsumoto AM & Bremner WJ (1984) Modulation of pulsatile gonadotropin secretion by testosterone in man. *Journal of Clinical Endocrinology and Metabolism* **58**: 609–614.

McCann SM, Lumpkin MD, Mizunuma H et al (1984) Peptidergic and dopaminergic control of prolactin release. *Trends in Neurosciences* **21**: 109–116.

Meites JL, Lu KH, Wuttke W et al (1972) Recent studies on functions and control of prolactin secretion in rats. *Recent Progress in Hormone Research* **28**: 471–516.

Midgley AR & Jaffe RB (1971) Regulation of human gonadotrophins: X. Episodic fluctuation of LH during the menstrual cycle. *Journal of Clinical Endocrinology and Metabolism* **33**: 962–969.

Miyake A, Kawamura Y, Aono T & Kurachi K (1980) Changes in plasma LRH during the normal menstrual cycle in women. *Acta Endocrinologica* **93**: 257–263.

Morel G, Besson J, Rosselin G & Dubois PM (1982) Ultrastructural evidence for endogenous vasoactive intestinal peptide-like immunoreactivity in the pituitary gland. *Neuroendocrinology* **34**: 85–89.

Morrell JI, McGinty JF & Pfaff DW (1985) A subset of β-endorphin- or dynorphin-containing neurons in the medial basal hypothalamus accumulates estradiol. *Neuroendocrinology* **41**: 417–426.

Naftolin F, Yen SSC & Tsai CC (1972) Rapid cycling of plasma gonadotrophins in normal men as demonstrated by frequent sampling. *Nature* **236**: 92–93.

Nakai Y, Ochiai H, Kitazawa S, Shioda S & Watanabe T (1985) Electron microscopic cytochemistry of the relationship between catecholaminergic axons and peptidergic neurons in the rat hypothalamus. In Kobayashi H (ed.) *Neurosecretion and the Biology of Neuropeptides*, pp 121–129. Tokyo: Japan Scientific Societies Press. Berlin: Springer-Verlag.

Nankin HR & Troen P (1971) Repetitive luteinizing hormone elevations in serum of normal men. *Journal of Clinical Endocrinology and Metabolism* **33**: 558–560.

Neill JD (1980) Neuroendocrine regulation of prolactin secretion. In Martini L & Ganong WF (eds) *Frontiers in Neuroendocrinology*, vol. 6, pp 129–155. New York: Raven Press.

Neill JD, Patton JM, Dailey RA, Tsou RC & Tindall GT (1977) Luteinizing hormone releasing hormone (LH-RH) in pituitary stalk blood of rhesus monkeys: relationship to levels of LH release. *Endocrinology* **101**: 430–434.

O'Donahue TL, Chronwall BM, Pruss RM et al (1985) Neuropeptide and peptide YY neuronal and endocrine systems. *Peptides* **6**: 755–768.

Pavasuthipaisit K, Hess DL, Norman RL et al (1981) Dopamine: effects on prolactin and luteinizing hormone secretion in ovariectomized rhesus macaques after transection of the pituitary stalk. *Neuroendocrinology* **32**: 42–49.

Pert CB, Kuhar MJ & Snyder SH (1976) Opiate receptor: autoradiographic localisation in rat brain. *Proceedings of the National Academy of Sciences (USA)* **73**: 3729–3733.

Petraglia F, Locatelli V, Penalva A et al (1984) Gonadal steroid modulation of naloxone-induced LH secretion in the rat. *Journal of Endocrinology* **101**: 33–39.

Piva F, Limonta P, Maggi R & Martini L (1986) Stimulatory and inhibitory effects of the opioids on gonadotropin secretion. *Neuroendocrinology* **42**: 504–512.

Quigley ME & Yen SS (1980) The role of endogenous opiates on LH secretion during the menstrual cycle. *Journal of Clinical Endocrinology and Metabolism* **51**: 179–181.

Quigley ME, Ropert JF & Yen SSC (1981) Acute prolactin release triggered by feeding. *Journal of Clinical Endocrinology and Metabolism* **52**: 1043–1045.

Rahe CH, Owens RE, Fleeger ML, Newton JT & Harms PG (1980) Patterns of plasma luteinizing hormone in the cyclic cow: dependence upon the period of the cycle. *Endocrinology* **107**: 498–503.

Ramirez VD, Feder HH & Sawyer CH (1984) The role of brain catecholamines in the regulation of LH secretion: a critical inquiry. In Martini L & Ganong WF (eds) *Frontiers in Neuroendocrinology*, pp 27–84. New York: Raven Press.

Reeves JJ, Arimura A & Schally AV (1971) Pituitary responsiveness to purified luteinizing hormone-releasing hormone (LH-RH) at various stages of the estrous cycle in sheep. *Journal of Animal Science* **32**: 123–126.

Reymond MJ, Speciale SG & Porter JC (1983) Dopamine in plasma of lateral and medial hypophysial portal vessels: evidence for regional variation in the release of hypothalamic dopamine into hypophysial portal blood. *Endocrinology* **112**: 1958–1963.

Ropert JF, Quigley MR & Yen SSC (1981) Endogenous opiates modulate pulsatile luteinizing hormone release in humans. *Journal of Clinical Endocrinology and Metabolism* **52**: 583–585.

Said SI & Porter JC (1979) Vasoactive intestinal polypeptide: release into hypophysial portal blood. *Life Sciences* **24**: 227–230.

Santen RJ (1975) Is aromatization of testosterone to estradiol required for inhibition of luteinizing hormone secretion in man? *Journal of Clinical Investigation* **56**: 1555–1563.

Santen RJ & Bardin CW (1973) Episodic luteinizing hormone secretion in man. *Journal of Clinical Investigation* **52**: 2617–2628.

Sarkar DK, Chiappa SA, Fink G & Sherwood NM (1976) Gonadotrophin-releasing hormone surge in pro-oestrous rats. *Nature* **264**: 461–463.

Sawchenko PE, Swanson LW, Grzanna AR et al (1985) Colocalization of neuropeptide Y immunoreactivity in brainstem catecholaminergic neurons that project to the paraventricular nucleus of the hypothalamus. *Journal of Comparative Neurology* **241**: 138–153.

Sawyer CH (1952) Stimulation of ovulation in the rabbit by the intraventricular injection of epinephrine or norepinephrine. *Anatomical Record* **51**: 385.

Sawyer CH (1963) Neuroendocrine blocking agents and gonadotropin release. In Nalbandov AV (ed.) *Advances in Neuroendocrinology*, pp 444–459. Urbana: University of Illinois Press.

Schanbacher BD (1984) Regulation of luteinizing hormone secretion in male sheep by endogenous estrogen. *Endocrinology* **115**: 944–950.

Schanbacher BD & Ford JJ (1976) Seasonal profiles of plasma luteinizing hormone, testosterone and estradiol in the ram. *Endocrinology* **99**: 752–757.

Schillo KK, Leshin LS, Kuehl D & Jackson GL (1985) Simultaneous measurement of luteinizing hormone-releasing hormone and luteinizing hormone during estradiol-induced
luteinizing hormone surges in the ovariectomized ewe. *Biology of Reproduction* **33**:
644–652.

Shangold MM, Gatz ML & Thysen B (1981) Acute effects of exercise on plasma concentrations
of prolactin and testosterone in recreational women runners. *Fertility and Sterility* **35**:
699–702.

Shimatsu A, Kato Y, Matsushita N et al (1981) Immunoreactive vasoactive intestinal polypeptide in rat hypophysial portal blood. *Endocrinology* **108**: 395–398.

Shin SH & Reifel CW (1981) Adenohypophysis has an inherent property for pulsatile prolactin
secretion. *Neuroendocrinology* **32**: 139–144.

Silverman AJ, Antunes JL, Abrams GM et al (1982) The luteinizing hormone-releasing
hormone pathways in rhesus (*Macaca mulatta*) and pigtailed (*Macaca nemestrina*)
monkey: new observations on thick, unembedded sections. *Journal of Comparative
Neurology* **211**: 309–317.

Soper BD & Weick RF (1980) Hypothalamic and extrahypothalamic mediation of pulsatile
discharges of luteinizing hormone in the ovariectomized rat. *Endocrinology* **106**: 348–355.

Stewart JK, Clifton DK, Koerker DJ et al (1985) Pulsatile release of growth hormone and
prolactin from the primate pituitary in vitro. *Endocrinology* **116**: 1–5.

Stumpf WE & Jennes L (1984) The A–B–C (allocortex–brainstem–core) circuitry of
endocrine–autonomic integration and regulation. A proposed hypothesis on the
anatomical–functional relationships between estradiol sites of action and peptidergic–
aminergic neuronal systems. *Peptides* **5**: 221–226.

Sylvester PW, van Vugt DA, Aylsworth CA, Hanson EA & Meites J (1982) Effects of
morphine and naloxone on inhibition by ovarian hormones of pulsatile release of LH in
ovariectomized rats. *Neuroendocrinology* **34**: 269–273.

Tan YM, Steele PA & Judd SJ (1986) The effect of physiological changes in ovarian steroids on
the prolactin response to gonadotrophin releasing factor. *Clinical Endocrinology* **24**:
71–78.

Thiery JC & Pelletier J (1981) Multiunit activity in the anterior median eminence and adjacent
areas of the hypothalamus of the ewe in relation to LH secretion. *Neuroendocrinology* **32**:
217–224.

Thiery JC, Pelletier J & Signoret JP (1978) Effect of hypothalamic deafferentation on LH and
sexual behaviour in ovariectomized ewe under hormonally induced oestrous cycle.
Annales de Biologie Animale, Biochemie, Biophysique **18**: 1413–1426.

Thomas GB, Cummins JT, Cavanagh L & Clarke IJ (1986) A transient elevation of prolactin
secretion following hypothalamo-pituitary disconnection in the ewe during two seasons.
Journal of Endocrinology (in press).

Tyson JE, Friesen HG & Anderson MS (1972a) Human lactational and ovarian response to
endogenous prolactin release. *Science* **177**: 897–900.

Tyson JE, Hwang P, Guyda H & Friesen H (1972b) Studies of prolactin secretion in human
pregnancy. *American Journal of Obstetrics and Gynecology* **113**: 14–20.

Van Dieten JAMJ, Steijsiger J, Dullaart J & Van Rees GP (1974) The effect of estradiol
benzoate on the pituitary responsiveness to LH-RH in male and female rats. *Neuroendocrinology* **15**: 182–188.

Van Vugt DA, Bakst G, Dyrenfurth I & Ferin M (1983) Naloxone stimulation of luteinizing
hormone secretion in the monkey: influence of endocrine and experimental conditions.
Endocrinology **113**: 1858–1864.

Veldhuis JD, Evans WS, Rogol AD et al (1984) Intensified rates of venous sampling unmask
the presence of spontaneous, high-frequency pulsations of luteinizing hormone in man.
Journal of Clinical Endocrinology and Metabolism **59**: 96–102.

Vetekemans M & Robyn C (1975) The influence of exogenous estrogen on the circadian
periodicity of circulating prolactin in women. *Journal of Clinical Endocrine Metabolism*
40: 886–889.

Vijayan E, Samson WK, Said SI & McCann SM (1979) Vasoactive intestinal peptide: evidence
for a hypothalamic site of action to release growth hormone, luteinizing hormone and
prolactin in conscious ovariectomized rats. *Endocrinology* **104**: 53–57.

Walters DL, Schams D & Schallenberger E (1984) Pulsatile secretion of gonadotrophins, ovarian steroids and ovarian oxytocin during the luteal phase of the oestrous cycle in the cow. *Journal of Reproduction and Fertility* **71:** 479–491.

Weitzman ED, Boyar RM, Kapen S & Hellman L (1975) The relationship of sleep and sleep stages to neuroendocrine secretion and biological rhythm in man. *Recent Progress in Hormone Research* **31:** 399–446.

Wilson RC, Kesner JS, Kaufman JM et al (1984) Central electrophysiologic correlates of pulsatile luteinizing hormone secretion in the rhesus monkey. *Neuroendocrinology* **39:** 256–260.

Yen SSC, Rebar R, Vandenberg G et al (1972) Synthetic luteinizing hormone releasing hormone: a potent stimulation of gonadotropin release in men. *Journal of Clinical Endocrinology and Metabolism* **34:** 671–675.

Yen SSC, Vandenberg G & Siler TM (1974) Modulation of pituitary responsiveness to LRF by estrogen. *Journal of Clinical Endocrinology and Metabolism* **39:** 170–177.

Yen SSC & Lein A (1976) The apparent paradox of the negative and positive feedback control system on gonadotropin secretion. *American Journal of Obstetrics and Gynecology* **126:** 942–954.

Yen SSC (1982) Neuroendocrine regulation of gonadotropin and prolactin secretion in women: disorders in reproduction. In Vaitukaitis JL (ed.) *Clinical Reproductive Neuroendocrinology*, pp 137–176. New York: Elsevier.

2

Pulsatility of reproductive hormones:
applications to the understanding of puberty
and to the treatment of infertility

C. G. D. BROOK
H. S. JACOBS
R. STANHOPE
J. ADAMS
P. HINDMARSH

In this article we discuss some of the implications of the pulsatility of gonadotrophin secretion. We consider studies of spontaneous secretion and of secretion induced by treatment with pulsatile luteinizing hormone releasing hormone (LHRH) in an attempt to determine to what extent spontaneous reproductive function can be mimicked by therapy.

PUBERTY

Puberty, defined as the acquisition of reproductive capability, is attained through a series of physical changes which have their onset in more than 50% of boys and girls by their 12th birthday. Considering breast development in girls to be equivalent to genital development in boys, the sequence of acquisition of pubertal characteristics differs between the sexes in only one major aspect, that is in the timing of the adolescent growth spurt. In girls, as breast development starts and as pubic hair appears, the growth rate increases and reaches a peak at Tanner stage 3 breast maturation. Growth rate begins to decline with the acquisition of stage 4 breast development and menarche occurs during this period of diminishing height velocity. By contrast, in boys, the prepubertal growth rate, with its slow deceleration, is maintained during early stages of genital and pubic hair development and starts to rise only when a testicular volume of 10 ml has been reached. Thus, at the age that girls are beginning to slow down in their growth, the rate in boys increases dramatically and they finally stop growing about 1 year later than girls (Largo et al, 1978).

The mechanism by which puberty is brought about is the subject of much controversy. The hypothalamic–pituitary–gonadal axis is fully functional in the fetus and newborn, but a decade passes before secondary sexual characteristics appear. Some form of inhibition has been postulated to account for the apparent quiescence of gonadal activity during the first decade of life, but the search for an inhibitor of pubertal development or for a hormone whose primary function is to initiate pubertal development has been unavailing. Our studies on the use of pulsatile gonadotrophin releasing hormone (LHRH) to induce puberty in boys and girls have indicated that the likely mechanism for puberty in man, just as in the rhesus monkey (Knobil, 1980), is a gradually increasing amplitude of pulsatile LHRH secretion with advancing years. The studies described here have necessarily been drawn from a patient population. Fortunately, since ultrasound is a non-invasive method of investigating ovarian morphology, we have concomitant data in normal subjects which encourage us to believe that what we observe in pathological situations mirrors normality.

STUDIES IN NORMAL SUBJECTS

The work of Peters et al (1981) indicated that prepubertal ovaries, obtained from autopsies of victims of road accidents in Denmark, were far from quiescent. We have used ultrasound examination of normal girls to confirm that ovarian follicular development is common throughout childhood (Stanhope et al, 1985a). The size and number of follicles increase with age,

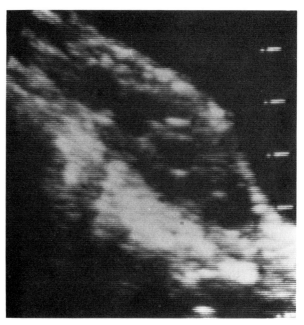

Figure 1. Ovarian ultrasound image in sagittal section from a 9-year-old girl with no signs of puberty. The dark area at the top is the bladder. 1 cm markers are shown on the vertical scale. The ovary contains more than six 'cysts' of 4 mm or greater in diameter—a multicystic morphology.

but it is not until pubertal signs begin to appear, indicating a progressively rising level of oestradiol secretion, that uterine dimensions start rapidly to increase.

The appearance of the active prepubertal ovary (Figure 1), as seen on ultrasound, is seen whenever pulsatile gonadotrophin secretion occurs without the modulating effect of oestrogen-mediated positive feedback, which appears later and enables normal ovulatory menstrual cycles to be achieved. The multicystic appearance is seen not only in prepuberty, but also in patients recovering from anorexia nervosa (Adams et al, 1985; Treasure et al, 1985), as well as in patients presenting with normal secondary sexual characteristics, but with amenorrhoea (see below).

At menarche, we have been able to discern two distinct patterns of ovarian morphology. In some girls a dominant ovarian follicle which suppresses other ovarian follicular development is found, as in the normal menstrual cycle. In others, several large follicles may be seen, one of which may be larger than the others. We have termed this a 'lead' (as opposed to a dominant) follicle, because it has not suppressed the other follicles in that ovary. If an LH surge occurs during a menarcheal cycle, ovulation may occur from either dominant or lead follicles. In normal women the LH surge lasts 24–36 hours, but in pubertal children pulsatile gonadotrophin secretion is usually confined to the night (Boyar et al, 1972), so most of the early postmenarcheal cycles of girls with either form of ovarian morphology are anovulatory. Ovulatory cycles consequent upon oestrogen-mediated positive feedback and an LH surge require pulsatile gonadotrophin secretion throughout 24 hours.

EXPERIMENTAL PUBERTY

Subjects and methods

We have administered LHRH in a pulsatile fashion to 35 patients (18 male, 17 female) with delayed puberty in an attempt to define the minimum endocrine support needed for the initiation and maintenance of human puberty. Because it is difficult to distinguish patients with 'constitutional' delay of growth and puberty from those who have a true deficiency of LHRH, we treated patients who presented to us with significant delay of puberty (more than 2 standard deviations from the mean for the patient's chronological age) and only later assigned to them a diagnosis, which we based on the course of pubertal development after the treatment with LHRH was discontinued. Using a miniature pulsatile infusion pump as a hypothalamic prosthesis, we have been able to reproduce the physical and endocrine changes of normal puberty, including the consonance of the adolescent growth spurt and sexual development in both sexes.

We have so far discontinued treatment in 11 males and 12 females, of whom three and five respectively were subjects with simple delay of puberty, whereas the remainder have varying degrees of LHRH insufficiency. On follow-up, we have been able to observe in some of the former their own spontaneous subsequent progress through puberty after our treatment was discontinued, thus reproducing the results obtained by Knobil (1980) in monkeys. In that study Knobil's group showed that pubertal changes could be induced in the immature rhesus monkey by the pulsatile administration of LHRH, that the changes regressed when treatment was discontinued, but that they subsequently reappeared at the appropriate age. From the present data we are able to offer the following account of human puberty.

Sequence of pubertal development

The ovarian ultrasonographic appearance and pretreatment gonadotrophin

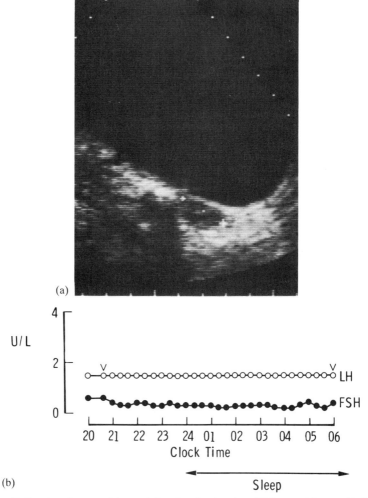

Figure 2. Ovarian ultrasound image (a) and endocrine data (b) from a 16-year-old girl with hypogonadotrophic hypogonadism. The pretreatment ovary was small and contained two small follicles; there was no pulsatile gonadotrophin secretion.

profile of a girl of 16 who had no signs of puberty are shown in Figure 2. Her treatment was commenced with nocturnal administration of 2 μg pulses of LHRH subcutaneously at 90 minute intervals over 8 hours. By 6 weeks of this treatment her overnight gonadotrophin profile had changed dramatically (Figure 3). At this stage, her ovarian morphology had the multicystic

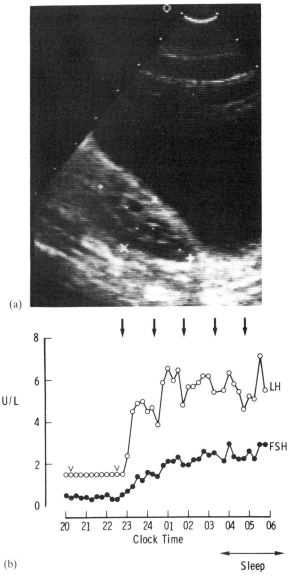

(a)

(b)

Figure 3. Ovarian ultrasound (a) and endocrine data (b) from the same patient as shown in Figure 2 after one week of therapy with 2 μg pulses of LHRH (vertical arrows) subcutaneously every 90 minutes at night only. The pulsatile gonadotrophin secretion is accompanied by a multicystic appearance of the ovary.

appearance indistinguishable from that shown in Figure 1, which we now recognize as characteristic of the girl with the pulsatile gonadotrophin secretion that occurs only at night in early puberty. The gonadotrophin data obtained from this patient (Figure 3) are superimposable on those obtained in normal females in spontaneous early puberty by Boyar et al (1972).

In all our female patients, as pulsatile gonadotrophin secretion was induced by pulsatile LHRH administration, we were able to demonstrate a marked change in growth hormone (GH) pulsatility (Stanhope et al, 1985b). We believe that this early change in GH secretion is responsible for the immediate increase in height velocity that accompanies the appearance of pubertal characteristics in girls. We have observed an immediate increase in growth rate in all the girls whom we have treated in this fashion.

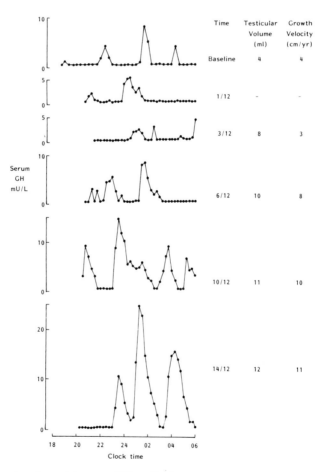

Figure 4. A series of overnight serum GH profiles from a 14-year-old boy with arrested puberty on treatment with pulsatile LHRH. Growth velocity increased and the attainment of a 10 ml testicular volume was coincident with an increase in GH pulse amplitude and the area under the pulse. As GH secretion progressively increased, growth acceleration occurred.

In the boys larger doses of LHRH per pulse were required to maintain adequate progress through puberty and if LHRH therapy was not administered throughout 24 hours, the patients did not obtain a testicular volume of 10 ml or a peak plasma testosterone of 12 nmol/l. As in normal boys, it was not until those conditions were achieved that we regularly observed the adolescent increase in growth rate, which as mentioned above occurs later in the sequence of pubertal development in males than in females.

In the boys, as in the girls, we have been able to observe the effect of increasing sex hormone concentrations on profiles of GH secretion (Figure 4). These data demonstrate why the growth spurt in normal males occurs so much later in the sequence of pubertal development than it does in girls. They also confirm the dependence of growth in puberty on GH secretion, which complements our observations on the same subject in childhood. In a series of 24-hour GH profiles obtained on 54 prepubertal children of short stature, we have been able to demonstrate a direct relationship between the rate at which a child grows and the amount of GH that the child secretes (Hindmarsh et al, 1986). Height velocity standard deviation score is related to GH secretion by an asymptotic regression (Figure 5). From these data we conclude that height velocity is controlled by the amplitude of the GH pulse.

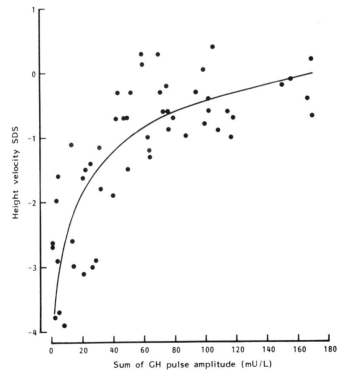

Figure 5. The relationship between height velocity standard deviation score (SDS) and GH secretion is indicated by the sum of GH pulse amplitudes in 54 short children.

Menarche

We have continued treatment with LHRH in our female patients for up to 18 months. Most have needed to change from nocturnal to 24-hour treatment in order to maintain progression of pubertal development beyond the attainment of stage 3 breast development. In those in whom we have induced menarche, we have, as mentioned above, observed two patterns of ovarian morphology. The ovarian morphology and endocrine profiles of two such patients during their first induced menstrual cycles are shown in Figure 6. They are very similar, but one patient had a single dominant follicle and the other had three follicles, the largest of which ovulated. In both patients, progesterone concentrations were elevated after the LH surge and a corpus luteum was seen on ultrasound. We conclude that the selection of a domi-

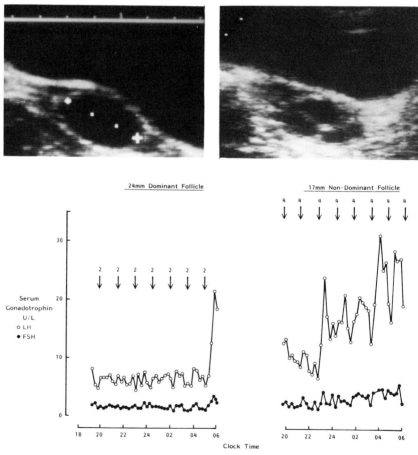

Figure 6. Comparison of the pelvic ultrasound and endocrinology of two ovulatory first menstrual cycles from a dominant 'lead follicle' on the left and non-dominant lead follicles on the right. In both cases the levels of FSH and the size of the first pulse of the LH surge are similar.

nant or lead follicle is primarily regulated from within the ovary and not by the pituitary.

Two of our patients with simple delay of puberty have been followed through their own spontaneous menarche following discontinuation of LHRH treatment. We have thus been able to compare in the same girls the gonadotrophin and ovarian events of menarche induced by pulsatile LHRH therapy with those occurring in spontaneous menarche. When pulsatile LHRH therapy was administered throughout the 24-hour period, menarche was ovulatory; during spontaneous menarche a gonadotrophin profile showed high amplitude gonadotrophin pulsatility confined to the night and the cycle was anovulatory.

DISORDERS OF PUBERTY

The use of the LHRH pump as a hypothalamic prosthesis, together with the increase in our understanding of the ovarian morphological changes in response to gonadotrophin secretion, has greatly improved our ability to manage patients with disorders of puberty.

Figure 7 shows the ovarian morphological appearance and the overnight gonadotrophin profile in a girl of 3 with idiopathic central precocious puberty. The parallel with the profiles and figures shown earlier is easy to see. The administration of an intranasal LHRH analogue (D-Ser^6) LHRH (Buserelin, Hoechst) induced the changes in ovarian morphology and endocrine profile shown in Figure 8. The important observation is that the absolute levels of gonadotrophins were not altered by the treatment but that their pulsatility was abolished, thus indicating how important is the pulsatility of gonadotrophin secretion to the progress of human reproductive function.

A corollary of this work is that it has become relatively easy to determine whether or not a female patient has pulsatile gonadotrophin secretion simply by evaluating the ultrasonographic appearance of the ovaries. This places the management of delayed and early puberty in female subjects in a very different clinical category from that of male subjects, in whom we remain very dependent on gonadotrophin sampling in order to define the presence or otherwise of an abnormality.

A final example indicates how important are the relative contributions made by LH and follicle stimulating hormone (FSH) to the successful acquisition of human secondary sexual characteristics. In Figure 9 the ovarian ultrasound appearance and overnight gonadotrophin profile of a girl with simple premature thelarche is shown (Stanhope et al, 1986). Here it is clear that the concentrations of FSH predominate over those of LH, in contrast to the findings in normal and precocious puberty. The high FSH levels induce follicular development with inadequate luteinization, just as happens in patients with primary hypothyroidism. In hypothyroidism the clinical concomitant is, as would be predicted, breast enlargement without the other changes of puberty. An equivalent of this situation almost certainly occurs in adult life (see below).

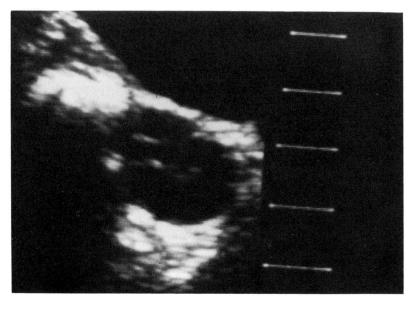

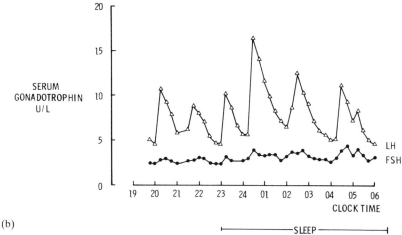

(b)

Figure 7. Ovarian ultrasound image (a) and overnight gonadotrophin profile (b) from a 3-year-old girl with central precocious puberty. The ovary is multicystic in response to high amplitude of pulsatile gonadotrophin secretion.

Conclusion

These results show that all the phenotypic events of normal puberty can be reproduced by a gradual increase in exogenous pulsatile LHRH stimulation. We hypothesize that normal puberty results from a gradual increase in the concentration of exogenous LHRH in the hypothalamopituitary portal circulation. There is no necessity to postulate changes in LHRH pulse

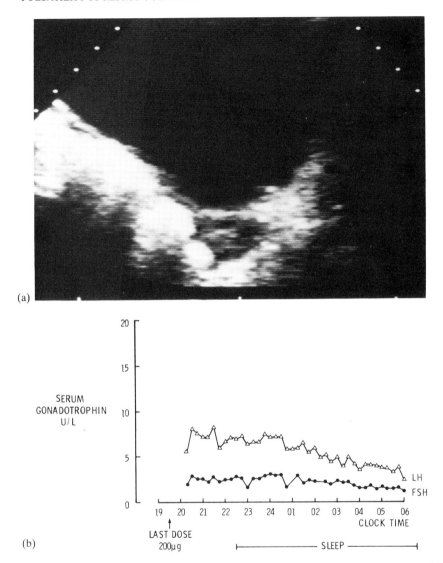

Figure 8. Ovarian ultrasound image and overnight gonadotrophin profile from the same girl shown in Figure 8 following 6 months of treatment with (D-Ser⁶) LHRH analogue (Buserelin). Pulsatile gonadotrophin secretion was abolished and in response the ovary had decreased in size and lost the multicystic morphology.

frequency, the presence of an inhibitor of gonadotrophin secretion, the concept of a changing feedback sensitivity of the pituitary, nor indeed of any stimulator of puberty other than LHRH. The duration of high amplitude pulsatile secretion changes from nocturnal to 24-hour secretion in order to achieve reproductive capability. We do not, however, know what is respon-

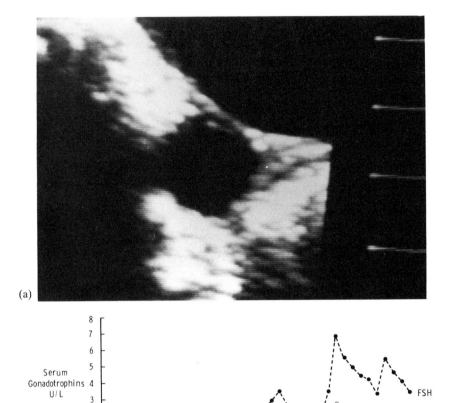

(a)

(b)

Figure 9. (a) Ovarian ultrasound image in sagittal section from a 2.3-year-old girl with isolated premature thelarche. A 15 ml isolated cyst is shown. The upper limit of size of ovarian cyst in normal girls at this age is 8 ml. (b) The overnight gonadotrophin profile from a 1.4-year-old girl with isolated premature thelarche. The predominant gonadotrophin secreted was FSH.

sible for the timing of the onset of the neuroendocrine signals or what determines their being present throughout the 24 hours.

If high-amplitude gonadotrophin pulses occur prematurely, precocious puberty results; this condition can be treated by reducing the pulsatility of gonadotrophin secretion. These studies of pulsatility shed light on the underlying neuroendocrinology of puberty and have been helpful in explaining the interaction of the pubertal growth spurt with the other events of puberty.

It has always been difficult to understand how hypogonadotrophic adults may achieve secondary sexual characteristics and yet not have intact ovulatory menstrual cycles. Our data strongly suggest that it is possible for the increase in LHRH stimulation of the pituitary to become arrested at any stage, so that patients with hypogonadotrophic hypogonadism may present in prepuberty, with arrested puberty or with a failure to attain reproductive maturity, depending simply on the degree and timing of their LHRH insufficiency. It is for this reason that the treatment of infertility using pulsatile LHRH necessarily complements our understanding of the control of the onset of puberty.

INFERTILITY

Numerous studies in adult women, succinctly summarized by Yen (1986), have shown that gonadotrophin secretion is pulsatile and that the pulse rate varies throughout the ovulation cycle, slowing from a follicular phase frequency of every 60–90 minutes to a luteal phase frequency of every 3–4 hours. One assumption implicit in this type of data is that each pulse of LH (and of FSH) represents a pulse of LHRH stimulation of the pituitary and that each pulse of LHRH represents the integrated discharge of neurons in the medial basal hypothalamus, as revealed by electrorecordings from that area simultaneously with measurements of LH in peripheral blood (Wilson et al, 1984).

In humans, precise details of the average LH(RH) pulse rate vary according to the methods of assessment, but representative data are shown in Table 1. For the clinician interested in using pulsatile administration of LHRH as a

Table 1. Characteristics of pulsatile LH secretion in normal women.

	Follicular phase			Luteal phase		
	Early	Mid	Late	Early	Mid	Late
Frequency (minutes)	113	73	83	109	265	339
Amplitude (U/l)	7.5	5.8	10.8	15.8	19.8	12.4

Data from Crowley et al (1985).

form of treatment, these data beg several important questions. Firstly, is the midcycle surge of LH dependent upon a change at hypothalamic level of the LHRH pulse amplitude (and/or frequency)? Secondly, are the low-frequency, high-amplitude pulses characteristic of the luteal phase critical for normal luteal function and thirdly, is an increase of the pulse rate from the luteal to the follicular phase required for the recruitment of follicles for the next cycle? Each of these questions has to some extent been answered by data generated from the therapeutic application of pulsatile LHRH. In our own studies for instance, the LHRH has been administered subcutaneously in a fixed dose (15 µg per pulse) at a fixed frequency (every 90 minutes) (Mason et al, 1984). The clinical efficacy of this regimen is exemplified by our finding a normal cumulative conception rate in 128 women treated with this fixed frequency and amplitude of LHRH: 82 have so far conceived, at a rate that has not been different from normal. Thus, no alterations in the fixed amplitude or frequency of the LHRH pulses were required to repair the reproductive defects from which these women suffered. Inspection of Figure 10 indicates the normal daily pattern of gonadotrophins obtained using this regimen. The results show that a normal preovulatory LH surge occurs in women subjected to an unvarying schedule of pulsatile LHRH stimulation. Since the cycles produced by this treatment were continuous and of normal duration, clearly no change in the LHRH pulse rate was required to recruit follicles for the ensuing cycle.

Studies in the luteal phase of these women showed that if the LHRH pulse frequency was not reduced from the rate of 1 per 90 minutes to the rate of 1 per 240 minutes, seen in the luteal phase of spontaneous cycles, although overall luteal function was normal, not every LH pulse was attended by a pulse of progesterone (Franks et al, 1984). When the pulse rate was reduced to 1 per 180 minutes, each LH (and LHRH) pulse was then associated with a pulse of progesterone. When the LHRH treatment was stopped progesterone and oestrogen secretion ceased and the women menstruated prematurely (Franks et al, 1984). Zeleznick and Hutchison (1986) have extended this experiment by application of pulsatile LHRH to hypothalamically lesioned monkeys. They showed that reapplication of LHRH early in an aborted luteal phase could rescue the corpus luteum but that reapplication later (in a cycle that had been aborted later) could not—that is, that despite its ability to rescue the corpus luteum from deficient endocrine support, treatment with LHRH could not extend the life of the corpus luteum beyond its genetically programmed duration. These studies strongly suggest that

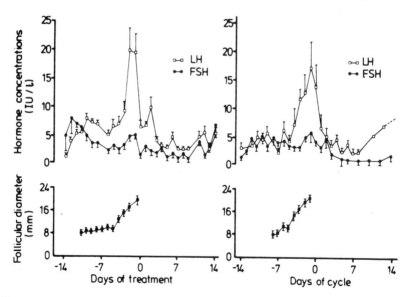

Figure 10. Serum gonadotrophin concentrations during treatment with pulsatile LHRH in subjects who ovulated but did not conceive (left) and subjects who conceived (right). From Mason et al (1984).

expression of the genetically programmed duration of luteal function is determined by pulsatile LH(RH) stimulation. One therefore anticipates clinical descriptions of intrinsic defects of the corpus luteum (producing perhaps a short luteal phase) and endocrine-mediated defects of the corpus luteum (producing perhaps an impaired luteal phase of normal duration). The therapeutic implications of the two types of disorder would of course be widely different.

ABNORMAL REPRODUCTIVE FUNCTION

When pulsatile secretion of LH and FSH and by implication of LHRH, ceases, hypogonadotrophic hypogonadism ensues and the patient develops amenorrhoea associated with small ovaries and a small uterus. The common clinical associations of hypogonadotrophic hypogonadism are organic hypothalamic pituitary disease, weight-related amenorrhoea and hyperprolactinaemia. In each of these situations the reproductive defect can be repaired by application of pulsatile LHRH therapy. Thus using LHRH we have induced ovulation and pregnancy in eight patients with organic pituitary disease (Morris et al, 1986), 19 patients with partially recovered weight-related amenorrhoea (Armar et al, 1986) and five patients with hyperprolactinaemic amenorrhoea (Polson et al, 1986). Figure 11 shows the normal gonadotrophin and steroid profile of a patient with hyperprolactin-

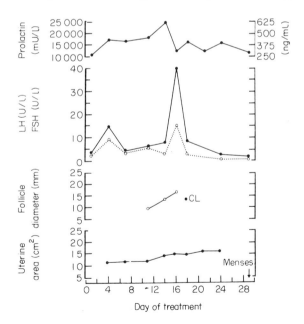

Figure 11. Plasma gonadotrophin and prolactin concentrations in a woman with hyperprolactinaemia during treatment with LHRH. The midluteal phase progesterone was 32 nmol/l. From Polson et al (1986).

aemic amenorrhoea during treatment with standard doses of LHRH. This study clarifies at last the nature of the reproductive defect in women with hyperprolactinaemia. It indicates that the mechanism of amenorrhoea is a reduction of pulsatile release of endogenous LHRH rather than a deleterious effect of prolactin on the ovary itself.

Although these studies of endogenous pulsatility and of therapeutic application of LHRH confirm the vital importance of pulsatility of gonadotrophin secretion to normal reproductive function, they do not indicate the degree of impairment required for the development of a clinically identifiable disorder. From the detailed studies of Filicori et al (1986) it does seem likely that the system is quite tolerant, since periods of complete neuroendocrine 'silence' may occur during night-time sleep in cycles that are otherwise perfectly normal. This is an area where one may anticipate useful clinical information from studies in which the intervals between therapeutic pulses are systematically extended at different stages of artifically induced cycles. Such studies may provide the neurophysiological background to the spectrum of disorders thought to underlie the blanket diagnosis of hypogonadotrophic hypogonadism.

Cystic ovaries

As mentioned earlier, multifollicular cystic ovaries (or multicystic ovaries) may be observed as a feature of women with amenorrhoea. In our experience patients with ovaries with this ultrasound appearance almost always have weight-related amenorrhoea, induced by starvation either self-imposed (Treasure et al, 1985) or disease-imposed (Stead et al, 1986). A few of the patients have exercise-related amenorrhoea, although we emphasize that other ultrasound patterns are more frequently seen in such subjects. As the nutrition of the patient with weight-related amenorrhoea improves, so the ovarian ultrasound pattern returns to normal (Treasure et al, 1985). We think the abnormality in these patients is impaired gonadotrophic stimulation of the ovaries, caused by a reduction in LHRH pulse amplitude. When treatment with exogenous LHRH is used, gonadotrophin pulse amplitude naturally increases, a dominant follicle emerges (together with normal suppression of the other follicles) and ovulation and conception rates are normal. At present the mechanism by which subnormal nutrition impairs endogenous LHRH pulse amplitude is unknown.

Polycystic ovaries

Patients with polycystic ovaries, as diagnosed by ultrasound (Adams et al, 1985), have been extensively studied with respect to analysis of endogenous gonadotrophin pulse frequency and in response to treatment with exogenous LHRH. No clear defect of endogenous pulsatility has emerged, although the amplitude of the LH pulses is usually greater than normal. Treatment with LHRH further exaggerates the increased LH pulse amplitude; Abdulwahid et al (1985) found that the mean follicular phase LH concentrations in ovulatory cycles induced with LHRH were higher in patients with polycystic ovaries than in any of the other groups of patients that they studied. The rate of ovulation in these subjects was lower than normal and was less than that seen in the other groups treated in the same way (Armar et al, 1986). When these patients did ovulate, however, they conceived at a completely normal rate. These data indicate that administration of pulsatile LHRH is not the optimal form of treatment for patients with polycystic ovaries. The data are also consistent with the idea that the ovulatory defect in patients with polycystic ovaries is not caused by a defect in hypothalamic LHRH production but is sited within the ovary itself. Finally the data show that, since there is no disparity in the rates of ovulation and conception, the essential cause of infertility in this syndrome is failure of ovulation.

Solitary ovarian cysts

The syndrome of recurrent solitary ovarian cysts is well recognized in the gynaecological literature (Stone and Swartz, 1979). Typically, when these patients are treated with oral contraceptives the cysts regress, but withdrawal of therapy frequently permits the development of single or multiple solitary ovarian cysts. In the past at least, these cysts were often treated surgically. Many of the patients ended up undergoing frequent operations and became sterile, either because of pelvic adhesions consequent upon the operations or from eventual extirpation of their ovaries.

We have studied the development of solitary ovarian cysts in 11 patients treated with LHRH, none of whom had polycystic or multicystic ovaries (Abdulwahid et al, 1986). During treatment with LHRH, provided ovulation did not also occur, development of a cyst was associated with elevated concentrations of circulating oestradiol, normal concentrations of circulating LH, but elevated concentrations of FSH. The parallel with the endocrine findings in children with premature thelarche (Figure 9) is striking. Although the long-term outcome of this syndrome when it is first seen in children is not well known, one of our adult patients with recurrent solitary ovarian cysts gave a history of precocious breast development (aged 8) but a normal age of development of pubic and axillary hair and of menarche. At present it is uncertain whether isolated thelarche in small children and recurrent solitary cyst formation in adults represent extremes of a continuum, but it is intriguing that, in addition to the parallels in their patterns of endogenous hormones, they also both show relative resistance to the suppressive effect of treatment with the superactive LHRH agonist Buserelin. An attractive hypothesis to explain the disorder is that the essential defect is excessive production of one of the recently described peptide stimulators of FSH secretion (Ling et al, 1986; Vale et al, 1986) (see also Chapter 5). Such an excess would be expected to result in high circulating FSH concentrations, the inappropriate stimulation by FSH leading to the formation of ovarian cysts that produce high circulating concentrations of oestradiol (which themselves have not suppressed the excessive FSH secretion). Such a mechanism would be consistent with the resistance of FSH secretion to suppression by the LHRH analogue described above, since the FSH stimulatory peptides have been shown in vitro to act via a pathway that is independent of LHRH receptors and therefore independent of suppression by LHRH analogues (Vale et al, 1986).

It is clear from the foregoing that analysis of endogenous gonadotrophin pulses and of the response to exogenous pulsatile LHRH treatment is beginning to yield data in both adults and children of considerable value to our understanding of the development and maintenance of the reproductive process. Results hitherto inexplicable, such as those obtained in patients with isolated premature thelarche and with recurrent solitary cyst formation, are becoming understandable by interpreting the dynamics of in vivo gonadotrophin secretion in the light of recently acquired in vitro data.

REFERENCES

Abdulwahid NA, Tucker M, Armar NA et al (1985) Recurrent ovarian cysts and infertility: evidence for an ovarian defect. Submitted for publication.

Abdulwahid NA, Adams J & Van der Spuy ZM (1986) Gonadotrophin control of follicular development. *Clinical Endocrinology* 23: 613–626.

Adams J, Franks S, Polson DW et al (1985) Multifollicular ovaries; clinical and endocrine features and response to pulsatile gonadotrophin releasing hormone. *Lancet* ii: 1375–1379.

Armar NA, Adams J & Jacobs HS (1986) Induction of ovulation with gonadotrophin releasing hormone. *Recent Advances in Obstetrics and Gynaecology* 15: 259–277.

Boyar RM, Finkelstein R, Roffwarg H et al (1972) Synchronisation of augmented luteinising hormone secretion with sleep during puberty. *New England Journal of Medicine* 287: 582–586.

Crowley WF Jr, Filicori M, Spratt DI & Santiro NF (1985) The physiology of gonadotropin releasing hormone (GnRH) secretion in men and women. *Recent Progress in Hormone Research* 41: 473–531.

Filicori M, Santoro N, Merriam GR & Crowley WF Jr (1986) Characterization of the physiological pattern of episodic gonadotrophin secretion throughout the human menstrual cycle. *Journal of Clinical Endocrinology and Metabolism* 62: 1136–1144.

Franks S, Van der Spuy ZM, Mason WP, Adams J & Jacobs HS (1984) Luteal function after ovulation induction by pulsatile LHRH. In Jeffcoate SC (ed.) *The Luteal Phase*, pp 89–100, Chichester: John Wiley.

Hindmarsh P, Smith PJ, Brook CGD & Matthews DR (1986) The relationship between height velocity and growth hormone secretion in short prepubertal children. Submitted for publication.

Knobil E (1980) The neuro-endocrine control of the menstrual cycle. *Recent Progress in Hormone Research* 36: 53–88.

Largo RH, Gasser T, Prader A, Stuetzle W & Huber PJ (1978) Analysis of the adolescent growth spurt using smoothing spline functions. *Annals of Human Biology* 5: 421–434.

Ling N, Shao-Yao SY, Ueno N et al (1986) Pituitary FSH is released by a heterodimer of the β-subunits from the two forms of inhibin. *Nature* 321: 779–782.

Mason P, Adams J, Morris DV et al (1984) Induction of ovulation with pulsatile luteinising hormone releasing hormone. *British Medical Journal* 288: 181–185.

Morris DV, Abdulwahid NA, Armar NA & Jacobs HS (1986) Induction of fertility in patients with organic hypothalamic pituitary disease: response to treatment with LHRH. *Fertility and Sterility* (in press).

Peters H, Byskov AG & Grinster J (1981) The development of the ovary during childhood in health and disease. In Coutts JRT (ed.) *Functional Morphology of the Human Ovary*, pp 26–34. Lancaster: MTP Press.

Polson DW, Sagle M, Mason HD et al (1986) Ovulation and normal luteal function during LHRH treatment in women with hyperprolactinaemic amenorrhoea. *Clinical Endocrinology* 24: 531–537.

Stanhope R, Adams J, Jacobs HS & Brook CGD (1985a) Ovarian ultrasound assessment in normal children, idiopathic precocious puberty and during low dose pulsatile GnRH therapy of hypogonadotrophic hypogonadism. *Archives of Disease in Childhood* **60:** 116–119.

Stanhope R, Pringle PJ & Brook CGD (1985b) Alteration in the nocturnal pulsatile release of growth hormone during the induction of puberty using low dose pulsatile LHRH. *Clinical Endocrinology* **22:** 117–120.

Stanhope R, Abdulwahid NA, Adams J & Brook CGD (1986) Studies of gonadotrophin pulsatility and pelvic ultrasound examinations distinguished between isolated premature thelarche and central precocious puberty. *European Journal of Pediatrics* **145:** 190–194.

Stead RJ, Hodson ME, Batten JC, Adams J & Jacobs HS (1986) Amenorrhoea in cystic fibrosis. *Clinical Endocrinology* (in press).

Stone SC & Swartz WJ (1979) A syndrome characterised by recurrent symptomatic functional ovarian cysts in young women. *American Journal of Obstetrics and Gynecology* **134:** 310–314.

Treasure JL, Gordon PAL, King EA, Wheeler M & Russell JFM (1985) Cystic ovaries; a phase of anorexia nervosa. *Lancet* **ii:** 1379–1381.

Vale W, Rivier J, Vaughan J et al (1986) Purification and characterization of an FSH releasing protein from porcine ovarian follicular fluid. *Nature* **321:** 776–779.

Wilson RC, Kesner JS, Kaufman JM et al (1984) Central electrophysiological correlates of pulsatile luteinising hormone secretion in the rhesus monkey. *Neuroendocrinology* **39:** 256–262.

Yen SSC (1986) The human menstrual cycle. In Yen SSC & Jaffe RB (eds) *Reproductive Endocrinology*, 2nd Edition. pp 200–236. Philadelphia: WB Saunders.

Zeleznick AJ & Hutchison JS (1986) The use of pulsatile GnRH treatment to investigate the regulation of the primate corpus luteum. In Coelingh Bennink HJT, Dogterom AA, Lappohn RE, Rolland R & Schoemaker J (eds) *Pulsatile GnRH*, Proceeding of the 3rd Ferring Symposium, 1985, pp 71–78. Haarlem: Ferring.

3

Clinical applications of LHRH analogues

HAMISH M. FRASER
DAVID T. BAIRD

In both men and women the gonads secrete steroid hormones which stimulate target organs throughout the body. Many clinical disorders of these tissues therefore are dependent on the secretion of steroid hormones and can be alleviated by suppressing production. Compounds such as aminoglutethimide and epostane can be used to inhibit the synthesis of steroids, but because they also affect steroid synthesis in the adrenal they have limited use for benign conditions. Gonadal activity can be inhibited directly by administering synthetic steroids which themselves have androgenic, oestrogenic or gestagenic activity. In hormone-dependent conditions these properties are a disadvantage and administration may cause undesirable side-effects. Hence any method of suppressing gonadal activity temporarily by medical means could have attractions both as a contraceptive and as a means of treating clinical problems. In this chapter we review the clinical applications of agonists and antagonists of luteinizing hormone releasing hormone (LHRH or GnRH (gonadotrophin releasing hormone)). It will become obvious that there are many more published clinical studies in women than in men. We do not think that this is due to male chauvinism; rather it reflects the difficulty of suppressing spermatogenesis without interfering with the secretion of testosterone and hence diminishing libido. Moreover women are prone to a much wider range of disorders of the reproductive system than men due, no doubt, to the complex range of functions that the female reproductive system is required to fulfil.

Following the isolation and identification of the structure of LHRH in 1971 by the groups of Schally and Guillemin it was hoped that it could be used to treat hypogonadal states in which the anterior pituitary was present but receiving inadequate hypothalamic stimulation. A variety of long-acting analogues were developed which, by virtue of substitution of one or more amino acids, were relatively resistant to enzymatic degradation and therefore produced prolonged release of gonadotrophins. However, somewhat surprisingly, when they were used repeatedly they produced inhibition rather than stimulation of gonadal activity. In this chapter we review the status of the current applications of LHRH agonists which have developed rapidly from these fundamental observations. Almost every area of clinical reproductive biology has been influenced ranging from contraception to in

Table 1. Examples of LHRH agonists in clinical use and the forms of administration.

Structure	Proprietary name	Form of administration	Company
(D-Leu^6,Pro^{9}NEt)LHRH	Leuprolide/Leuprorelin	Injection	Takeda–Abbott Products
(D-Trp^6)LHRH	Tryptorelin	Injection, injectable polymer microspheres	De Biopharm/Lederle
(D-Ser(tBu)^6,Pro^{9}NEt)LHRH	Buserelin	Injection, nasal spray, polymer implant	Hoechst
(D-Ser(tBu)^6,Aza-Gly^{10})LHRH	Zoladex	Injection, polymer implant	ICI
(D-Trp^6,Pro^{9}NEt)LHRH		Injection	Salk Institute
(D-Nal(2)^6,Aza-Gly^{10})LHRH	Nafarelin	Nasal spray, injectable polymer microspheres	Syntex
Antagonist			
(N-Ac-D-Nal(2)^1,D-pCl-Phe^2,D-Trp^3,D-hArg(Et$_2$)^6,D-Ala^{10})LHRH		Injection	Syntex

The agonists are listed in order of potency, starting with the least potent.
The amino acid substitutions in a LHRH antagonist are shown for comparison.
Adapted in part from Vickery (1986).

vitro fertilization, and from treatment of precocious puberty to hormone-dependent tumours. For earlier references, the reader is referred to the bibliography by Fraser and Dewart (1985).

LHRH AGONISTS: MECHANISM OF ACTION

In both men and women, normal reproductive activity is totally dependent on the anterior pituitary and hypothalamus. In response to an increase in electrical activity of the hypothalamic neurons, pulses of LHRH are released into the hypothalamic–hypophyseal portal blood at intervals of approximately 1–2 h. The mechanism underlying this pulsatile discharge is not fully understood, but the pulsatile nature appears to be essential to stimulate the secretion of gonadotrophins from the anterior pituitary. If a continuous infusion of LHRH is given, the pituitary very rapidly becomes insensitive to further stimulation (desensitization) and the levels of gonado-trophins fall (Belchetz et al, 1978; Sandow, 1982). The development of agonists free of side-effects by relatively simple modifications of the LHRH decapeptide (Table 1) led to rapid clinical application of this approach to suppress the pituitary–gonadal axis. The more logical approach of blocking the pituitary LHRH receptor by LHRH antagonists has required the synthesis of some 2000 compounds (Karten and Rivier, 1986). Those currently in use have five substituted synthetic amino acids (Table 1) and need to be used in higher doses than do agonists. The resulting higher costs of treatment indicate that the antagonists will only be employed when agonists are not effective or for short-term use (Vickery, 1986).

Continued daily administration of LHRH agonists blocks ovulation and prevents normal follicular development in women and suppresses testo-sterone secretion and sperm production in men. The degree of suppression of the pituitary–gonadal axis is affected by dose and route of administration, but also by individual variation. Minimal effective doses allow some fol-licular growth and hence oestradiol secretion in the majority of women. LHRH analogues are inactivated if taken orally, but are effective if administered by intranasal spray (Petri et al, 1984). If a greater and more consistent suppression of oestradiol is required or it is desired to cause oligospermia and low testosterone secretion in men (Table 2) the agonist may be injected, more frequent nasal administration used, or the agonist may be infused or released continuously from a depot formulation implanted subcutaneously (s.c.) or injected intramuscularly (i.m.).

Low doses/minimal effective dose

It is important to consider in detail the endocrine effects of these different regimens. When the agonist buserelin is used by once daily nasal administration for contraception, an initial surge of LH and follicle stimulating hormone (FSH) release of 8–12 h duration occurs (Lemay et al, 1983). Although pituitary responsiveness decreases after repeated administration, significant responses lasting several hours continue to be observed after each

Table 2. Suppression of the pituitary–gonadal axis by LHRH agonists: indications.

Degree of suppression	Indication
Partial	Inhibition of ovulation
Medium	Premenstrual syndrome
	Menorrhagia
	Endometriosis
↓	Fibromyomata
Total	Polycystic ovary syndrome
	Male contraception
Total	Ovulation induction with gonadotrophins
	Precocious puberty
	Prostatic cancer
	Breast cancer

administration (Schmidt-Gollwitzer et al, 1981, 1984). During the first treatment cycle when therapy is commonly commenced during the early follicular phase, serum oestradiol concentrations will rise due to the development of a number of follicles (Bergquist and Lindgren, 1983), but these do not ovulate and oestradiol secretion subsequently falls (Schmidt-Gollwitzer et al, 1981; Bergquist et al, 1982b; Nillius et al, 1984). It is likely that normal development of a dominant follicle fails to occur due to the drastic disturbance in the pattern of secretion of LH and FSH following repeated administration of the agonist. Some workers have described a preferential suppression of basal serum FSH concentrations (Kuhl et al, 1984). This, together with the elevations in serum LH produced after agonist administration, could have a deleterious effect on follicular development. Although the pituitary continues to release a large quota of gonadotrophin in response to agonist (Kuhl et al, 1984), the normal preovulatory LH surge does not occur (Fraser et al, 1980).

As daily treatment is continued, subsequent follicular development will be suppressed in some women, although the majority will continue to have fluctuations in the concentration of oestradiol associated with intermittent follicular development which become less frequent or pronounced as treatment progresses (Schmidt-Gollwitzer et al, 1981; Nillius et al, 1984). Why should follicles in some women continue to mature during agonist treatment? In women in whom follicular development is completely inhibited it is likely that the pituitary response to agonist and to endogenous LHRH is most impaired; the levels of FSH are too low to initiate development of large antral follicles as is observed in the more suppressed state induced by higher doses of agonist (DeFazio et al, 1983). When follicular development continues, the gonadotrophin drive is more like the first treatment cycle but the exact nature of the stimulus and the relative contributions of elevated gonadotrophins produced after agonist administration and endogenous pulses produced between doses are difficult to determine.

There is evidence for a change in the nature of the LH produced during chronic agonist treatment from measurements using some radioimmunoassays. Use of these radioimmunoassays combined with in vitro bioassays for LH revealed a decreasing bioreactive/immunoreactive ratio as agonist treatment progressed, due in part to an increase in the α subunit concentrations of LH while the β subunit concentrations decreased (Meldrum et al, 1984; Santen et al 1984b; Bhasin and Swerdloff, 1986), and studies in rat pituitaries suggest that there is a decline in the expression of the β subunit gene parallel with the concentrations of bioactive LH (Barden et al, 1985). There is also evidence that the LH immunoreactivity may represent a deglycosylated molecule or an altered state of glycosylation of a free subunit. It should be noted that the magnitude of these differences will decline as the specificity of the antisera for biologically active LH increases. There are indications that the nature of FSH released may also be altered by agonist treatment. In some, but not all studies, an unexplained rise in serum FSH concentrations has been observed after an initial suppression in men with prostate cancer being treated with agonist injections (Santen et al, 1984a). We have also observed a gradual increase in serum FSH concentrations in some perimenopausal women after several months of exposure to LHRH agonist by infusion or slow-release implant (Healy et al, 1986; West and Baird, 1987).

Surprisingly, LHRH agonists were found to exert direct actions via high-affinity LHRH receptors on the rat gonad, initially stimulating steroidogenesis, whereas after 24 h exposure they inhibited gonadotrophin-stimulated steroidogenesis (Hseuh and Jones 1981). There is an early report of LHRH agonist having an inhibitory action on steroidogenesis by human granulosa cells in long-term culture (Tureck et al, 1982) but more detailed studies failed to confirm these observations (Casper et al, 1984). LHRH receptors have not been identified on human gonadal tissue although low affinity binding sites are present (Bramley et al, 1985). The role of these binding sites, perhaps receptors for a paracrine LHRH-like molecule, requires further investigation but it is reasonable to assume they would not be activated by the doses of agonist in clinical use (Fraser et al, 1986b).

It seems likely from the changes in LH and FSH described above and the fact that administration of oestrogen fails to induce positive feedback (Fraser, 1981; Bergquist et al, 1982b) that the primary mechanism of the long-term suppression of ovulation by daily agonist administration is at the pituitary level.

High doses and slow-release implants

A more marked and consistent suppressive effect is obtained by increasing pituitary exposure to agonist either by using agonists of increasing potency, by daily s.c. injections of high doses (1 mg), by repeated nasal administration 3–6 times per day (Hardt and Schmidt-Gollwitzer, 1984), by infusion by means of pumps (Akhtar et al, 1983; Healy et al, 1986) (Figure 1), or by using slow-release depots (Walker et al, 1984, 1986).

In these situations pituitary responsiveness is rapidly severely reduced and it is the suppression of gonadotrophins and absence of pulsatile release which prevent gonadal stimulation (Akhtar et al, 1983; Healy et al, 1986; Walker et al, 1986). Studies in rodents and sheep have demonstrated that infusions of LHRH agonist lead to a rapid reduction in the numbers of

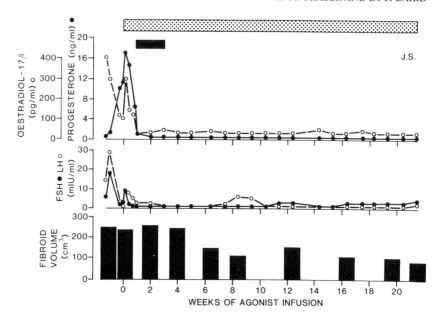

Figure 1. Inhibition of ovulation, as evidenced by low serum progesterone values, and suppression of oestradiol secretion and gonadotrophin release in a woman receiving 200 µg buserelin per day by s.c. infusion for 20 weeks. Horizontal bar shows menstrual bleeding. This patient had a uterine fibromyoma and the bottom column shows shrinkage of the fibroid during treatment as measured by ultrasound. Similar results can now be obtained using s.c. implants. From Healy et al (1986), with permission.

pituitary LHRH receptors and pituitary content of LH and FSH, changes not found when daily injections are given over the same period (Clayton, 1982; Sandow, 1982).

The development of slow-release depot preparations of LHRH agonists has resulted in a more convenient mode of administration giving a more effective suppression at a much reduced cost and obviating problems of patient compliance and variance introduced by frequent self-administration. For example, 1–3 mg agonist can be incorporated into a poly(D,L-lactide-co-glycolide) co-polymer to form a rod which, when injected s.c., slowly hydrolyses and is effective for a 4-week period (Walker et al, 1984, 1986). Alternatively, the agonist can be encapsulated in the same material and the microcapsules injected i.m. (Sanders et al, 1984; Roger et al, 1986). The duration of release may be controlled by appropriate adjustment of the composition and molecular weight of the polymer. Apparently, the polymer has no toxicological problems (Petri et al, 1984; Sanders et al, 1984). It is a linear polyester which hydrolyses in vivo to produce successively smaller polymeric units. The final L-lactic and glycolic acids produced are found endogenously and poly(D,L-lactide-co-glycolide) is an established bio-degradable suture material.

Optimization of therapy and 'combination' treatment

Since the majority of indications for agonist therapy are tumours dependent for their growth on the steroid sex hormones (Table 2) it is important to consider how the influence of sex steroids remaining during agonist treatment can be reduced.

When agonist therapy is commenced during the follicular phase of the menstrual cycle the initial rises in gonadotrophins can stimulate development of maturing follicles with resulting elevations in serum oestradiol for 1–3 weeks. The degree of stimulation is reduced by initiating treatment as early as possible during the follicular phase (Meldrum, 1985) or eliminated by starting treatment during the luteal phase (Fleming et al, 1982; Fraser and Sandow, 1985; Healy et al, 1986). The latter approach causes an initial rise in both progesterone and oestradiol, but when the corpus luteum regresses the pituitary is already desensitized and the rise in FSH required for follicular maturation fails to occur (Figure 1).

In the male such a strategy is not possible, but an alternative approach to overcome the biological effects of the initial stimulation of testosterone, e.g. in prostatic cancer, is to combine the treatment with either a specific steroid synthetase inhibitor, a steroid receptor blocker or a steroid having inhibitory metabolic effects at the target tissue (Table 3). This combined treatment may be used continuously and a similar approach could be applied to the female with inhibitors of oestrogen action.

Table 3. Effects of LHRH agonists and receptor blockers on gonads, pituitary and target organs.

	Gonad		Anterior pituitary	Target organ	
	Testis (testosterone)	Ovary (oestradiol)	LH/FSH	Prostate	Uterus/breast
Agonist (A)	↓	↓	↓	↓	↓
Receptor blocker (R)					
Antioestrogen[1]	—	↑	↑	—	↓
Antiandrogen[2]	↑	—	↑	↓	—
Combination (A + R)	↓	↓	↓	↓↓	↓↓
Gonadotrophin inhibitors/receptor blocker[3]	↓	↓	↓	↓	?
Combination (A + CA)	↓↓	↓↓	↓↓	↓↓	↓↓

Examples: 1 = tamoxifen, 2 = flutamide, 3 = cyproterone acetate (CA). Note that CA has strong gestagenic as well as antigonadotrophic activity.

SIDE-EFFECTS OF LHRH ANALOGUES

Side-effects can be divided into those directly due to the analogue and those due to change in hormonal milieu. Minor problems associated with use of LHRH agonist nasal spray, including occasional headaches, nasal irritation or presence of a bad taste in the mouth, are probably related to the presence of a preservative. Although LHRH agonists can be classed as 'foreign' peptides there are no reports to date of antibody formation (e.g. Fraser et al, 1983; Boepple et al, 1986). If antibodies are produced, the immunochemical differences between agonists and LHRH are such that they should not interfere with the action of endogenous LHRH (Fraser et al, 1983).

Certain LHRH antagonists, particularly those with D-Arg or other basic side chains in position 6, when administered in high doses s.c. to rats produce transient oedema of the face, feet and tail (Schmidt et al, 1984; Karten and Rivier, 1986), an effect attributed to a change in vascular permeability. This appears to involve a histamine response and erythema and some transient induration may be observed after s.c. administration in humans. Chemists have now developed alternative antagonists with similar biological potency but with considerably reduced side-effects. These observations of side-effects of some antagonists, although mild, have been sufficient to curtail proposed clinical trials.

Hormonal side-effects

Toxicity trials and clinical evaluation of agonists have demonstrated the absence of secondary hormone effects, e.g. on adrenal steroid biosynthesis, very good biological tolerance, and the absence of metabolic side-effects frequently observed with synthetic steroids (Sandow et al, 1986). However, the effects resulting from changes in ovarian oestrogen production and testicular testosterone production require careful evaluation.

The degree of gonadal suppression required for a therapeutic effect depends on the clinical condition (Table 2). When used for contraceptive purposes in women it is sufficient to suppress ovulation and retain a degree of follicular activity. However, the presence of fluctuating serum oestradiol concentrations unopposed by progesterone is likely to lead to endometrial hyperplasia, which might eventually predispose to malignant change (Schmidt-Gollwitzer et al, 1981; Balmaceda et al, 1984). Although a more detailed study after long-term treatment demonstrated a predominance of inactive or weak proliferative glands with slightly atrophic stroma and no signs of hyperplasia (Bergquist et al, 1981) the occurrence of oestradiol fluctuations associated with irregular bleeding during long-term contraceptive use would make it difficult to completely eliminate concern that an abnormality had arisen.

When complete inhibition of oestradiol secretion is required, e.g. in breast cancer, the complications will be due more to the long-term hypo-oestrogenic state. The first symptom of oestrogen withdrawal is the experience of hot flushes which begins a few weeks after the start of therapy (e.g. DeFazio et al, 1983; Hardt and Schmidt-Gollwitzer, 1984). These occur in the majority of women but are generally mild and can be tolerated. It has been suggested that they may be treated with low dose clonidine, a centrally acting α_2-receptor agonist prescribed at non-hypotensive doses (Sandow et al, 1986) although the benefits of this drug have yet to be established. Concomitant administration with a gestagen should reduce the incidence and severity of flushes and when treating oestrogen-dependent uterine tumours may have the additional advantage of counteracting the action of oestradiol on the target tissue (Meldrum, 1985). Ten to twenty per cent of women receiving agonist to fully suppress ovarian function complain of vaginal dryness and/or dyspareunia (Lemay et al, 1984; Schriock et al, 1985) due to vaginitis. Such symptoms could be treated with local vaginal application of a low dose oestrogen, but significant absorption into the systemic circulation could partially negate the therapeutic effect of the agonist treatment. Some patients with very low oestrogen experience decreased libido and slight agitation and depression as is also associated with the perimenopause (Klijn et al, 1984; Lemay et al, 1984; Schriock et al, 1985; Bancroft et al, 1986).

A more serious concern over the use of these agents in the long term is that the hypo-oestrogenic state will predispose to osteoporosis by inducing accelerated loss of calcium from the skeleton (Aitken et al, 1973). It is known that, following castration, about 1% of skeletal calcium is lost every year, mainly from the vertebrae, and women who have a premature menopause or who have been surgically castrated have a higher incidence of pathological bone fractures due to osteoporosis (Johansson et al, 1975). Similar loss of bone mineral occurs in women with hypothalamic amenorrhoea and hyperprolactinaemia (Klibanski et al, 1980; Koppelman et al, 1984). It seems unlikely that this will be a significant clinical problem following short-term treatment (less than 12 months) because, under natural conditions, women experience similar prolonged periods of amenorrhoea during lactation when there are increased demands on body calcium as well as very low levels of oestrogen. It is important, therefore, that it has been demonstrated that loss of bone can be reversed by oestrogen therapy provided it is commenced within 3 years of ovariectomy or the menopause (Abdalla et al, 1984). Thus, return of ovulatory cycles after therapy or contraception for less than 3 years should result in restoration of bone mineral.

A higher incidence of ischaemic heart disease has been described in women whose ovaries have failed or been removed prior to the age of 35 years (Oliver and Boyd, 1959; Rosenberg et al, 1981). It should be remembered, however, that cessation of ovarian activity is likely also to have some beneficial effects. A number of studies have demonstrated that removal of the ovaries protects against breast cancer, the incidence of which falls to 30% that of control women in those who have their ovaries removed before the age of 35 years (Trichopoulos et al, 1972; Doll, 1975). As 5% of the population in Western countries will be affected by breast cancer and the mortality is relatively high in young women, it may be that the risk of subsequently developing osteoporosis in old age is balanced by the reduction in death rate for sex hormone-dependent tumours, e.g. breast and endometrial carcinoma.

When investigated in men as a contraceptive, LHRH agonist induced reduction in serum testosterone, led to decreased libido, impotence and even hot flushes (Linde et al, 1981) and its application without testosterone replacement has been precluded. Men receiving LHRH agonist for treatment of prostate cancer also suffer these side-effects, but in this indication they are considered acceptable.

CONTRACEPTION

Agonist in the female

The simplest approach for contraception in women is to administer LHRH analogues daily throughout the cycle to prevent ovulation. The use of LHRH agonist buserelin nasal spray given continuously for up to 2 years has been the subject of two phase 2 trials on 140 women in Sweden and West Germany (Schmidt-Gollwitzer et al, 1981, 1984; Bergquist et al, 1982a; Nillius et al, 1984). Ovulation was suppressed as indicated by absence of serum progesterone rises. Small rises in progesterone in a few women, occurring mostly in the first few months of therapy, were attributed to luteinized unruptured follicles or deficient corpora lutea. No pregnancies occurred in either study. Bleeding patterns were similar in both studies ranging from amenorrhoea (25%) to regular menstrual-like bleeds (37%) to oligomenorrhoea (38%) although none had clinical symptoms of dysfunctional uterine bleeding (Nillius et al, 1984). After cessation of agonist treatment ovulatory cycles returned without significant delay, the women with amenorrhoea during treatment taking slightly longer to have their first menstruation than those who had fairly regular bleedings. No significant side-effects were observed in the Swedish study (Bergquist et al, 1982a) whereas three women in the German study developed symptoms of oestrogen deficiency.

When the more potent agonist nafarelin was administered by nasal spray in a lower dose during a 6 month study, suppression of oestrogen was sufficient to cause hot flushes in 19 of 47 women (Gudmundsson et al, 1986) suggesting that more prolonged use might cause further symptoms of oestrogen deficiency.

The individual variation in response to the contraceptive doses of agonist poses practical problems in bleeding patterns. Irregular bleeding is unacceptable to women, whereas absence of bleeding removes an important index which assures the woman she is not pregnant. However, amenorrhoea could be acceptable to many women once contraceptive efficacy was established and the women appropriately informed. If there is concern about the long-term effects of low oestrogen, then it would be logical to titre the dose of agonist if symptoms of oestrogen deficiency were apparent. Unfortunately, it seems that symptoms of hot flushes, although the most common side-effect, are not always observed when serum oestrogen concentrations are low. Thus it is essential to evaluate whether the levels of oestrogen observed do put the women at significant risk of osteoporosis.

One way of maintaining both oestrogen production and regular menstrual bleeds is to combine the agonist with a progestagen in a cyclic regimen (e.g. buserelin nasal spray for days 1–21, and a progestagen for days 16–22 of the treatment cycle for secretory transformation of the endometrium). Follicular maturation occurs in the treatment-free interval of 7 days before starting the next contraceptive cycle. This would prevent any risk of osteoporosis, whereas the progestagen would establish regular menses and remove any risk of unopposed oestrogen causing endometrial hyperplasia. Trials of this regimen have been encouraging (Hardt et al, 1984; Kuhl et al, 1984; Lemay et al, 1985, Sandow et al, 1986) although the method does detract from the concept of avoiding administration of steroids. Another simpler approach may be to prevent ovulation using a long-acting agonist implant releasing agonist at a dose which does not completely suppress oestrogen secretion and to administer a progestagen at intervals to obtain a withdrawal bleed.

The development of LHRH agonists for contraception should not be looked upon as providing a replacement for steroid contraception but rather as offering an alternative for women in whom steroids are contraindicated, e.g. women over the age of 35, particularly smokers, who run the most significant risk. Another indication would be in lactating women. Although lactation has a suppressive effect on ovulation, the introduction of solid feeds and reduction in duration of breast feeding result in a variable reinitiation of ovulatory cycles and a fertile cycle may occur before a menstruation. The combined pill cannot be taken during lactation since it decreases milk yield and the progestagen only pill may cause irregular bleeding and is unacceptable to some women. LHRH agonist could be used to suppress ovulation during the period of lactation, e.g. from 6 to 18 months post partum reinforcing the lactational amenorrhoea which some mothers who fully breast feed experience naturally. The duration of treatment would be short enough to prevent any long-term consequences of low oestrogen production. Interestingly, it has been suggested that during lactation plasma vitamin D levels are elevated as a protective mechanism to optimize calcium absorption from the gut (Kumar et al, 1979). Although the duration of treatment is short, because on a global scale lactation prevents more pregnancies than any contraceptive, the number of women benefiting by increasing birth spacing would be considerable. Studies are currently being conducted on lactating women using agonist nasal spray and these have demonstrated that small amounts of agonist appearing in the breast milk are without biological effect, presumably because of inactivation in the infant's gut (Dewart et al, 1986). If successful, use of long-acting implants could be envisaged.

The second approach to female contraception, using LHRH agonists at selected periods of follicular or luteal development, has yielded some interesting observations without providing a viable practicable method of ensuring an infertile cycle (see Fraser and Dewart, 1985 for references).

For example, a single administration of agonist during the midluteal phase will induce an increase followed by a premature decline in serum progesterone concentrations and premature menstruation (Lemay et al, 1982). It appears that the agonist causes an abnormally high level of LH release followed by decreased pituitary responsiveness to endogenous LHRH resulting in a period of lowered LH release. However, it seems unlikely this approach could be effective as a contraceptive because effect can be obliterated by exogenous human chorionic gonadotrophin (hCG). High dose agonist treatment during early pregnancy failed to induce abortion or alter serum concentrations of oestradiol, progesterone or hCG (Casper et al, 1980).

Antagonists in the female

LHRH antagonists would be unlikely to be used for contraception in the continuous mode, because of higher dose requirements than for agonists, higher costs, and because it is unlikely that they would solve the problems of obtaining optimum oestrogen secretion as seen with agonists. Nevertheless continued high doses should effectively suppress oestradiol secretion (Balmaceda et al, 1984; Abbasi and Hodgen, 1986; Kenigsberg et al, 1986). Antagonists are, however, being studied for their potential to interfere with specific gonadotrophin-dependent events in the cycle when administered intermittently and at the same time are providing valuable information on hypothalamic–pituitary–ovarian interrelationships. To date, most published observations have been made on non-human primates since antagonists still have to be given in milligram doses by s.c. injection, have only recently been developed in sufficient potency for clinical studies and have troublesome local side-effects.

One suggestion is to allow the follicular phase to proceed to the stage of selection of the dominant follicle (days 5–7) and at this time administer a single high dose of antagonist, depriving the follicle of gonadotrophin support and leading to its ablation. This approach has been proved success-ful when antagonist was administered at intervals of 7 days for 4 weeks in monkeys by Kenigsberg and Hodgen (1986) who suggest periodic progestin (progesterone) supplementation to cause shedding of proliferated endo-metrium if such a regimen were developed for contraception. There have been reports that administration of LHRH antagonist can prevent ovulation when administered during the late follicular phase (Balmaceda et al, 1981; Zarate et al, 1981), but in our experience in macaques it appears that the pituitary–ovarian axis is relatively resistant to antagonist during this period (Fraser, 1987).

Progesterone secretion by the corpus luteum is also susceptible to antagonist-induced gonadotrophin withdrawal even during the early luteal phase (Fraser et al, 1985, 1986a) and earlier suggestions that the primate corpus luteum functioned independently of the pituitary gland were prob-ably due to incomplete suppression of LH (Balmaceda et al, 1983). Three consecutive daily injections of LHRH antagonist during any stage of the luteal phase in macaques will cause a sustained fall in serum progesterone concentrations to follicular phase levels for the remainder of the luteal phase. Administration of hCG from day 7 of the luteal phase to mimic the additional luteal support observed during a fertile cycle will induce a rise in serum progesterone in antagonist-treated monkeys, but only 20% of that observed in control animals. However if antagonist treatment is not initiated until the mid-luteal phase the hCG can 'rescue' the corpus luteum (Fraser, 1987). Thus, the 'window' of susceptibility may be too narrow for the antagonist to act as a postovulatory contraceptive. Although these observa-tions provide valuable information on the pituitary–ovarian axis, any hormonal contraceptive which depends upon the woman knowing the exact stage of her ovulatory cycle is unlikely to have widespread application.

Agonists and antagonists in the male

For male contraception, the goal is to suppress FSH release and hence spermatogenesis without significantly reducing LH stimulation of testicular testosterone production. Unfortunately, the use of both LHRH agonist and antagonist analogues suppresses both hormones causing a decrease in circulating testosterone levels leading to decreased libido and impotence (Linde et al, 1981; Weinbauer et al, 1984). Androgens must, therefore, be replaced if LHRH analogues are to be made acceptable for male fertility regulation. This in turn presents a problem in that replacement testosterone reduces the suppressive effect of agonist on spermatogenesis even when the replacement is delayed as long as possible (Doelle et al, 1983; Schurmeyer et al, 1984; Swerdloff and Bhasin, 1984; Michel et al, 1985). Although agonist therapy of men with prostate cancer results in marked suppression of testosterone production and spermatogenesis, younger healthy men are more resistant and it is rare that azoospermia is achieved. Although it may not be necessary to induce complete azoospermia for effective male contraception it seems unlikely that use of agonist plus testosterone will have a sufficiently suppressive effect on spermatogenesis.

Continued administration of LHRH antagonists to male monkeys has a more profound inhibitory effect upon spermatogenesis (Weinbauer et al, 1984) and although testosterone replacement is likely to counteract this effect to some degree it may be that the suppressive effect is sufficient to achieve an acceptable suppression of fertility (Vickery, 1986).

In conclusion, although LHRH analogues plus testosterone replacement do not appear very encouraging possibilities for male contraception, the dearth of other leads should allow continued research in this area and, hopefully, progress can be made eventually.

THERAPEUTIC APPLICATIONS

Endometriosis

Endometriosis is one of the commonest clinical conditions associated with infertility. In addition, it causes considerable morbidity in the form of dysmenorrhoea, lower abdominal pain and menorrhagia. It has been suggested that retrograde menstruation leads to deposits of endometrium on the ovaries, uterosacral ligaments and pouch of Douglas although it may be situated anywhere in the abdominal cavity.

The deposits of ectopic endometrium are sensitive to ovarian hormones and bleed in response to fluctuations in the levels of oestradiol and progesterone. Much of the pain and subsequent formation of scar tissue is due to this cyclical bleeding. When cyclical ovarian function is suppressed during pregnancy and lactation, endometriosis remains quiescent and resolution of existing deposits may take place. Although localized areas may be treated by surgical excision or destroyed by diathermy, it may even be necessary to remove the ovaries to control widespread disease in which deposits are infiltrating bowel, ureter, etc.

It is clear, therefore, that a means of temporarily suppressing secretion of ovarian steroids, i.e. 'medical castration', could have important clinical use (Meldrum et al, 1982; Meldrum, 1985). A large number of clinical trials on the effects of agonists on endometriosis are currently in progress. Recently, Lemay et al (1984) treated 10 patients using buserelin 200 µg s.c. twice daily for 5 days followed by 400 µg three times per day by nasal spray, for 25–31 weeks, whereas Schriock et al (1985) treated eight women with 500 µg nafarelin intranasally every 12 h for 8 months. After the first month, oestradiol concentrations were markedly suppressed and the patients then experienced near complete relief of painful symptoms of endometriosis and at the end of treatment a significant improvement in endometrial deposits was observed. A major constraint on evaluation of the optimal dose, duration and mode of administration is the necessity for repeated laparoscopies to assess objectively the response to treatment. It is doubtful whether it is ethically justifiable to subject women to repeated, potentially hazardous surgical investigations merely in order to assess response to treatment. As the objective of treating endometriosis is often to restore fertility, studies evaluating treatment as compared to placebo in terms of subsequent pregnancy rates are necessary.

Other medical means of treating endometriosis involving the induction of amenorrhoea with large doses of synthetic steroids, e.g. danazol and gestrinone, are associated with various side-effects, e.g. acne, weight gain and metabolic changes. It appears that medical ovariectomy using LHRH agonists will induce regression of endometriosis in the majority of women with fewer side-effects and its use, probably in the form of a slow-release implant, may become the method of choice for treatment of this disease. It may be that combination with steroids, e.g. gestagens, may alleviate side-effects and produce a more effective treatment (Meldrum, 1985). Clinical trials comparing efficacy and side-effects of these forms of medical treatment are awaited with interest.

Fibromyomata

Fibromyomata (fibroids) of the uterus are the commonest benign tumour occurring in women. Although many remain asymptomatic, they are found with increasing frequency as women age and may give rise to infertility, pain and heavy menstrual bleeding. Being dependent on oestrogen, growth is accelerated during pregnancy and regression occurs after the menopause. Current treatment is entirely surgical and, particularly if associated with pelvic inflammatory disease, operation may be difficult and potentially liable to complications such as haemorrhage. Even conservative treatment by myomectomy may impair subsequent fertility.

Initial studies have demonstrated that rapid regression, as measured by serial ultrasound, occurs in most patients following suppression of ovarian activity with LHRH agonist as an intermittent s.c. injection (Fillicori et al, 1983; Maheux et al, 1985), continuous infusion (Figure 2) (Healy et al, 1986) or by slow-release implant. Heavy irregular menstrual bleeding was alleviated and, although all the patients experienced hot flushes, none wished to discontinue the treatment.

Although it has now been shown that treatment with LHRH agonist is an effective means of treating fibroids at least in the short term, a number of questions remain to be answered before its place in their clinical management can be agreed. In most patients studied so far there has been a rapid regrowth of the fibroid as ovarian activity returns following cessation of treatment. However, in those women who have finished their child bearing, treatment with LHRH agonist may allow postponement of surgery until the natural menopause occurs. It may be that the shrinkage in size of the fibromyata during medical treatment may restore fertility, due to the decrease in the distortion of the uterine cavity and tube. The shrinkage is probably associated with a reduced blood supply. Treatment for periods of up to 6 months preoperatively will alleviate symptoms by reducing or abolishing blood loss. Any subsequent surgery (myomectomy or hysterectomy) should be technically easier.

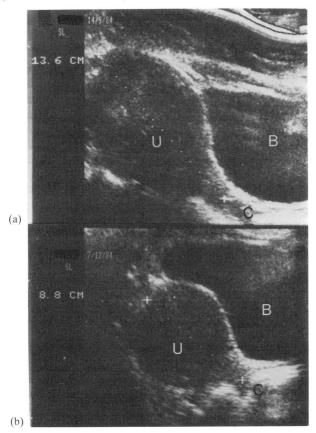

(a)

(b)

Figure 2. Sagittal ultrasound scan of uterus (a) before and (b) after 3 months' treatment with buserelin 200 μg per day subcutaneously. A single intramural fibroid was confirmed at hysterectomy some months later. (Scan by courtesy of Dr S. Lawson.) U = uterus, B = bladder, C = cervix.

Menorrhagia and dysmenorrhoea

Disorders of menstruation are the commonest reason why women consult their doctor in the reproductive years. Excessive and/or irregular menstruation is not only socially inconvenient, but may lead to morbidity associated with anaemia. Although the pattern of menstruation may usually be controlled by therapy with cyclical oestrogens and gestagens, in many circumstances induction of a hypogonadal state and amenorrhoea would be desirable. Shaw and Fraser (1984) showed that menstrual blood loss could be reduced in four women with dysfunctional uterine bleeding treated with buserelin 200 μg three times per day by nasal spray. However, the response was variable and the pattern of bleeding unpredictable. A more consistent suppression of ovarian activity, by slow-release implant, would probably induce amenorrhoea which could certainly be useful to control excessively heavy bleeding, at least in the short term. Because of the long-term effect on demineralization of bone, its use will probably be restricted to acute episodes in adolescence or prior to the menopause.

Polycystic ovary syndrome and hirsutism

It is now established that in the majority of patients with polycystic ovary syndrome (PCO) excessive ovarian secretion of testosterone and androstenedione result in varying degrees of hirsutism and probably perpetuate the anovulatory condition. Suppression of the chronically raised levels of LH found in this condition results in a lowering of the ovarian androgen secretion. Paradoxically, the mean concentration of LH as measured by radioimmunoassay during treatment with LHRH agonist may be actually further raised, although there is reduced pulsatile secretion and the bioactive LH is markedly reduced (Chang et al, 1983; Meldrum, 1985).

It seems unlikely, however, that suppression of androgen secretion alone will be sufficient to cause a reduction of hair growth in women with PCO. Experience with other agents, such as medroxyprogesterone acetate and oestrogen–gestagen oral contraceptives, has demonstrated that antagonism of any residual androgen at the target organ by an antiandrogen is required to produce clinical improvement. It may be that the combination of an antiandrogen together with an LHRH agonist may be a useful and more acceptable alternative to the usual combination of ethinyloestradiol and cyproterone acetate. However, LHRH agonist treatment may be of greater value to induce a hypogonadal state prior to induction of ovulation with exogenous gonadotrophins in women with PCO (see below).

Induction of ovulation for infertility and in vitro fertilization (IVF)

Induction of ovulation with exogenous gonadotrophins is a highly successful form of treatment for infertility due to hypogonadotrophic hypogonadism. However, in other anovulatory conditions associated with a disturbance rather than a deficiency of gonadotrophins, treatment with human menopausal gonadotrophin (hMG) is much more difficult to manage due to release of endogenous LH and FSH (Kenigsberg et al, 1986). Fleming and

Coutts (1986) have approached this problem by inducing a hypogonado-trophic state by administration of LHRH agonist for up to 21 days prior to commencing therapy with gonadotrophins. Multiple follicular development could be induced with daily injections of hMG and ovulation timed by injection of hCG. Positive feedback is suppressed, thus preventing prema-ture discharge of LH before maturation of the follicles was optimal. There were seven pregnancies in 12 cycles of this combination therapy in eight patients with anovulation who had failed to conceive following at least 12 months treatment with clomiphene citrate in a dose of up to 200 mg/day (Fleming et al, 1985). Ovarian enlargement and premature luteinization occurred in the majority of cycles treated with hMG alone. This combined treatment of LHRH agonist and gonadotrophin has been applied to women with PCO, unexplained infertility and to induce multiple follicular develop-ment during IVF and embryo transfer (Porter et al, 1984). This latter application will be particularly useful in women whose cycles are abandoned because of persistent premature discharge of endogenous LH. The period of gonadotrophin therapy can be prolonged almost indefinitely until optimal follicular development has been achieved before hCG is given prior to elective recovery of the eggs.

Premenstrual syndrome

The premenstrual syndrome (PMS) is manifested by a complex of signs and symptoms such as irritability, depression, tiredness, feelings of abdominal bloating, tender swollen breasts, headaches, appetite changes, especially carbohydrate craving, changes in bowel and bladder function, allergic reactions, acne, reduced resistance to infections and others. The symptoms are usually confined to the second half of the cycle, declining soon after the onset of menstruation. Current therapies with vitamin B_6, progesterone supplementation or diuretics are empirical and it has been difficult to demonstrate improvement over placebo. The phenomenon is poorly under-stood and its investigation is important because of its high incidence (30% of women of reproductive age) and its theoretical relevance to the interaction between the hypothalamic–pituitary–ovarian axis and central modulators of mood.

Although there is no simple relationship between oestradiol or progester-one concentrations and the level of symptoms, use of daily LHRH agonist administration has been utilized to prevent ovulation and determine whether symptoms depend on the presence of luteal progesterone.

Results of two studies have been reported, with somewhat different experimental design and results. Muse et al (1984) treated eight women with agonist for 3 months in a placebo-controlled regimen. Since a potent agonist was given at a 50 μg dose by the s.c. route, after the initial stimulatory phase, oestradiol and progesterone secretion were uniformly suppressed throughout treatment. Physical premenstrual symptoms were significantly reduced during the first and subsequent months of agonist treatment, but not by placebo. Psychological symptoms were suppressed during the second and third months.

Bancroft et al (1986) have treated 20 women for periods up to 2 years. These patients had failed to respond to other forms of therapy. Using 600 μg buserelin intranasally, ovulation was inhibited but the degree of suppression of oestradiol was variable. In 10 women, cyclical symptoms were effectively reduced on treatment for 5–15 months. The other 10 women discontinued treatment after 10 weeks or less, seven of these because 'premenstrual' symptoms both intensified and were made persistent. The treatment induced an adverse effect on cyclical acne in one of these women and on cyclical eczema in another. One woman experienced relief of premenstrual symptoms but stopped treatment because of loss of sexual interest.

Thus, symptoms of PMS can occur in the absence of luteal steroids and it was noted that the failures were not related to degree of suppression of oestradiol. According to Bancroft et al (1986), since the principal symptoms which failed to respond were psychological symptoms, either depression or irritability, it may be that these states are related to the ovarian cycle simply in terms of the 'ovarian clock' and are not *caused* by ovarian factors.

Since the majority of women in the two studies overall benefited from the agonist-induced suppression of ovarian steroid production it seems that agonist could prove a useful treatment in some women with PMS, the non-responders perhaps representing a subgroup in this disorder.

Breast cancer

Approximately one-third of human breast carcinomas are hormone responsive, the most important stimulators being the steroid hormones, particularly oestrogens. Endocrine intervention therefore represents a major treatment option for advanced breast cancer, especially against tumours which are rich in oestrogen receptors. In premenopausal women, therapy usually takes the form of castration which classically is achieved by surgical or radiotherapeutic ablation of the ovaries.

Use of LHRH agonist as a non-surgical method of suppressing oestrogen in these women has been explored in three trials with different agonists in the USA, The Netherlands and in the UK. To gain maximum suppression, agonist has been injected s.c. (Nicholson et al, 1986; Manni et al, 1986) or given by infusion or injection followed by nasal spray for maintenance of suppression (Klijn et al, 1984) and more recently by slow-release implant (Walker et al, 1986). Over 70 women have been treated in these studies and clinical outcome has been similar to surgical removal of the ovaries with a similar duration of response and an objective tumour regression in about 40% of patients.

Although s.c. injections of 1 mg of the agonist leuprolide produced uniform sustained suppression of oestradiol, with higher doses having no additional benefit (Manni et al, 1986), six of 10 patients using nasal spray administration of 400 μg buserelin three times daily showed transient peaks of oestradiol (Klijn et al, 1984). Since reliable suppression of oestrogen is essential, there is little doubt that for this type of therapy long-acting depot formulations will be used in the future.

Although ovariectomy is irreversible, it is a surgical procedure with very little morbidity and, because of the age-related incidence of breast cancer, the operation is usually being performed in late premenopausal women. This means that many patients already have the children they desire and, in the face of potentially life-threatening disease, irreversible loss of reproductive function becomes a minor consideration. As it stands, therefore, agonist therapy is unlikely to have a major impact in treatment of breast cancer.

The concept of using LHRH agonist in combination with an oestrogen receptor blocker such as tamoxifen is being seen as of potential advantage. Although tamoxifen is used in treatment of breast cancer, its administration to premenopausal women can stimulate the pituitary–ovarian axis by virtue of blockade of oestrogen receptors in the brain and pituitary (Table 3). The resulting inhibition of negative feedback causes an increased production of oestrogen. A combination with LHRH agonist or antagonist should prevent the rise in peripheral oestrogen by preventing gonadotrophin release while the tamoxifen should block the action of residual oestrogen present after agonist.

When tamoxifen was introduced in patients already receiving buserelin by nasal spray, three of five actually showed increased ovarian activity, so it will be important to ensure that the optimal conditions for dual treatment are established (Klijn et al, 1984). It is likely when more profound pituitary suppression is obtained by slow-release implants that tamoxifen will be unable to stimulate pituitary function.

Because the concept of using the agonist as a form of medical castration would preclude benefits in women without ovarian function, less attention has been given to the use of LHRH agonists in postmenopausal patients. However, there are indications that some tumours in postmenopausal women respond to agonist. Harvey et al (1984) treated 72 postmenopausal patients with advanced breast cancer with leuprolide and reported that 10% obtained a partial response and 22% experienced stabilization of progressive disease with therapy. In a further investigation (Nicholson et al, 1986), two of nine postmenopausal patients responded to Zoladex injections. The importance of these investigations in postmenopausal women is that they indicate the possibility of obtaining antitumour effects with LHRH agonists in patients without overtly functioning ovaries and in whom treatment does not significantly change circulating oestrogens (Nicholson et al, 1986). In order to explain the mechanism by which beneficial effects are achieved it is necessary to look beyond the pituitary–ovarian axis and consider more direct effects on the tumour itself.

Cell lines form useful systems in which to study regulation of cell growth. In particular, MCF-7 human breast cancer cells have been well characterized. Growth of MCF-7 cells in culture is stimulated by oestrogen, and inhibited by the antioestrogen, tamoxifen. When incubated with low doses of buserelin growth of these cells is suppressed in comparison with control cells. These inhibitory effects were dose-related and overcome by addition of LHRH antagonist (Miller et al, 1985). The action of the agonist is not a non-specific effect on the growth of cells in general since it has no, or minimal, effect on the growth of two other cell lines. These findings suggest that LHRH-like molecules may be capable of exerting direct effects on some human breast tumours, although what proportion of tumours might respond, and the nature of the response, remain to be determined.

Precocious puberty

The treatment of central precocious puberty by down-regulation of the pituitary gonadotroph by LHRH agonists is an optimal strategy since this disorder is brought about by premature stimulation of LHRH from the hypothalamus. Previous therapies, dependent on suppressing gonado-trophin release via medroxyprogesterone acetate, cyproterone acetate or danazol, can have unwanted endocrine side-effects and have not always been successful in obtaining uniform suppression. LHRH agonist appears to be becoming established as the method of treatment of this rare disorder, being effective and free of side-effects, and a number of studies are being conducted in several countries involving several hundred children. Current findings of the longest-running studies have been recently reviewed (Comite et al, 1984a; Boepple et al, 1986). Boepple et al (1986) administered $(D-Trp^6)$LHRH ethylamide by daily s.c. injection to 74 children for up to 5 years. A dose of agonist 8 μg/kg per day is uniformly effective, this being higher than the corresponding adult dose, so it appears that the pituitaries of these children are particularly difficult to suppress. These authors empha-size the importance of avoiding lower dose regimens which produce in-adequate suppression in some patients; this is particularly undesirable in treating this disorder. Effective dosages result in suppression of basal gonadotrophins and marked reduction in response to an LHRH test. Clinically, the treatment results in a fall in serum concentrations of gonadal sex steroids to the prepubertal range and halting or regression of sexual development and cessation of menses. Growth velocity and bone matu-ration are slowed and epiphyseal fusion can be held in check. Although longer observations are required before the effects on adult height can be evaluated, the findings to date look most encouraging. Cessation of short-term therapy results in reactivation of the pituitary–gonadal axis but the effects of many years treatment on the outcome of puberty and gonadal function at normal age remain to be evaluated.

Although high dose buserelin nasal spray is more acceptable to both children and parents (Luder et al, 1984; Stanhope et al, 1985) there is greater individual variability in degree of suppression. It is likely that agonist will be administered by slow-release formulations for treatment of this disorder and successful application of monthly i.m. injections of agonist microcapsules have been described (Roger et al, 1986).

Agonist therapy is without significant benefit in patients with gonadotrophin-independent precocity in whom gonadal activation appears autonomous, as in girls with McCune–Albright syndrome (Comite et al, 1984a,b). This disorder requires treatment to prevent gonadal steroidogenesis such as with aromatase inhibitors.

Prostate cancer

Cancer of the prostate is the third largest cause of death due to cancer in man. Growth of the prostate is dependent upon the presence of circulating androgens and the drastic reduction in androgen after orchiectomy or administration of oestrogens results in a response in 60–80% of patients. Eventually, however, further tumour growth will occur which is thought to be hormone insensitive. The existing therapy of castration is unacceptable to many patients whereas oestrogen treatment can cause side-effects, in particular cardiovascular complications.

LHRH agonist therapy has been studied widely as an alternative therapy in patients with prostate cancer and has proved more acceptable, but not any more effective, than conventional treatment. Daily s.c. injections of 1–10 mg leuprolide have induced marked suppression of testosterone (Santen et al, 1984a). A number of different regimens have been investigated in order to obtain a sustained and profound suppression of testosterone production using buserelin by the more acceptable intranasal route (Faure et al, 1984; Wenderoth and Jacobi, 1984). The initial stimulatory phase in testosterone secretion lasting 5–10 days with its potential to cause disease 'flare' has been a cause for concern for some (Labrie et al, 1986) but not all clinicians. In order to obtain a more rapid suppression of testosterone, buserelin is now administered s.c. at a dose of 500 µg every 8 h for the first 7 days of treatment followed by a maintenance dose of 100 µg six times daily intranasally. Again, slow-release implants will probably replace other routes of administration and treatment of patients with prostate cancer with s.c. Zoladex is in progress (Walker et al, 1984).

The use of LHRH agonist in treatment of prostate cancer has precipitated considerable debate and controversy as to the role of a combined therapy with an antiandrogen. Prevention of action of this androgen should prevent any adverse effects of the initial agonist-induced testosterone stimulation, inhibit the action of the low amounts of residual testosterone produced by the testis or adrenal glands and prevent the action of intraprostatic androgen (Table 3) (Santen et al, 1984b; Labrie et al, 1986).

Combined therapy has been suggested using ketoconazole, an antifungal agent, which blocks androgen biosynthesis (Santen et al, 1984b), flutamide, a non-steroidal pure antiandrogen, which blocks the androgen receptor (Labrie et al, 1986) but also elevates gonadotrophin secretion, or cyproterone acetate which will block both the androgen receptor and, because of its progestagenic nature, also prevent pituitary gonadotrophin release (Knuth et al, 1984; Klijn et al, 1985).

There is ample logic behind the combined approach, particularly use of receptor blockade. Any risk from 'flare' following initial testosterone should be removed, and prevention of adrenal steroid involvement is valid since it has been shown that adrenalectomy or adrenal suppression using aminoglutethimide can result in objective regression in some castrate men (Santen et al, 1984b). More controversial, are the claims by Labrie et al (1986) that low levels of testosterone present after castration or LHRH agonist therapy are of crucial importance in the development of tumour growth. They emphasize the danger of high intraprostatic concentrations of dihydrotestosterone that remain after castration. Furthermore they propose that, contrary to previous belief, most of the tumours which were termed androgen-resistant because of their lack of response to castration are in fact androgen-supersensitive, since they respond to further blockade with anti-androgen. They claim that, when exposed for some time to low levels of adrenal androgens, tumours will eventually become androgen-insensitive or autonomous. The logical treatment is therefore to use a combined LHRH agonist and androgen receptor blocker as the first line treatment. Their data on 88 patients treated with a combination therapy of LHRH agonist and flutamide show that death rate at 2 years is 10.9% as compared to 50% after standard hormone therapy. However, the death rate calculated at 2 years was increased by as much as four-fold in patients where the combination therapy was delayed and given as a second treatment at the time of disease progression. These claims have given rise to considerable debate. The need for evaluation by other centres has been recognized and findings are awaited with interest.

Other indications

As the onset of menopausal flushes is temporally associated with the initiation of pulsatile LH release by the pituitary, it is of interest to examine the effects of altering the pattern of pituitary LH release by agonist. As already described, treatment of premenopausal women with high dose agonist will induce hot flushes because serum oestradiol concentrations are suppressed (DeFazio et al, 1983). In both this situation and in postmenopausal women treated with LHRH agonist, flushes occur in the absence of LH pulses (Casper and Yen, 1981; Shaw et al, 1985). Furthermore, there are no indications that the pattern of flushes is modified by the different patterns of LH release induced in relation to the time after daily agonist administration. Thus, while flushes are caused by the withdrawal of oestrogen mediated via oestrogen-sensitive neurons linked to the control of pulsatile LHRH secretion and thermoregulation, it is clear that: (1) pulsatile LH release from the pituitary is not causally related to flush onset, (2) variations in LH pattern of release are not related to flush magnitude, (3) after agonist administration there is no evidence of a short-loop feedback of LH suppressing thermoregulatory centres, and (4) there is no direct effect of agonist on the thermoregulatory centres.

It has been suggested that suppression of testicular function by LHRH analogues might protect against testicular toxicity caused by cancer chemotherapy, allowing return of normal spermatogenesis after cessation of chemotherapy. However, current results have not substantiated this hypothesis (Vickery, 1986).

SUMMARY

What is the current state of clinical application of inhibition of gonadal activity with LHRH agonists or antagonists? It seems unlikely in the short term that antagonists will be widely applied due to the short-acting nature of the present compounds and their troublesome side-effects. In contrast clinical studies with a number of agonists have demonstrated their efficacy in producing a hypogonadal state safely with rapid recovery following cessation of therapy. Although nasal administration may be suitable for short-term suppression (up to 28 days) it seems likely that long-acting depot preparations will be useful for more prolonged suppression.

Perhaps the easiest application to determine will be the profound suppression required to produce medical castration in hormone-dependent tumours. The combination of agonist and receptor blocker is attractive particularly when the receptor blocker like cyproterone acetate also suppresses the release of LH, FSH and adrenocorticotrophic hormone. In cancer of the prostate and breast the side-effects due to inhibition of secretion of testosterone and oestradiol are tolerable although the only benefit over castration is the avoidance of minor surgery.

The agonists should improve significantly the existing treatment for precocious puberty, endometriosis, uterine fibroids, polycystic ovary syndrome (PCO) and induction of ovulation although large scale trials comparing different therapies and doses are required. Finally, the concept of combination therapies to block further the influence of steroid hormones suggests challenging possibilities for even more effective therapy.

REFERENCES

Abbasi R & Hodgen GD (1986) Predicting the predisposition to osteoporosis. Gonadotropin-releasing hormone antagonist for acute estrogen deficiency test. *Journal of the American Medical Association* **255:** 1600–1604.

Abdalla H, Hart DM & Lindsay RL (1984) Differential bone loss and effects of long-term estrogen therapy after oophorectomy. In Christiansen et al (eds) *Osteoporosis*, vol. 2, pp 621–623. Stittsbottrykkeri: Aalborg.

Aitken JM, Hart DM & Lindsay R (1973) Oestrogen replacement therapy for prevention of osteoporosis after ovariectomy. *British Medical Journal* **iii:** 515–518.

Akhtar BF, Marshall GR, Wickings EJ & Nieschlag E (1983) Reversible induction of azoo-spermia in rhesus monkeys by constant infusion of a gonadotropin-releasing hormone agonist using osmotic minipumps. *Journal of Clinical Endocrinology and Metabolism* **56:** 534–540.

Balmaceda JP, Schally AV, Coy D & Asch RH (1981) The effects of an LH-RH antagonist ([N-Ac-D-Trp1,3, D-*p*-Cl-Phe2, D-Phe6,D-Ala10]-LH-RH) during the preovulatory period in the rhesus monkey. *Contraception* **24:** 275–281.

Balmaceda JP, Borghi MR, Coy DH, Schally AV & Asch RH (1983) Suppression of post-ovulatory gonadotropin levels does not affect corpus luteum function in rhesus monkeys. *Journal of Clinical Endocrinology and Metabolism* **57:** 866–868.

Balmaceda JP, Borghi MR, Burgos L et al (1984) The effects of chronic administration of LHRH agonists and antagonists on the menstrual cycle and endometrium of the rhesus monkey. *Contraception* **29:** 83–90.

Bancroft J, Boyle H & Fraser HM (1986) The use of an LHRH agonist in the treatment and investigation of the premenstrual syndrome. In Kerns KW, Fink G & Harmar AJ (eds) *Proceedings of 13th Annual Meeting of International Foundation for Biochemical Endocrinology*, Edinburgh, 1985, pp 456–473. New York: Plenum Press.

Barden N, Chin WW, St-Arnaud R & Guay J (1985) Pituitary levels of glycoprotein hormone alpha subunit mRNAs following long term treatment with an LHRH agonist in the rat. *Program of the 67th Annual Meeting of The Endocrine Society*, Baltimore, 1985, p 281 (abstract 1123).

Belchetz PE, Plant TM, Nakai Y, Keogh EJ & Knobil E (1978) Hypophyseal responses to continuous and intermittent delivery of hypothalamic gonadotropin releasing hormone (GnRH). *Science* **202**: 631–633.

Bergquist C & Lindgren PG (1983) Ultrasonic measurement of ovarian follicles during chronic LRH agonist treatment for contraception. *Contraception* **28**: 125–133.

Bergquist C, Nillius SJ, Wide L & Lindgren A (1981) Endometrial patterns in women on chronic luteinizing hormone-releasing hormone agonist treatment for contraception. *Fertility and Sterility* **36**: 339–342.

Bergquist C, Nillius SJ & Wide L (1982a) Long-term intranasal luteinizing hormone-releasing hormone agonist treatment for contraception in women. *Fertility and Sterility* **38**: 190–193.

Bergquist C, Nillius SJ & Wide L (1982b) Failure of positive feedback of oestradiol during chronic intranasal luteinizing hormone-releasing hormone agonist treatment. *Clinical Endocrinology* **16**: 147–151.

Bhasin S & Swerdloff RS (1986) Mechanism of gonadotropin-releasing hormone agonist action in the human male. *Endocrine Reviews* **7**: 106–114.

Boepple PA, Mansfield MJ, Wierman ME et al (1986) Use of a potent, long acting agonist of gonadotropin-releasing hormone in the treatment of precocious puberty. *Endocrine Reviews* **7**: 24–33.

Borghi MR, Niesvisky R, Balmaceda JP, Coy DH & Schally AV (1983) Administration of LHRH analogs delays ovulation without affecting the luteal function in rhesus monkeys. *Fertility and Sterility* **40**: 678–682.

Bramley TA, Menzies GS & Baird DT (1985) Specific binding of gonadotrophin-releasing hormone and an agonist to human corpus luteum homogenates: characterization, properties and luteal phase levels. *Journal of Clinical Endocrinology and Metabolism* **61**: 834–841.

Casper RF & Yen SSC (1981) Menopausal flushes: effect of pituitary gonadotropin desensitization by a potent luteinizing hormone releasing factor agonist. *Journal of Clinical Endocrinology and Metabolism* **51**: 1056–1058.

Casper RF, Sheehan KL & Yen SSC (1980) Chorionic gonadotropin prevents LRF-agonist-induced luteolysis in the human. *Contraception* **21**: 471–478.

Casper RF, Erickson GF & Yen SSC (1984) Studies on the effect of gonadotropin-releasing hormone and its agonist on human luteal steroidogenesis in vitro. *Fertility and Sterility* **42**: 39–43.

Chang RJ, Lauffer LR, Meldrum DR et al (1983) Steroid secretion in polycystic ovarian disease after ovarian suppression by a long-acting gonadotropin-releasing hormone agonist. *Journal of Clinical Endocrinology and Metabolism* **56**: 897–903.

Clayton RN (1982) GnRH modulation of its own pituitary receptors: evidence for biphasic regulation. *Endocrinology* **111**: 152–161.

Comite F, Pescovitz OH, Foster CM et al (1984a) LHRH analog effect on pubertal development, growth and maturation in precocious puberty. In Labrie F, Belanger A & Dupont A (eds) *LHRH and its Analogues*, pp 438–454. Amsterdam: Elsevier.

Comite F, Shawker TH, Pescovitz OH, Loriaux DL & Cutler GA (1984b) Cyclical ovarian function resistant to treatment with analogue of LHRH in McCune–Albright syndrome. *New England Journal of Medicine* **311**: 1032–1035.

DeFazio J, Meldrum DR, Laufer L et al (1983) Induction of hot flushes in premenopausal women with a long-acting GnRH agonist. *Journal of Clinical Endocrinology and Metabolism* **56**: 445–448.

Dewart PJ, McNeilly AS, Smith SK et al (1986) LHRH agonist buserelin as a post-partum contraceptive: lack of biological activity of buserelin in breast milk. *Acta Endocrinologica* (in press).

Doelle GC, Alexander AN, Evans RM et al (1983) Combined treatment with an LHRH agonist and testosterone in man. *Journal of Andrology* **4**: 298–302.

Doll R (1975) The epidemiology of cancers of the breast and reproductive system. *Scottish Medical Journal* **20**: 305–313.

Faure N, Lemay A, Tolis G et al (1984) Buserelin therapy for prostate carcinoma. In Vickery BH, Nestor JJ Jr & Hafez ESE (eds) *LHRH and Its Analogs: Contraceptive and Therapeutic Applications*, pp 337–349. Lancaster: MTP Press.

Fleming R & Coutts JRT (1986) Induction of multiple follicular growth in normally menstruating women with endogenous gonadotropin suppression. *Fertility and Sterility* **45**: 226–230.

Fleming R, Adam AH, Barlow DH et al (1982) A new systemic treatment for infertile women with abnormal hormone profiles. *British Journal of Obstetrics and Gynaecology* **89:** 80–83.

Fleming R, Haxton MJ, Hamilton MPR et al (1985) Successful treatment of infertile women with oligomenorrhoea using a combination of an LHRH agonist and exogenous gonadotrophins. *British Journal of Obstetrics and Gynaecology* **92:** 369–373.

Filicori M, Hall DA, Lughlin JS, Rivier J & Vale W (1983) A conservative approach to the management of uterine leiomyoma: pituitary desensitization by a luteinizing hormone-releasing hormone analogue. *American Journal of Obstetrics and Gynecology* **147:** 726–727.

Fraser HM (1981) Effect of oestrogen on gonadotrophin release in stumptailed monkeys (*Macaca arctoides*) treated chronically with an agonist analogue of LHRH. *Journal of Endocrinology* **91:** 525–530.

Fraser HM (1987) LHRH antagonists and female reproductive function. In Vickery BH & Nestor JJ Jr (eds) *LHRH and its Analogs: Contraceptive and Therapeutic Applications*, part 2. Lancaster: MTP Press.

Fraser HM & Dewart PJ (1985) Control of the menstrual cycle by LHRH and its analogues. *Bibliography of Reproduction* **46**(6): C1–C12.

Fraser HM & Sandow J (1985) Suppression of follicular maturation by infusion of a luteinizing hormone releasing hormone agonist starting during the late luteal phase in the stumptailed macaque monkey. *Journal of Clinical Endocrinology and Metabolism* **60:** 579–584.

Fraser HM, Laird NC & Blakeley DM (1980) Decreased pituitary responsiveness and inhibition of the luteinizing hormone surge and ovulation in the stumptailed monkey (*Macaca arctoides*) by chronic treatment with an agonist of luteinizing hormone-releasing hormone. *Endocrinology* **106:** 452–457.

Fraser HM, Sandow J & Krauss B (1983) Antibody production against an agonist analogue of luteinizing hormone releasing hormone: evaluation of immunochemical and physiological consequences. *Acta Endocrinologica* **103:** 151–157.

Fraser HM, Baird DT, McRae GI, Nestor JJ & Vickery BH (1985) Suppression of luteal progesterone secretion in the stumptailed macaque by an antagonist analogue of luteinizing hormone releasing hormone. *Journal of Endocrinology* **104:** R1–R4.

Fraser HM, Abbott M, Laird NC et al (1986a) Effects of an LHRH antagonist on the secretion of LH, FSH, prolactin and ovarian steroids at different stages of the luteal phase in the stumptailed macaque (*Macaca arctoides*). *Journal of Endocrinology* **111:** 83–90.

Fraser HM, Bramley TA, Miller WR & Sharpe RM (1986b) Extra pituitary actions of LHRH analogues in tissues of the human female and investigation of the existence and function of LHRH-like peptides. In Chadha DR & Rolland R (eds) *Gonadotropin Down-regulation in Gynaecological Practice*. New York: Alan R Liss.

Gudmundsson JA, Nillius SJ & Bergquist C (1986) Intranasal peptide contraception by inhibition of ovulation with the gonadotropin-releasing hormone superagonist nafarelin: six months' clinical results. *Fertility and Sterility* **45:** 617–623.

Hardt W & Schmidt-Gollwitzer M (1984) Sustained gonadal suppression in fertile women with the LHRH agonist buserelin. *Clinical Endocrinology* **19:** 613–617.

Hardt W, Genz T & Schmidt-Gollwitzer M (1984) Antifertility by discontinuous treatment with buserelin in women. In Vickery BH, Nester JJ Jr & Hafesz ESE (eds) *LHRH and Its Analogs: Contraceptive and Therapeutic Applications*, pp 235–242. Lancaster: MTP Press.

Harvey HA, Lipton A & Max DT (1984) LHRH analogs for human mammary carcinoma. In Vickery BH, Nestor JJ Jr & Hafesz ESE (eds) *LHRH and Its Analogs: Contraceptive and Therapeutic Applications*, pp 329–336. Lancaster: MTP Press.

Healy DL, Lawson SR, Abbott M, Baird DT & Fraser HM (1986) Towards removing uterine fibroids without surgery: subcutaneous infusion of a luteinizing hormone-releasing hormone agonist commencing in the luteal phase. *Journal of Clinical Endocrinology and Metabolism* **63:** 619–625.

Hsueh AJ & Jones PBC (1981) Extrapituitary actions of the gonadotropin-releasing hormone. *Endocrine Reviews* **2:** 437–461.

Johansson BW, Kaij L, Kullander S et al (1975) On some late effects of bilateral oophorectomy in the age range 15–30 years. *Acta Obstetrica et Gynecologica Scandinavica* **54:** 449–461.

Karten MJ & Rivier JE (1986) Gonadotropin-releasing hormone analog design. Structure-function studies toward the development of agonists and antagonists: rationale and perspective. *Endocrine Reviews* **7:** 44–66.

Kenigsberg D & Hodgen GD (1986) Ovulation inhibition by administration of weekly gonadotropin-releasing hormone antagonist. *Journal of Clinical Endocrinology and Metabolism* **62:** 734–736.

Kenigsberg D, Littman BA & Hodgen GD (1986) Induction of ovulation in primate models. *Endocrine Reviews* **1:** 34–43.

Klibanski A, Neer RM, Beitins IZ et al (1980) Decreased bone density in hyperprolactinaemic women. *New England Journal of Medicine* **303:** 1511–1514.

Klijn JGM, De Jong FH, Blankenstein MA et al (1984) Anti-tumour and endocrine effects of chronic LHRH agonist treatment (buserelin) with or without tamoxifen in premenopausal metastatic breast cancer. *Breast Cancer Research and Treatment* **4:** 209–220.

Klijn JGM, De Voogt HJ, Schröder FH & De Jong FH (1985) Combined treatment with buserelin and cyproterone acetate in metastatic prostatic carcinoma. *Lancet* **ii:** 493.

Knuth UA, Hano R & Nieschlag E (1984) Effect of flutamide or cyproterone acetate on pituitary and testicular hormones in normal men. *Journal of Clinical Endocrinology and Metabolism* **59:** 963–969.

Koppelman MCS, Kurtz DW, Morrish KA et al (1984) Vertebral body bone mineral content in hyperprolactinaemic women. *Journal of Clinical Endocrinology and Metabolism* **59:** 1050–1053.

Kuhl H, Jung C & Taubert H-D (1984) Contraception with an LHRH agonist: effect on gonadotrophin and steroid secretion patterns. *Clinical Endocrinology* **21:** 179–188.

Kumar R, Cohen WR, Silva P and Epstein FH (1979) Elevated 1,25-dihydroxyvitamin D plasma levels in normal human pregnancy and lactation. *Journal of Clinical Investigation* **63:** 343–344.

Labrie F, Dupont A, Bélanger A et al (1986) Treatment of prostate cancer with gonadotropin-releasing hormone agonists. *Endocrine Reviews* **7:** 67–74.

Lemay A, Faure N & Labrie F (1982) Sensitivity of pituitary and corpus luteum responses to single intranasal administration of (D-Ser(TBU)6-des-Gly-NH$_2$10)LHRH ethylamide (buserelin) in normal women. *Fertility and Sterility* **37:** 193–200.

Lemay A, Metha AE, Tolis G, Faure N & Labrie F (1983) Gonadotropins and estradiol responses to a single intranasal or subcutaneous administration of a luteinizing hormone-releasing hormone agonist in the early follicular phase. *Fertility and Sterility* **39:** 668–673.

Lemay A, Maheux R, Faure N, Clement J & Fazekas ATA (1984) Reversible hypogonadism induced by a luteinizing hormone-releasing hormone (LHRH) agonist (buserelin) as a new therapeutic approach for endometriosis. *Fertility and Sterility* **41:** 863–871.

Lemay A, Faure N, Labrie F & Fazekas ATA (1985) Inhibition of ovulation during discontinuous intranasal luteinizing hormone-releasing hormone agonist dosing in combination with gestagen-induced bleeding. *Fertility and Sterility* **43:** 868–877.

Linde R, Doelle GC, Alexander N et al (1981) Reversible inhibition of testicular steroidogenesis and spermatogenesis by a potent gonadotropin-releasing hormone agonist in normal men. *New England Journal of Medicine* **305:** 663–667.

Luder AS, Holland FJ, Costigan DC et al (1984) Intranasal and subcutaneous treatment of central precocious puberty in both sexes with a long-acting analog of luteinizing hormone-releasing hormone. *Journal of Clinical Endocrinology and Metabolism* **58:** 966–972.

Maheux R, Guilloteau C, Lemay A, Bastide A & Fazekas TA (1985) Luteinising hormone-releasing hormone agonist and uterine leiomyoma: a pilot study. *American Journal of Obstetrics and Gynecology* **152:** 1035–1039.

Manni A, Santen R, Harvey H, Lipton A & Max D (1986) Treatment of breast cancer with gonadotropin-releasing hormone. *Endocrine Reviews* **7:** 89–94.

Meldrum DR (1985) Clinical management of endometriosis with luteinizing hormone-releasing hormone analogues. *Seminars in Reproductive Endocrinology* **3:** 371–375.

Meldrum DR, Chang RJ, Lu J et al (1982) 'Medical oophorectomy' using a long-acting GnRH agonist—a possible new approach to the treatment of endometriosis. *Journal of Clinical Endocrinology and Metabolism* **54:** 1081–1083.

Meldrum DR, Tsao Z, Monroe SE, Braunstein GD & Sladek J (1984) Stimulation of LH fragments with reduced bioactivity following GnRH agonist administration in women. *Journal of Clinical Endocrinology and Metabolism* **58:** 755–757.

Michel E, Bents H, Akhtar FH et al (1985) Failure of high-dose sustained release luteinizing hormone releasing hormone agonist (buserelin) plus oral testosterone to suppress male fertility. *Clinical Endocrinology* 23: 663–675.

Miller WR, Scott WN, Morris R, Fraser HM & Sharpe RM (1985) Growth of human breast cancer cell line inhibited by a luteinizing hormone-releasing hormone agonist. *Nature* 313: 231–233.

Muse KN, Cetel NS, Futterman LA & Yen SSC (1984) The premenstrual syndrome. Effects of 'medical ovariectomy'. *New England Journal of Medicine* 311: 1345–1449.

Nicholson RI, Walker KJ, Turkes A et al (1986) The British experience with the LHRH agonist Zoladex (ICI 118630) in the treatment of breast cancer. In Klijn JGM (ed.) *Hormonal Manipulation of Cancer: Peptides, Growth Factors and New (Anti) Steroidal Agents*. New York: Raven Press.

Nillius SJ, Bergquist C, Gudmundsson JA & Wide L (1984) Superagonists of LHRH for contraception in women. In Labrie F, Belanger A & Dupont A (eds) *LHRH and Its Agonists*, pp 261–274. Amsterdam: Elsevier.

Oliver MF & Boyd GS (1959) Effect of bilateral ovariectomy on coronary artery disease and serum lipid levels. *Lancet* ii: 690–694.

Petri W, Seidel R & Sandow J (1984) A pharmaceutical approach to long-term therapy with peptides. In Labrie F, Belanger A & Dupont A (eds) *LHRH and Its Analogues*, pp 63–76. Amsterdam: Elsevier.

Porter RN, Smith W, Craft IL & Abdulwahid NA (1984) Letter. Induction of ovulation for in-vitro fertilization using buserelin and gonadotropins. *Lancet* ii: 1284–1285.

Roger M, Chaussain JL, Berlier P et al (1986) Long term treatment of male and female precocious puberty by periodic administration of a long-acting preparation of D-Trp[6]-luteinizing hormone-releasing hormone microcapsules. *Journal of Clinical Endocrinology and Metabolism* 62: 670–677.

Rosenberg L, Hennekens CH, Rosner B et al (1981) Early menopause and the risk of myocardial infarction. *American Journal of Obstetrics and Gynecology* 139: 47–51.

Sanders LM, McRae GI, Vitale KM, Vickery BH & Kent JS (1984) An injectable biodegradable controlled release delivery system for nafarelin acetate. In Labrie F, Belanger A & Dupont A (eds) *LHRH and Its Analogues*, pp 53–62. Amsterdam: Elsevier.

Sandow J (1982) Inhibition of pituitary and testicular function by LHRH analogues. In Jeffcoate SL & Sandler M (eds) *Progress Towards a Male Contraceptive*, p 19. Chichester: John Wiley.

Sandow J, Fraser HM & Geisthövel F (1986) Pharmacology and experimental basis of therapy with LHRH agonists in women. In Rolland R & Chadha D (eds) *Gonadotropin Down-regulation in Gynaecological Practice*, New York: Alan Liss.

Santen RJ, Demers LM, Max DT et al (1984a) Long term effects of administration of a gonadotropin-releasing hormone superagonist analog in men with prostate carcinoma. *Journal of Clinical Endocrinology* 58: 397–400.

Santen RJ, English HF & Warner BF (1984b) GnRH superagonist treatment of prostate cancer: hormonal effects with and without an androgen biosynthesis inhibitor. In Labrie F, Belanger A & Dupont A (eds) *LHRH and Its Analogues*, pp 336–348. Amsterdam: Elsevier.

Schmidt F, Sandaram K, Thau R & Bardin CW (1984) [Ac-D-NAL(2)1,4FD-Phe2,D-Trp3,D-Arg6]-LHRH, a potent antagonist of LHRH, produced transient edema and behavioral changes in rats. *Contraception* 29: 283–288.

Schmidt-Gollwitzer M, Hardt W & Schmidt-Gollwitzer K (1984) Risks and benefits of LHRH agonists as antifertility agents. In Vickery BH, Nestor JJ Jr & Hafesz ESE (eds) *LHRH and Its Analogs: Contraceptive and Therapeutic Applications*, pp 243–254. Lancaster: MTP Press.

Schmidt-Gollwitzer M, Hardt W & Schmidt-Gollwitzer K (1981) Influence of the LHRH analogue buserelin on cyclic ovarian function and on endometrium. A new approach to fertility control? *Contraception* 23: 187–195.

Schriock E, Monroe SE, Henzl M & Jaffe RB (1985) Treatment of endometriosis with a potent agonist of gonadotropin-releasing hormone (nafarelin). *Fertility and Sterility* 44: 583–588.

Schürmeyer TH, Knuth UA, Freischem CW et al (1984) Suppression of pituitary and testicular function in normal men by constant gonadotrophin-releasing hormone agonist infusion. *Journal of Clinical Endocrinology and Metabolism* 59: 19–24.

Shaw RW & Fraser HM (1984) Use of a superactive LHRH agonist in the treatment of menorrhagia. *British Journal of Obstetrics and Gynaecology* 91: 913–916.

Shaw RW, Kerr-Wilson RHJ, Fraser HM et al (1985) Effect of an intranasal LHRH agonist on gonadotrophins and hot flushes in post-menopausal women. *Maturitas* **7:** 161–167.

Stanhope R, Adams J & Brook CGD (1985) The treatment of central precocious puberty using an intranasal LHRH analogue (buserelin). *Clinical Endocrinology* **22:** 795–806.

Swerdloff RS & Bhasin S (1984) Hormonal effects of GnRH agonist in the human male: an approach to male contraception using combined androgen and GnRH agonist treatment. In Labrie F, Belanger A & Dupont A (eds) *LHRH and Its Analogues*, pp 287–301. Amsterdam: Elsevier.

Trichopoulos P, MacMahon B & Cote P (1972) Menopause and breast cancer. *Journal of the National Cancer Institute* **48:** 605–613.

Tureck RW, Mastroianni L, Blasco L & Strauss JF (1982) Inhibition of human granulosa cell progesterone secretion by a gonadotrophin-releasing hormone agonist. *Journal of Clinical Endocrinology and Metabolism* **54:** 1078–1080.

Vickery BH (1986) Comparison of the potential for therapeutic utilities with gonadotropin-releasing hormone agonists and antagonists. *Endocrine Reviews* **7:** 115–124.

Walker KJ, Turkes AO, Turkes A et al (1984) Treatment of patients with advanced cancer of the prostate using a slow-release (depot) formulation of the LHRH agonist ICI 118630 (Zoladex). *Journal of Endocrinology* **103:** R1–R4.

Walker KJ, Turkes A, Williams MR, Blamey RW & Nicholson RI (1986) Preliminary endocrinological evaluation of a sustained-release formulation of the LH-releasing hormone agonist D-Ser(Bu^r)^6 Azgly^{10}LHRH in premenopausal women with advanced breast cancer. *Journal of Endocrinology* **111:** 349–353.

Weinbauer GF, Surmann FJ, Bint-Akhtar F et al (1984) Reversible inhibition of testicular function by a gonadotrophin hormone-releasing hormone antagonist in monkeys (*Macaca fascicularis*). *Fertility and Sterility* **42:** 906–914.

Wenderoth UK & Jacobi GH (1984) Three years experience with the GnRH-analogue buserelin in 100 patients with advanced prostatic cancer. In Labrie F, Belanger A & Dupont A (eds) *LHRH and Its Analogues*, pp 349–358. Amsterdam: Elsevier.

West C & Baird DT (1987) Suppression of ovarian activity by Zoladex depot (ICI 118630), a long acting LHRH agonist analogue. *Clinical Endocrinology* (in press).

Zarate A, Canales ES, Sthory I et al (1981) Anovulatory effect of a LHRH antagonist in women. *Contraception* **24:** 315–320.

4

Endocrinology of the hypothalamic–pituitary–testicular axis with particular reference to the hormonal control of spermatogenesis

ALVIN M. MATSUMOTO
WILLIAM J. BREMNER

The endocrine control of testicular function involves a complex, finely regulated interaction between the central nervous system (CNS) (in particular the hypothalamus), the anterior pituitary gland, and the testis (Figure 1). The testis consists of two structurally and functionally distinct compartments, each of which is responsible for one of the two major physiological functions of the testis:

1. The seminiferous tubules produce and transport spermatozoa, which determine a man's ability to conceive children (i.e. fertility);

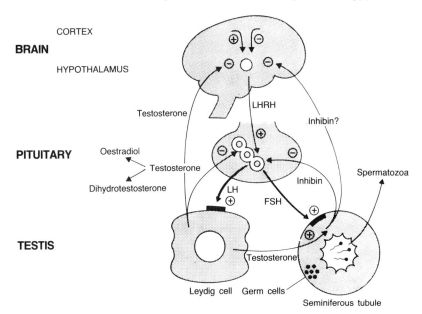

Figure 1. Diagram of the normal physiology of the hypothalamic–pituitary–testicular axis.

2. The interstitial or Leydig cells produce and secrete sex steroid hormones, primarily testosterone (T), that mediate the development and maintenance of primary and secondary sexual characteristics and normal sexual behaviour and potency, as well as playing an important role in the initiation and maintenance of spermatogenesis.

Although the two compartments of the testis are structurally and functionally distinct, there is considerable evidence for intercompartmental paracrine regulatory mechanisms. Details of intragonadal regulatory mechanisms are discussed in Chapter 11.

Knowledge of the normal physiological regulation of testicular function provides the basis for understanding the pathophysiology and treatment of testicular disorders and for formulating strategies to alter testicular function, such as suppressing T production in the treatment of prostate cancer and suppressing sperm production in male contraceptive development.

NORMAL PHYSIOLOGY OF THE HYPOTHALAMIC–PITUITARY– TESTICULAR AXIS

Hypothalamic regulation of pituitary gonadotrophin secretion

Testicular function is primarily under the control of the gonadotrophins, luteinizing hormone (LH) and follicle stimulating hormone (FSH) secreted by the anterior pituitary gland (Figure 1). Both LH and FSH are glycoprotein hormones. Like thyroid stimulating hormone and human chorionic gonadotrophin (hCG), they are composed of two polypeptide subunits (the α and β subunits). Alpha and β subunits are synthesized separately, assembled, and glycosylated prior to secretion from the pituitary. The α subunits for all four glycoprotein hormones are identical and biologically inactive, whereas the β subunits are unique for each hormone and determine their immunological and biological distinctiveness. However, the α and β subunits must be bound together (non-covalently) to exert biological activity. With the recent availability of sensitive in vitro bioassays for LH (VanDamme et al, 1974) and FSH (Jia et al, 1986), it is being appreciated that circulating gonadotrophin levels measured by radioimmunoassay may not always reflect the levels of biologically active hormone (Evans et al, 1984). The relationship between biological and immunological LH activity is discussed in Chapter 8.

LH and (to a lesser extent) FSH are secreted into the peripheral circulation by the anterior pituitary gland in an episodic fashion (Santen and Bardin, 1973). The physiological significance of pulsatile gonadotrophin secretion in the regulation of testicular function is presently not known. However, the realization that levels of gonadotrophins, particularly LH, fluctuate markedly in blood has influenced blood sampling regimens to determine normal values of these hormones. The biological significance of pulsatile hormone secretion is discussed in further detail in Chapter 1.

The pulsatile secretion of gonadotrophins is regulated primarily by the episodic stimulation of the pituitary gland by luteinizing hormone releasing hormone (LHRH). LHRH is a decapeptide which is synthesized by hypothalamic neurons and secreted episodically into the hypothalamo-hypophyseal portal system, where it is carried to the anterior pituitary gland. LHRH binds to specific receptors on the plasma membrane of pituitary gonadotrophs and stimulates the release of both LH and FSH by a calcium-dependent mechanism (Figure 1). Studies by Knobil (1980) in non-human primates demonstrated that a pulsatile, as opposed to a continuous, pattern of LHRH stimulation of the pituitary was essential for induction and maintenance of normal gonadotrophin secretion.

There is also good evidence that the pulsatile pattern of LHRH stimulation is important to normal pituitary gonadotroph function in humans. Administration of low dosage pulsatile LHRH has been used successfully to induce normal testicular development and function in patients with hypogonadotrophic eunuchoidism, who presumably lack endogenous LHRH (Hoffman and Crowley, 1982). By contrast, administration of high dosage, continuous LHRH or superactive LHRH agonists has been demonstrated to severely suppress gonadotrophin and testicular function (Labrie et al, 1986), and has been used as a method to medically castrate patients with androgen-dependent tumours, such as prostate cancer. Clinical applications of LHRH agonists are discussed in greater detail in Chapter 3.

Hypothalamic LHRH neurons are regulated by numerous stimulatory and inhibitory neurotransmitter (e.g. catecholamine, serotonin, and amino acid) and neuropeptide (e.g. opioid) systems. Many of these neuromodulatory systems participate in the regulation of LHRH-secreting neurons by higher neural centres (e.g. the limbic system and cerebral cortex) and by testicular steroids. Therefore, the hypothalamic LHRH neuronal system serves an important integrative function in the regulation of testicular function (Figure 1). It receives input from higher CNS centres and from testicular negative feedback factors to alter LHRH output; alterations in LHRH secretion regulate pituitary gonadotrophin secretion which, in turn, controls testicular function. Knowledge of the neurotransmitter regulation of LHRH secretion has helped increase our understanding of effects, such as those of pharmacological agents (e.g. catecholaminergic and opiate drugs) and malnutrition, on testicular function.

Gonadotrophin regulation of testicular function

LH binds to specific, high affinity membrane receptors on Leydig cells of the testis and stimulates testicular steroidogenesis via a cyclic adenosine monophosphate (AMP)-mediated process. LH receptor stimulation accelerates cholesterol transport into the mitochondria of Leydig cells and increases the activity of the cholesterol 20,22 desmolase/side-chain cleavage enzyme complex which enhances the conversion of cholesterol to pregnenolone, the rate-limiting step in T biosynthesis. Ultimately, LH stimulation leads to increased secretion of T, the major steroid product of the testis (Figure 1). T secretion occurs both locally within the testis and into the peripheral circulation.

The majority of T that is secreted into the blood stream by the testis is bound to plasma proteins, primarily sex hormone-binding globulin (SHBG) and albumin. It has been thought that only the non-protein-bound or free fraction of T is physiologically active. However, recent studies have suggested that albumin-bound T may also be available to act as an androgen in many target organs (Pardridge, 1981). Protein binding of T in the peripheral circulation is believed to serve as a buffer or reservoir for free T. In certain clinical situations (e.g. hepatic cirrhosis, obesity, and thyroid dysfunction) alterations in SHBG levels result in abnormal total T measurements, although free T levels remain normal.

Normal levels of T are necessary for sexual differentiation of male internal and external genitalia during embryogenesis, development and maintenance of secondary sexual characteristics at the time of puberty, maintenance of sexual functioning and behaviour, other aspects of behaviour (such as aggressiveness), and negative feedback regulation of gonadotrophin secretion in adults. In addition to increasing secretion of T into blood, LH also stimulates high local production of T within the testis, which is thought to be important in initiating and maintaining spermatogenesis.

Knowledge of the differing roles of T during development has resulted in an appreciation that the clinical presentation of androgen deficiency differs depending on the stage of sexual development during which the deficiency occurs (Odell and Swerdloff, 1978). T deficiency occurring during embryogenesis results in varying degrees of ambiguous genital development, from phenotypically female to nearly normal male (i.e. male pseudohermaphroditism). T deficiency that occurs before puberty results in failure of development of secondary sexual characteristics with infantile genitalia and testis, lack of androgen-dependent hair growth, high-pitched voice, poor muscular development, persistence of prepubertal fat distribution, and increased long bone growth (i.e. eunuchoidism). Finally, androgen deficiency in adults is characterized by reduced libido and potency, infertility, behavioural changes, weakness and fatigue, and loss of androgen-dependent hair (i.e. adult male hypogonadal syndrome).

In many androgen-dependent target tissues, circulating T is converted intracellularly to a more potent androgen, dihydrotestosterone (DHT), by the enzyme 5α-reductase. In peripheral tissues (including the hypothalamus and pituitary gland) and to a lesser extent within the testis, T is also aromatized to oestradiol (E_2). Although the extent to which these intracellular metabolites of T contribute to androgen action in specific tissues is unclear, both 5α-reduction and aromatization are important in the biological effects of T on target tissues. For example, patients with 5α-reductase deficiency fail to develop normal male external genitalia in utero and are born and usually raised as phenotypic females (Wilson et al, 1981).

Circulating T and its active metabolites bind to intracellular androgen (T and DHT) or oestrogen (E_2) receptors which interact with the genome to stimulate DNA transcription, messenger RNA translation and protein synthesis, resulting in expression of androgen action. Quantitative or qualitative alterations in androgen receptors result in varying degrees of male pseudohermaphroditism (Wilson et al, 1983).

High intratesticular T concentrations are maintained within the seminiferous tubules, in part, by the binding of T to androgen binding protein (ABP). ABP is produced by Sertoli cells under the influence of T and FSH. A high local concentration of T within the testis is thought to be important in the initiation and maintenance of normal spermatogenesis. However, the mechanism by which T affects spermatogenesis and the actual quantity of T necessary in the seminiferous tubules to maintain normal sperm production and fertility are not well defined.

FSH binds to specific receptors on the plasma membrane of Sertoli cells and probably spermatogonia of the seminiferous tubule compartment of the testis. FSH receptor binding results in stimulation of adenylate cyclase activity, increase in intracellular cAMP and protein kinase, and production of a variety of proteins that may be important in regulating spermatogenesis (e.g. ABP and transferrin), feedback control of FSH (inhibin), and possibly modulation of Leydig cell function (Figure 1). Developing spermatogenic cells are enveloped in the cytoplasmic processes of the Sertoli cells which are thought to nurture and coordinate the completion of sperm maturation in the seminiferous tubule. Presumably through its action on Sertoli cells, FSH is thought to play an important role in spermatid maturation (spermiogenesis) and the initiation of spermatogenesis at the time of puberty. However, the role of FSH in the maintenance of sperm production in adults is less well understood (see below).

Testicular feedback regulation of gonadotrophin secretion

An important component in the regulation of the hypothalamic–pituitary–testicular axis is the negative feedback control of gonadotrophin secretion exerted by the testis (Figure 1). Both steroidal (T and E_2) and non-steroidal (inhibin) testicular products are involved in negative feedback. T (and its active metabolites E_2 and DHT) exerts a profound suppressive effect on both LH and FSH secretion. The site of the negative feedback effect of T on gonadotrophin secretion is not clear, but indirect evidence exists for an effect of T at both the hypothalamic and pituitary level. Inhibin is a non-steroidal, glycoprotein product of the Sertoli cell that selectively inhibits FSH secretion at the pituitary gland. The physiological significance of inhibin secretion is poorly understood. However, with the recent isolation and characterization of inhibin (Robertson et al, 1986) and cloning of the inhibin gene (Mason et al, 1985; Forage et al, 1986), human inhibin preparations should soon be available for clinical studies aimed at clarifying its physiological role in man. The development of sensitive radioimmunoassays to measure inhibin in human serum (McLachlan et al, 1986) will also help clarify the physiological role of this substance in man (see Chapter 5).

HORMONAL CONTROL OF SPERMATOGENESIS

The hormonal milieu necessary for the initiation and maintenance of spermatogenesis in man is poorly understood. It is well established that in

man sperm production requires the stimulatory actions of pituitary gonadotrophins. Spermatogenesis is not initiated in prepubertal hypogonadotrophic patients (e.g. hypogonadotrophic eunuchoidism or Kallmann's
syndrome) and not maintained in men who acquire gonadotrophin deficiency as adults (e.g. hypopituitarism as a result of hypophysectomy or
pituitary tumour). However, the specific roles played by LH and FSH and
the relative contribution of each in regulating human spermatogenesis are
unclear.

Previous studies investigating the hormonal requirements for initiation
and maintenance of sperm production in man have studied gonadotrophin
replacement requirements in men with hypogonadotrophic hypogonadism.
The majority of these studies have been performed in men with deficiency of
both gonadotrophins. Studies of spermatogenesis before and after selective
gonadotrophin treatment in the rare cases of selective LH or FSH deficiency
have not been performed. Most of the studies in hypogonadotrophic men
have been difficult to interpret because of uncertainties in the degree of
gonadotrophin deficiency present in these men and the lack of pure gonadotrophin preparations used for replacement therapy.

With the recent development of highly sensitive and specific assays for
measurement of gonadotrophins and the availability of highly purified
gonadotrophin preparations for clinical use, the specific roles of LH and
FSH in the control of human spermatogenesis can now be better investigated. Recently, we have performed several studies of selective gonadotrophin replacement using highly purified gonadotrophin preparations in
normal men in whom experimental gonadotrophin deficiency was induced
(by administration of either exogenous T or hCG). The following sections
will review studies we and others have performed in men with experimen-
tally induced and spontaneously occurring hypogonadotrophism that have
increased our understanding of the hormonal control of human spermatogenesis.

Gonadotrophin replacement studies in experimental hypogonadotrophic hypogonadism

As described above, normal testicular function requires the stimulatory
actions of the pituitary gonadotrophins, LH and FSH. While LH is clearly
required for stimulating steroidogenesis, the role of FSH is less clear. FSH
has been thought to be responsible for controlling spermatogenesis, but
there have been clinical and experimental reports of spermatogenesis in the
apparent absence of FSH (Johnsen, 1978).

We have performed a series of studies in normal men designed to assess
the role of FSH in the control of human spermatogenesis (Bremner et al,
1981; Matsumoto et al, 1983, 1984, 1986; Matsumoto and Bremner, 1985).
Several of these studies were designed to determine whether normal blood
levels of FSH are necessary for human spermatogenesis and, if so, to what
extent (Bremner et al, 1981; Matsumoto et al, 1983, 1984, 1986; Matsumoto
and Bremner, 1985). Our assumption was that this basic physiological
information would be useful in designing gonadotrophin replacement regi-

mens for men with hypogonadotrophic disease and in determining optimal strategies for male contraceptive development.

Our initial work made use of the earlier observation that approximately 50% of normal men become azoospermic when they receive T enanthate 200 mg intramuscularly weekly (Swerdloff et al, 1977). By its inhibitory effect on the hypothalamus and pituitary, T leads to a marked suppression of LH and FSH production and therefore to a loss of sperm production. We used this paradigm to test the effects on spermatogenesis of selective replacement regimens of LH (or the LH-like hormone, hCG) and FSH. In this unique situation, the specific effects of the two gonadotrophins on sperm production can be tested separately or together in men who are known to have normal testicular responsiveness since they demonstrated normal sperm counts prior to initiating T suppression.

In the first study (Bremner et al, 1981), following suppression of gonado-trophin and sperm production by the administration of T to five normal men, hCG (5000 IU intramuscularly three times weekly) was added to the T (Figure 2). Despite undetectable FSH levels in serum (and urinary excretion rates for FSH in the prepubertal range), sperm production increased markedly in all men, reaching mean values between 25×10^6 and 50×10^6/ml. These results demonstrated that normal levels of FSH were not an absolute requirement for spermatogenesis to occur. However, the dosage of hCG used was markedly supraphysiological in terms of LH-like activity.

To assess the issue of the effect of a physiological level of LH stimulation on sperm production, a second study was performed (Matsumoto et al, 1984). Gonadotrophin secretion and sperm production were again suppressed by the administration of T. Then human LH (1100 IU sub-cutaneously daily) was added to the T, yielding normal blood levels of LH and undetectable FSH (Figure 3). In this hormonal milieu, sperm pro-duction again increased markedly, implying that FSH deficiency does not totally eliminate sperm production in man, even when the level of the LH replacement is held within the physiological range.

In other studies, we determined that hCG led to reinitiation of spermato-genesis even following 9 months of gonadotrophin suppression by T (Matsu-moto and Bremner, 1985). Interestingly, however, we were also able to demonstrate a stimulatory effect of FSH on spermatogenesis when admin-istered in the absence of LH to normal men whose sperm production had been suppressed by T (Matsumoto et al, 1983).

In all studies of reinitiation of spermatogenesis by LH or FSH alone, we were never able to achieve sperm counts in the control range for the men studied. Instead, sperm counts increased to the range of 20×10^6 to 50×10^6/ml. This led us to wonder whether both LH and FSH together are required for quantitatively normal spermatogenesis.

To assess this issue, we used a different method of achieving a selective FSH deficiency (Matsumoto et al, 1986). We administered hCG alone (5000 IU intramuscularly twice weekly) to eight normal men, without additional T. This dosage of hCG leads to stimulation of T and E_2 production which secondarily inhibits endogenous FSH secretion. In this setting of high LH-like activity in serum due to the administered hCG and low FSH levels, sperm production was partially suppressed, again to the level of 20×10^6 to 50×10^6/ml (Matsumoto et al, 1986). Thus, in the hormonal milieu of normal or high LH, and very low FSH levels, mean sperm counts are in the range of 20×10^6 to 50×10^6/ml whether this is achieved by stimulating sperm counts from azoospermic levels or by suppression from normal levels (depending on the various experimental paradigms used).

The decrease in sperm counts during administration of hCG alone could have been due to the associated FSH deficiency or to a direct down-regulatory effect of hCG on testicular function (Cusan et al, 1982), possibly exerted through the high levels of E_2 produced. To differentiate between these possibilities and also to provide more information as to the normal role of FSH in spermatogenesis, we replaced FSH in four men while continuing

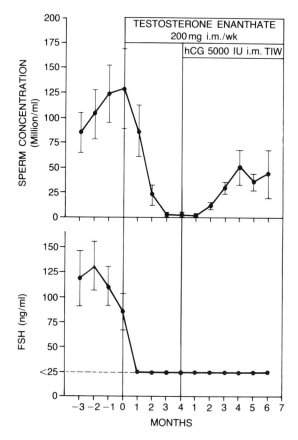

Figure 2. Monthly sperm concentrations and serum FSH levels (mean ± standard error of the mean (SEM)) in five normal men during a control period, T administration alone, and hCG plus T administration. T administration alone induced a profound suppression of gonado-trophin levels and sperm concentrations. Selective replacement of LH-like activity with the addition of hCG to T resulted in an increase in sperm concentration, despite undetectable serum FSH levels. TIW = three times per week. From Bremner et al (1981).

the administration of hCG (Figure 4). The FSH used for replacement was in the form of human FSH (100 IU subcutaneously daily) or human menopausal gonadotrophin (hMG) (75 IU subcutaneously daily). Both regimens returned serum FSH levels into the normal range. With the replacement of the FSH deficiency, sperm production returned into the control range for each man (Figure 4). These results demonstrated that the suppressive effect of hCG, administered by itself, on spermatogenesis was due to the FSH deficiency produced by this regimen, not to a direct down-regulatory effect of hCG on the testis.

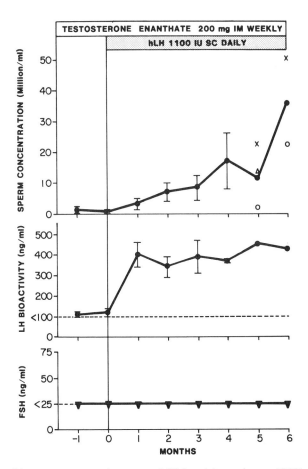

Figure 3. Monthly sperm concentrations, serum LH bioactivity, and serum FSH levels (mean ± SEM) in four normal men during the last 2 months of T-induced suppression of gonadotrophins and sperm production and during human LH (hLH) plus T administration. In the last 2 months of hLH plus T administration, individual mean monthly sperm concentrations are presented for each subject remaining in the study (×,△,○). Sperm concentrations and serum LH bioactivity were severely suppressed and serum FSH levels were undetectable during T suppression. The addition of hLH to T increased LH bioactivity into the physiological range and stimulated sperm production, despite continued undetectable FSH levels. From Matsumoto et al (1984).

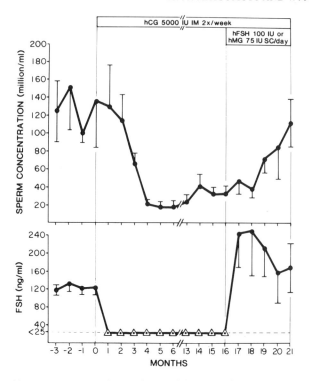

Figure 4. Monthly sperm concentrations and serum FSH levels (mean ± SEM) in four normal men during a control period, hCG administration, and hCG plus FSH (human FSH (hFSH) or hMG) administration. Chronic hCG administration resulted in partial suppression of sperm production for 13 months and reduction of serum FSH to undetectable levels for 16 months. The addition of FSH to hCG resulted in an increase in FSH levels and stimulation of sperm production to control levels. From Matsumoto et al (1986).

This series of studies demonstrates that normal serum levels of FSH are not required for *qualitatively* normal spermatogenesis in man since sperm counts in the range of 20×10^6 to 50×10^6/ml were typically found in a variety of hormonal milieus, which included severely suppressed FSH levels. However, to achieve *quantitatively* normal levels of sperm production, FSH replacement was required. This implies that the physiological role of FSH in men is the quantitative stimulation of spermatogenesis.

Treatment of hypogonadotrophic hypogonadism

The goals of treatment of hypogonadotrophic hypogonadism are to induce or restore and maintain virilization and fertility. Normal adult levels of T may be achieved and virilization may be induced either by exogenous administration of T (in the form of a long-acting ester such as T enanthate or cypionate) or stimulation of endogenous T production by administration of hCG, which contains LH-like activity almost exclusively. Because of the ease of administration (biweekly for T compared with one to three times weekly for hCG) and lower expense, the majority of hypogonadotrophic patients receive T treatment instead of hCG for the induction of virilization. T therapy does not impair subsequent testicular responses to gonadotrophin treatment (Burger et al, 1981; Ley and Leonard, 1985).

Despite occasional reports of induction of sperm production by T administration (Baranetsky and Carlson, 1980), when fertility is desired, exogenous T treatment is usually not adequate to stimulate spermatogenesis in gonadotrophin-deficient men. Exogenous administration of gonadotrophins or stimulation of endogenous gonadotrophin secretion with LHRH have been used successfully to induce sperm production in hypogonadotrophic hypogonadal men. The therapeutic use of gonadotrophins and LHRH has provided insight into the hormonal requirements necessary for the initiation and maintenance of spermatogenesis in man.

Initiation of sperm production in hypogonadotrophic hypogonadism of prepubertal onset (Figure 5) has generally required treatment with preparations of gonadotrophins containing both LH- and FSH-like activity, usually in the form of hCG and hMG, respectively. The levels of FSH activity required to initiate spermatogenesis are variable, but probably very low (Sherins et al, 1977). Occasionally, spermatogenesis is induced in prepubertal hypogonadotrophic patients with administration of hCG alone, which stimulates high intratesticular T levels (Sherins et al, 1977; Burger and Baker, 1984; Finkel et al, 1985; Ley and Leonard, 1985). These men usually have low levels of FSH that are indistinguishable from those of other

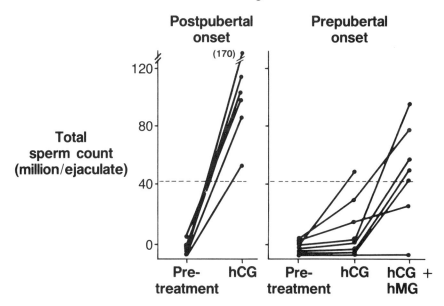

Figure 5. Effect of treatment with hCG alone and in combination with hMG on total sperm counts in men with hypogonadotrophic hypogonadism of postpubertal (left) and prepubertal (right) onset without cryptorchidism. In response to hCG alone, sperm counts increased to within the normal range (---) in all six patients with postpubertal onset of hypogonadism, but in only one of eight patients with prepubertal onset. From Finkel et al (1985).

patients with hypogonadotrophic hypogonadism. In addition, by stimulating gonadal steroid feedback, hCG administration results in suppression of endogenous FSH secretion (Reiter et al, 1972). Further evidence for the importance of high intratesticular T levels in the initiation of sperm production is found in the reports of stimulation of spermatogenesis in seminiferous tubules which lie adjacent to testicular Leydig cell tumours in prepubertal boys (Steinberger et al, 1973).

In contrast to the general requirement for both hCG and hMG treatment to stimulate sperm production in prepubertal patients, spermatogenesis can often be stimulated with hCG alone when hypogonadotrophic hypogonadism is acquired after puberty (Burger and Baker, 1984; Finkel et al, 1985; Ley and Leonard, 1985) (Figure 2). The course of patient J.P., whom we have seen in our clinics, serves as an example of this change in the requirement of FSH activity for the initiation of sperm production before and after puberty.

J.P. presented at age 20 with findings of hypogonadotrophic eunuchoidism and anosmia (Kallmann's syndrome). Pubertal development was induced by treatment with several courses of hCG alone. The patient was initially aspermic. With hCG treatment, ejaculates were induced but he remained azoospermic. Because fertility was desired, spermatogenesis was initiated and maintained with hCG and hMG treatment for a period of 4 years and two children were conceived. Gonadotrophin therapy was then stopped for 12½ years, during which time he received T enanthate to maintain virilization and sexual functioning (Figure 6). Then, because fertility was again desired, T treatment was stopped and hCG treatment alone was instituted. In contrast to initial courses of gonadotrophin therapy,

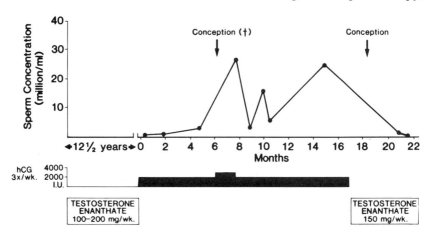

Figure 6. Response of sperm concentrations to hCG treatment alone in a patient J.P. with hypogonadotrophic eunuchoidism who had previously received combined hCG and hMG therapy to induce puberty and initiate spermatogenesis. Prior to hCG treatment, J.P. had received T enanthate for 12½ years. Sperm production was reinitiated and fertility was induced with hCG treatment alone, despite undetectable serum FSH levels (not shown). † denotes spontaneous abortion. From C. A. Paulsen A. M. Matsumoto and W. J. Bremner, 1986, unpublished observations.

spermatogenesis was reinitiated with hCG treatment alone (Figure 6), despite undetectable serum FSH levels.

In addition to the apparent differences in the requirement for FSH activity to initiate spermatogenesis in pre- and postpubertal hypogonadotrophic patients, there seem to be differences in the necessity for FSH in the initiation and maintenance of sperm production. Once sperm production is initiated with hCG and hMG in hypogonadotrophic hypogonadal men, it can often be maintained by treatment with hCG alone (Johnsen, 1978; Burger and Baker, 1984; Ley and Leonard, 1985).

Patient D.C. (Figure 7) was originally seen as a volunteer in a study design to characterize sperm production in normal young men. During this time, sperm counts, obtained twice monthly for 6 months, were normal and ranged between 80×10^6 and 250×10^6/ml. Four years later, he returned with complaints of infertility and diminished libido. He was found to have hypogonadotrophic hypogonadism and azoospermia as a result of haemochromatosis. Because he desired fertility, spermatogenesis was induced with hCG and hMG and conception occurred approximately 1 year after institution of gonadotrophin therapy. hMG was then discontinued and sperm production was maintained for over 3 years at the same level with hCG treatment alone. A second child was conceived at the end of the 3-year period of hCG treatment alone. Sperm concentrations during hCG treatment alone were lower than those obtained prior to the development of hypogonadotrophic hypogonadism. These findings suggest that, although hCG alone can maintain spermatogenesis in hypogonadotrophic men, sperm production induced by LH activity in the presence of markedly reduced FSH activity is not quantitatively normal.

These clinical experiences with gonadotrophin therapy of hypogonadotrophic hypogonadal patients re-emphasize the importance of gonadotrophin stimulation in the initiation and maintenance of spermatogenesis.

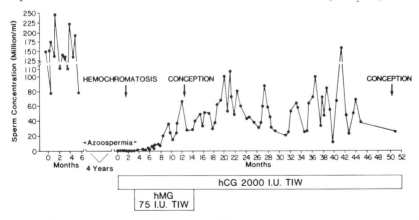

Figure 7. Sperm concentrations in a patient D.C. prior to and after the development of haemochromatosis and hypogonadotrophic hypogonadism 4 years later. Spermatogenesis and fertility were restored with combined hCG and hMG therapy and maintained with hCG treatment alone for over 3 years. From C. A. Paulsen A. M. Matsumoto and W. J. Bremner, 1986, unpublished observations.

Furthermore, they suggest that FSH is most important during the initiation of sperm production at the time of puberty and quantitatively less important in the reinitiation of spermatogenesis in patients who acquire hypogonadotrophic hypogonadism after puberty and in the maintenance of sperm production in adults.

In the absence of concomitant testicular disease (such as cryptorchidism), gonadotrophin therapy is very often successful in stimulating sperm production in men with hypogonadotrophic hypogonadism. However, spermatogenesis achieved with gonadotrophin treatment is usually not quantitatively normal, even with combined hCG and hMG therapy. Whether the inability to achieve quantitatively normal sperm production is related to the presence of testicular disease or to the unphysiological manner in which gonadotrophins are administered is not known.

Administration of LHRH to stimulate endogenous gonadotrophin secretion has also been successfully used to initiate and maintain spermatogenesis in patients with hypogonadotrophic hypogonadism (Figure 8). The theoretical advantage of this form of treatment is that it more closely mimics the normal physiological, pulsatile secretion of gonadotrophins than conventional gonadotrophin therapy. However, because this form of therapy requires the use of portable infusion pumps to deliver small doses of LHRH every few hours, it is a much more complex management problem than gonadotrophin therapy. Formal studies comparing the degree of spermatogenic stimulation of gonadotrophin and LHRH treatment in large numbers of hypogonadotrophic hypogonadal men are not available, but preliminary studies (Liu et al, 1986) suggest that the two forms of therapy are similar in their ability to stimulate spermatogenesis.

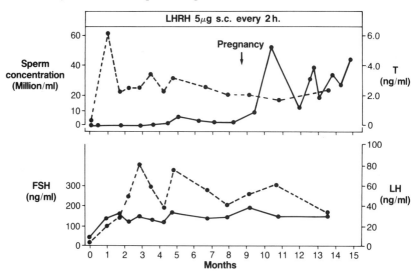

Figure 8. Stimulation of gonadotrophin and T secretion and subsequent initiation of spermatogenesis and induction of fertility by low dosage, pulsatile LHRH infusion in a patient with hypogonadotrophic eunuchoidism. From A. M. Matsumoto and W. J. Bremner, 1986, unpublished observations.

SUMMARY

The normal physiology of the hypothalamic–pituitary–testicular axis in man is reviewed. According to current concepts, LH plays an important role in the initiation and maintenance of spermatogenesis by stimulating Leydig cell production of high concentrations of T within the testes. FSH is thought to be important in spermatid maturation (spermiogenesis) during the initiation of spermatogenesis by stimulation of Sertoli cells.

Studies of selective gonadotrophin replacement in experimentally-induced hypogonadotrophic hypogonadal men demonstrate that *qualitatively* normal sperm production can be achieved by replacement of either LH or FSH alone, but both LH and FSH are necessary to maintain *quantitatively* normal spermatogenesis.

Studies of gonadotrophin replacement in spontaneously-occurring hypogonadotrophic men suggest that the requirement for FSH activity to stimulate sperm production is greatest during the initiation of sperm production at the time of puberty. The initiation of spermatogenesis in postpubertal men with acquired hypogonadotrophic hypogonadism and the maintenance of spermatogenesis after its initiation can often be achieved with LH activity alone.

Acknowledgements

We thank Elaine Rost and Anne Bartlett for their assistance in preparation of this manuscript. This work was supported in part by NIH Grant P50-HD-12629 and the Veterans Administration Medical Research Funds.

REFERENCES

Baranetsky NG & Carlson HE (1980) Persistence of spermatogenesis in hypogonadotropic hypogonadism treated with testosterone. *Fertility and Sterility* **34:** 477–482.

Bremner WJ, Matsumoto AM, Sussman AM & Paulsen CA (1981) Follicle-stimulating hormone and human spermatogenesis. *Journal of Clinical Investigation* **68:** 1044–1052.

Burger HG & Baker HWG (1984) Therapeutic considerations and results of gonadotropin treatment in male hypogonadotropic hypogonadism. *Annals of the New York Academy of Sciences* **438:** 447–453.

Burger HG, deKretser DM, Hudson B & Wilson JD (1981) Effects of preceding androgen therapy on testicular response to human pituitary gonadotropin (HPG) in hypogonadotropic hypogonadism (HH): a study of three patients. *Fertility and Sterility* **35:** 64–68.

Cusan L, Pelletier G, Bélanger A et al (1982) Inhibition of spermatogenesis and steroidogenesis during long-term treatment with hCG in the rat. *Journal of Andrology* **3:** 124–133.

Evans RM, Doelle GC, Lindner J et al (1984) A luteinizing hormone-releasing hormone agonist decreases biological activity and modifies chromatographic behavior of luteinizing hormone in man. *Journal of Clinical Investigation* **73:** 262–266.

Finkel DM, Phillips JL & Snyder PJ (1985) Stimulation of spermatogenesis by gonadotropins in men with hypogonadotropic hypogonadism. *New England Journal of Medicine* **313:** 651–655.

Forage RG, Ring JM, Brown RW et al (1986) Cloning and sequence analysis of cDNA species coding for the two subunits of inhibin from bovine follicular fluid. *Proceedings of the National Academy of Sciences (USA)* **83:** 3091–3095.

Hoffman AR & Crowley WF (1982) Induction of puberty in men by long-term pulsatile administration of low-dose gonadotropin-releasing hormone. *New England Journal of Medicine* **307**: 1237–1241.

Jia X-C, Kessel B, Yen SSC et al (1986) Serum bioactive follicle-stimulating hormone during human menstrual cycle and in hyper- and hypogonadotropic states: application of a sensitive granulosa cell aromatase bioassay. *Journal of Clinical Endocrinology and Metabolism* **62**: 1243–1249.

Johnsen SG (1978) Maintenance of spermatogenesis induced by hMG treatment by means of continuous hCG treatment in hypogonadotropic men. *Acta Endocrinologica* **89**: 763–769.

Knobil E (1980) The neuroendocrine control of the menstrual cycle. *Recent Progress in Hormone Research* **36**: 53–88.

Labrie F, Dupont A, Belanger A et al (1986) Treatment of prostate cancer with gonadotropin-releasing hormone agonists. *Endocrine Reviews* **7**: 67–74.

Ley SB & Leonard JM (1985) Male hypogonadotropic hypogonadism: factors influencing response to human chorionic gonadotropin and human menopausal gonadotropin, including prior androgens. *Journal of Clinical Endocrinology and Metabolism* **61**: 746–752.

Liu L, Chaudhari N & Sherins RJ (1986) Pulsatile gonadotropin-releasing hormone (GnRH) does not improve sperm production over that achieved with exogenous gonadotropins in men with Kallman's syndrome. *Proceedings of the Endocrine Society, 68th Annual Meeting*, Anaheim, CA, p 86 (Abstract 221).

Mason AJ, Hayflick JS, Ling N et al (1985) Complementary DNA sequences of ovarian follicular fluid inhibin show precursor structure and homology with transforming growth factor-β. *Nature* **318**: 659–663.

Matsumoto AM & Bremner WJ (1985) Stimulation of sperm production by human chorionic gonadotropin after prolonged gonadotropin suppression in normal men. *Journal of Andrology* **6**: 137–143.

Matsumoto AM, Karpas AE, Paulsen CA & Bremner WJ (1983) Reinitiation of sperm production in gonadotropin-suppressed normal men by administration of follicle-stimulating hormone. *Journal of Clinical Investigation* **72**: 1005–1015.

Matsumoto AM, Paulsen CA & Bremner WJ (1984) Stimulation of sperm production by human luteinizing hormone in gonadotropin-suppressed normal men. *Journal of Clinical Endocrinology and Metabolism* **59**: 882–887.

Matsumoto AM, Karpas AE & Bremner WJ (1986) Chronic human chorionic gonadotropin administration in normal men: evidence that follicle-stimulating hormone is necessary for the maintenance of quantitatively normal spermatogenesis in man. *Journal of Clinical Endocrinology and Metabolism* **62**: 1184–1192.

McLachlan RI, Robertson DM, Burger HG & deKretser DM (1986) The radioimmunoassay of bovine and human follicular fluid and serum inhibin. *Molecular and Cellular Endocrinology* **46**: 175–185.

Odell WD & Swerdloff RS (1978) Abnormalities of gonadal function in men. *Clinical Endocrinology* **8**: 149–180.

Pardridge WM (1981) Transport of protein-bound hormones into tissues in vivo. *Endocrine Reviews* **2**: 103–123.

Reiter EO, Kulin HE & Loriaux DL (1972) FSH suppression during short-term hCG administration is a gonadally mediated process. *Journal of Clinical Endocrinology and Metabolism* **34**: 1080–1084.

Robertson DM, deVos FL, Foulds LM et al (1986) Isolation of 31 kDa form of inhibin from bovine follicular fluid. *Molecular and Cellular Endocrinology* **44**: 271–277.

Santen RJ & Bardin CW (1973) Episodic luteinizing hormone secretion in man. Pulse analysis, clinical interpretation, physiologic mechanisms. *Journal of Clinical Investigation* **52**: 2617–2628.

Sherins RJ, Winters SJ & Wachslicht H (1977) Studies of the role of hCG and low dose FSH in initiating spermatogenesis in hypogonadotropic men. *Proceedings of the Endocrine Society, 59th Annual Meeting*, Chicago, IL, p 22 (Abstract 312).

Steinberger E, Root A, Ficher M & Smith KD (1973) The role of androgens in the initiation of spermatogenesis in man. *Journal of Clinical Endocrinology and Metabolism* **37**: 746–751.

Swerdloff RS, Palacios A, McClure RD et al (1977) Chemical evaluation of testosterone enanthate in the reversible suppression of spermatogenesis in the human male: efficacy, mechanism of action, and adverse effects. In Patenelli DJ (ed.) *Proceedings Hormonal*

Control of Male Fertility, pp 41–68. US Department of Health, Education and Welfare Publication No (NIH) 78-1097.

VanDamme MP, Robertson DM & Diczfalusy E (1974) An improved in vitro bioassay method for measuring luteinizing hormone (LH) activity using mouse Leydig cell preparations. *Acta Endocrinologica* **77:** 655–671.

Wilson JD, Griffith JE, George FW & Leshin M (1981) The role of gonadal steroids in sexual differentiation. *Recent Progress in Hormone Research* **37:** 1–39.

5

Inhibin—a non-steroidal regulator of pituitary follicle stimulating hormone

ROBERT I. McLACHLAN
DAVID M. ROBERTSON
DAVID DE KRETSER
HENRY G. BURGER

Over fifty years ago, a non-steroidal factor of gonadal origin was postulated to inhibit pituitary follicle stimulating hormone (FSH) (McCullagh, 1932). This substance, termed inhibin, is currently defined as a peptide factor that specifically or selectively lowers the rate of pituitary FSH secretion (Franchimont et al, 1979). Based on the inhibin hypothesis, it is postulated that diminished ovarian follicular or seminiferous tubule function results in decreased inhibin secretion. This diminished negative feedback upon the pituitary permits increased FSH release; in some instances at times of normal sex steroid and serum luteinizing hormone (LH) levels. There is strong indirect evidence for its existence in man based on various physiological and pathological states in which FSH and LH secretion are discordant and in which FSH secretion varies inversely with the adequacy of gametogenesis. Direct evidence for the existence of inhibin is plentiful in animal studies, whilst similar evidence in the human is limited. However, inhibin has recently been measured in the circulation and found to be stimulated by FSH-containing agents as proposed by the inhibin hypothesis (McLachlan et al, 1986a,b). Inhibin has now been purified from bovine follicular fluid (bFF) (Robertson et al, 1985, 1986a; Fukuda et al, 1986) and porcine follicular fluid (pFF) (Ling et al, 1985; Miyamoto et al, 1985; Rivier et al, 1985) and found to be a glycoprotein consisting of two disulphide-linked subunits. These peptides were subsequently cloned and sequenced (Mason et al, 1985; Forage et al, 1986). The sequence of inhibin is partially homologous to transforming growth factor β (TGF-β) (Derynck et al, 1985) and Mullerian inhibitory substance (MIS) (Cate et al, 1986). The sequence of human inhibin was derived by cloning techniques using complementary DNA (cDNA) probes derived from the sequences of porcine and bovine inhibin to identify the genes (Mason et al, 1986; Stewart et al, 1986). A recent surprising discovery was that dimers of the smaller (B) subunit of inhibin isolated from pFF stimulated FSH release from pituitary cells in vitro, in contrast to inhibin which inhibits FSH release (Ling et al, 1986; Vale et al, 1986). This rapidly advancing field of knowledge promises to broaden our horizons beyond the simple concept of inhibin as a single FSH-regulating peptide.

ASSAYS OF INHIBIN

All hormones are defined in terms of their biological activity and accordingly the vast majority of the inhibin literature is based on bioassay systems, both in vivo and in vitro. Radioimmunoassay (RIA) offers a more practicable and sensitive assay system, provided care is taken to ensure its specificity. Inhibin bioassay systems are based on a reduction in FSH secretion which can be detected by direct FSH measurement or indirectly by the measurement of the biological effect of FSH (see review by Baker et al, 1981). These methods have in common inhibitory end-points making them prone to non-specific effects. Much of the controversy regarding the nature and action of inhibin can be ascribed to the use of poorly characterized methods where any suppression of FSH or of its apparent biological activity is assumed to be due to inhibin (Baker et al, 1981).

In vivo bioassays

A number of in vivo bioassays which give an indirect measure of inhibin activity have been reported. These methods include the inhibition of the human chorionic gonadotrophin (hCG)-induced increase in ovarian or uterine weight (Chari et al, 1976; Ramasharma et al, 1979). A major disadvantage of these systems is the reported presence of non-inhibin substances in follicular fluid (FF) (Sluss and Reichert, 1984) and testicular homogenates (Reichert and Abou-Issa, 1977) that interfere with the binding of FSH to its ovarian receptors and thereby affect the estimation of inhibin activity. The direct measurement of FSH suppression in plasma has been used as a means of detecting inhibin bioactivity and studying its physiology. Such in vivo bioassays, although more specific than indirect bioassays, are semiquantitative at best, often difficult to reproduce and of poor practicability (Franchimont et al, 1979; Baker et al, 1981).

In vitro bioassays

Dispersed pituitary cell cultures (PCCs), particularly of rat cells, represent the most reliable bioassay system. End-points include the suppression of basal or LH releasing hormone (LHRH)-stimulated FSH release (de Jong et al, 1979; Eddie et al, 1979) or the suppression of FSH cell content (Scott et al, 1980). These methods are sufficiently precise (index of precision (λ) < 0.15) and sensitive for the measurement of inhibin activity in tissue extracts and during inhibin purification. In vitro systems are however prone to non-specific effects in the suppression of FSH but this can be minimized by: (1) the use of parallel line assay statistics to assess non-parallelism between sample and standard; (2) the simultaneous measurement of other pituitary hormones, usually LH (Scott et al, 1982; Robertson et al, 1986b) or prolactin and thyrotrophin (Franchimont et al, 1979) as these should not be suppressed by inhibin; (3) a graded morphological assessment of toxic changes (Scott et al, 1982); and finally (4) by the use of a ^{51}Cr release procedure from prelabelled pituitary cells as a sensitive technique for assessing cytotoxicity (Robertson et al, 1982).

Crude inhibin preparations have been observed to diminish LHRH-induced LH release whilst not affecting basal LH release or cell content (Scott et al, 1980). However, studies using purified inhibin have failed to show any inhibition of LHRH-stimulated LH release although the dose–response effects of LHRH and inhibin have yet to be explored (Robertson et al, 1986b).

In vitro bioassays have generally been too insensitive for measurement of circulating inhibin although rat PCCs (de Paolo et al, 1979b; Lee et al, 1983; Tsukamoto et al, 1986) and ovine PCCs (Tsonis et al, 1986) have been used to detect circulating inhibin under certain circumstances (see above).

Radioimmunoassay of inhibin

Inhibin was first purified in this laboratory from bFF (Robertson et al, 1985, 1986a) and shown to exist in both 58 kDa and 31 kDa forms. We have utilized this material in the development of a sensitive and specific RIA procedure for bFF and human follicular fluid (hFF) and serum inhibin (McLachlan et al, 1986a). An antiserum to purified 58 kDa inhibin was shown to neutralize maximal FSH-suppressing doses of bFF inhibin (crude and purified) and hFF inhibin bioactivity in vitro. Inhibin was iodinated using the chloramine T procedure and purified on Matrex Red A (Amicon) to a specific activity of approximately 40 µCi/µg. Using this tracer and antiserum, a second antibody RIA was developed which showed 30% cross-reactivity with hFF inhibin but low to undetectable levels of cross-reaction with inhibin in ovine FF, pFF, ovine rete testis fluid, and rat ovarian extract. The subunits of inhibin, TGF-β and MIS all showed less than 0.5% cross-reaction. This RIA was modified for the direct measurement of serum inhibin. Since iodinated 58 kDa inhibin was unstable in serum, the iodinated 31 kDa inhibin was used as tracer. Inhibin immunoactivity was not detectable in castrate bovine or human serum, or in serum of women with gonadal failure (postmenopausal, premature ovarian failure, Turner's syndrome), whilst detectable levels were found in cattle and human serum. Subsequently, improvements in assay sensitivity have allowed preliminary studies of circulating inhibin during the normal menstrual cycle and during ovarian hyperstimulation for in vitro fertilization where a marked increase in circulating levels was found (McLachlan et al, 1986b).

PHYSIOLOGICAL STUDIES OF INHIBIN

In vitro studies

Male

Extensive evidence supports the idea that Sertoli cells are the source of testicular inhibin. Rat Sertoli cell cultures (SCCs) have been shown to secrete inhibin which is active in dispersed pituitary cell culture systems (Steinberger and Steinberger, 1976; Le Gac and de Kretser, 1982; Verhoeven and Franchimont, 1983; Ultee-van Gessel et al, 1986). Inhibin secretion can be maintained for several weeks in culture. Spermatogenic cells, along with other testicular cell types, do not secrete inhibin (Steinberger, 1981) and, in fact, it has been suggested that spermatogenic cells diminish SCC inhibin production in coculture (Ultee-van Gessel et al, 1986). Dose-dependent enhancement of SCC inhibin secretion can be achieved with the addition of androgens which act presumably via the androgen receptor as their effect is blocked by cyproterone acetate (Verhoeven and Franchimont, 1983). This androgen effect was not confirmed by others who did report a stimulatory action of FSH upon SSC inhibin production (Steinberger, 1981; Le Gac and de Kretser, 1982; Ultee-van Gessel et al, 1986).

The physiological status of the rat from which the Sertoli cells have been isolated affects the ability of these cells to secrete inhibin. Hypophysectomy markedly impaired the secretion of inhibin by SCCs, whilst 10 days of replacement with testosterone and/or FSH prior to sacrifice restored this secretory capacity (Steinberger, 1981). These studies underline the trophic effects of FSH and testosterone on SCC inhibin production. Inhibition of inhibin production can be achieved by damaging the seminiferous tubule epithelium in vivo (Steinberger, 1981; Seethalakshmi and Steinberger, 1983).

Future studies will be needed to examine the synergism between FSH and testosterone. With the rapidly advancing knowledge of the structure of inhibin, messenger RNA (mRNA) levels for both inhibin subunits can be quantitated as a means of establishing the effects of these hormones on gene expression. The interaction between Sertoli cells, germ cells and peritubular myoid cells will also need further assessment. Currently it appears inhibin can be produced in the absence of other cell types; however, the validity of this culture system, which monitors inhibin production by Sertoli cells in isolation, needs to be questioned as regards its relevance to the in vivo state. For example, seminiferous peritubular cells have been shown to secrete a protein (P-Mol-5) under the influence of androgens which increases Sertoli cell production of androgen binding protein and transferrin (Skinner and Fritz, 1985). The existence of such paracrine factors indicates that future studies will need to examine the interaction of other testicular cell types in the hormonal control of inhibin production by Sertoli cells in vitro.

Female

Inhibin production in vitro has been demonstrated in ovarian granulosa cell cultures (GCCs) from many species including cattle (Henderson and Franchimont, 1981, 1983), pigs (Channing et al, 1982), humans (Channing et al, 1984a) and rats (Erickson and Hseuh, 1978; Hermans et al, 1982; Croze and Franchimont, 1984). Thecal and luteal cells on the other hand produced no detectable inhibin in vitro (Henderson and Franchimont, 1981, 1983; Channing et al, 1982).

During study of the control of inhibin production by bovine GCCs in vitro, spontaneous luteinization occurred, with a progressive increase in progesterone secretion and a reciprocal decline in inhibin secretion (Henderson and Franchimont, 1981). The addition of progesterone also inhibited inhibin secretion. These data agreed with the finding that corpus luteum cells in vitro did not secrete inhibin. Oestrogen had no effect on inhibin production whilst androgens (aromatizable, non-aromatizable or synthetic) were stimulatory possibly via the androgen receptor as the antiandrogen cyproterone acetate inhibited their effect (Henderson and Franchimont, 1983). It was suggested that follicular androgens and progesterone may be important opposing physiological regulators of inhibin production. It was speculated that thecal androgens could therefore directly enhance granulosa cell inhibin production as well as providing a substrate for aromatization to oestradiol. With the onset of luteinization, the increased progesterone levels would then inhibit further inhibin secretion. However, a recent study has identified the presence of mRNA coding for the A subunit of inhibin in the rat corpus luteum, raising questions as to its role (Davis et al, 1986).

FSH stimulates inhibin release from cultured rat granulosa cells in vitro (Erickson and Hseuh, 1978; Zhiwen et al, 1986). Both FSH and insulin-like growth factor I (IGF-I) promoted the release of inhibin in a dose-dependent manner from rat granulosa cells (Zhiwen et al, 1986). The physiological significance of IGF-I in the regulation of inhibin release is unknown, but it has recently been shown to be produced by ovarian granulosa cells, suggesting a possible autocrine role (Davoren and Hseuh, 1986). In addition, the FSH and IGF-I acted synergistically to enhance inhibin release from rat GCCs (Zhiwen et al, 1986). Recently, an inhibitory role for epidermal growth factor in the production of inhibin by GCCs has been proposed (Franchimont et al, 1986).

In vivo studies

Male

The obtaining of direct evidence relating to the in vivo control of inhibin production has been hampered by the inability to measure serum inhibin with available bioassays even in rat testicular venous blood (Au et al, 1984a). Indirect information has therefore been obtained (1) from the reciprocal relationship between serum FSH and the quantitative outcome of spermatogenesis, and (2) by the bioassay of testicular lymph, rete testis fluid and testis cytosol preparations as measures of inhibin production. The rat has been primarily used for such studies on the effects of spermatogenic damage (cryptorchidism, radiation, drugs, heat) or hormonal manipulation (e.g. hypophysectomy, hormone administration) on testicular inhibin production.

Indirect evidence in man includes the observation that in prepubertal boys the cumulative FSH response to LHRH administration (a measure of pituitary FSH reserve) is greater than that seen at sexual maturity, whereas a reverse pattern is observed with LH (Franchimont et al, 1975b). In the rat, pathological states studied, including cryptorchidism, pressure atrophy and heat treatment of the testis, show a marked reduction in testicular inhibin content and a reciprocal rise in serum gonadotrophins (Au et al, 1983, 1984b). Following surgical correction of cryptorchidism in childhood, some patients with oligospermia and normal Leydig cell function showed increased basal and LHRH-stimulated FSH (but not LH) release—indirect evidence in support of diminished inhibin production (Bramble et al, 1975). Similar observations have been made in irradiated mice and rats (Verjans and Eik-Nes, 1976; de Jong and Sharp, 1977), following exposure to chemotherapeutic agents which adversely affect spermatogenesis in rats (Gomes et al, 1973) and in man (Van Thiel et al, 1972), and following efferent duct ligation in which pressure atrophy of the seminiferous epithelium occurs (Au et al, 1984b). In men, comparison of testicular biopsies from patients with a range of seminiferous tubule disorders indicates an inverse relationship between serum FSH and the quantitative outcome of spermatogenesis (de Kretser et al, 1972; Franchimont et al, 1972).

Au et al (1985) reported that hypophysectomy in the rat was followed by a decrease in testicular inhibin content and production rates, the latter being assessed by the rate of inhibin accumulation in the testis following efferent duct ligation (Au et al, 1984a). FSH replacement (with or without testosterone) increased testicular inhibin content providing strong support for its trophic role in in vivo inhibin production (Figure 1), whilst no stimulation was obtained with testosterone alone. Testosterone implants inserted into hypophysectomized rats at the time of hypophysectomy were shown to maintain seminiferous tubule fluid production but only a partial restoration

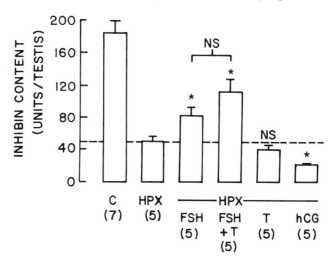

Figure 1. Changes in testicular inhibin content in adult rats hypophysectomized (HPX) for 30 days and given hormone replacement (FSH, testosterone (T) and human chorionic gonadotrophin (hCG)) for 3 days. The intact control (C) group and the HPX control group were injected with saline. Data represent the mean ± SEM with the number of animals shown in parentheses at the base of the column. *$P<0.01$ compared with HPX group (broken line: Student's t-test). NS = not significant. From Au et al (1986).

of inhibin production was achieved, even when circulating testosterone was maintained at high levels (Au et al, 1986). These data suggest a different regulation of these two aspects of Sertoli cell function.

Having been produced in the Sertoli cell, inhibin could leave the testis by several routes: (1) via the interstitial fluid/testicular lymph; (2) via seminiferous tubule fluid and eventually in semen, with the possibility of absorption in the rete testis or epididymis en route; and (3) by direct absorption into testicular venous blood. The relative importance of these routes is unclear. Inhibin levels are higher in testicular lymph and seminiferous tubule fluid than in testicular venous blood (Au et al, 1984b), although clearly this would be of little importance in terms of FSH regulation if the inhibin in these compartments did not reach the circulation. Absorption from the rete testis has been proposed as an important route (Le Lannou et al, 1979). However, the failure of FSH to rise immediately following efferent duct ligation in the rat (Au et al, 1984b) raises doubts as to the importance of this exit pathway.

It is therefore likely that bidirectional release of inhibin from the Sertoli cell occurs with secretion toward the lumen and the interstitium. Their relative importance is unclear but our understanding will be facilitated by the development of a sensitive RIA to be used in combination with surgical procedures in which tubular fluid secretion is modified or disrupted.

Female

Studies of the physiology of inhibin have been impeded until recently by the lack of sensitive methods for the detection of peripheral serum inhibin. Nonetheless, valuable information has been obtained using (1) indirect evidence correlating serum FSH with the quantitative outcome of oogenesis, (2) the effects on FSH and LH levels of inhibin administration, and (3) the bioassay of ovarian cytosolic extract and, in certain circumstances, of plasma inhibin.

Indirect evidence in humans comes from the observation that in perimenopausal women serum FSH increases before the rise in serum LH and the fall in serum oestradiol. At the menopause when follicular development ceases, serum FSH is elevated to several fold higher than serum LH. Such observations strongly suggest that oestradiol alone is insufficient to inhibit FSH secretion and they support the existence of other gonadal factors in the control of FSH secretion. The suppression of the postcastration rise of FSH in rats by steroid-free gonadal extracts is well described (Mader et al, 1977; Welschen et al, 1977). The restoration of normal gonadotrophin levels in castrate rats by intrasplenic ovarian transplantation is evidence for the ovarian origin of inhibin (Uilenbroek et al, 1978).

FF inhibin preparations also suppressed the pro-oestrous and oestrous peaks of FSH during the oestrous cycle of the rat (Schwarz and Channing, 1977; de Paolo et al, 1979a; Hoffman et al, 1979) and plasma FSH during the oestrous cycle of the sheep (Miller et al, 1982). Pulsatile FSH release in ovariectomized rats was inhibited in frequency, amplitude and response to LHRH by pFF administration whilst LH was unaffected (Lumpkin et al,

1984). Evidence that the active component in FF which inhibits FSH was inhibin was provided when pure 31 kDa bovine inhibin was administered to castrate ewes with an inhibition of FSH secretion (Findlay et al, 1987).

In primates, a reduction in the postcastration rise of gonadotrophins following pFF administration has been shown (Schenken et al, 1984). Administration of inhibin preparations to mature female rhesus monkeys resulted in disturbances of the menstrual cycles. Administration during the early follicular phase (days 1–3) suppressed serum FSH and oestradiol and this suppression was followed by a rebound hypersecretion of FSH and a normal midcycle surge (Stouffer and Hodgen, 1980). Luteal phase deficiencies were subsequently observed with deficient progesterone secretion in vivo and a diminished capacity of corpus luteum cells in vitro to produce progesterone. In a similar study during the early and late follicular phase, administration of pFF to monkeys led to a suppression of serum FSH and oestradiol, a deferral of new follicular growth equal to the period of inhibin administration and a failure of maturation of the preovulatory follicles (diZerega et al, 1981). These data indicate that the early follicular phase gonadotrophin profile is important for the subsequent development and function of the follicle and corpus luteum. These findings do not however constitute evidence for a physiological role for inhibin on their own as the inhibin preparations used were impure and measurements of circulating inhibin levels were not made.

FF inhibin concentrations, measured by in vitro bioassay in the normal human menstrual cycle, have been shown to increase in the follicular phase (Chappel et al, 1980) and to show a positive correlation with FF oestradiol (Marrs et al, 1984). In atretic or luteinized follicles, inhibin levels are low and show an inverse correlation with FF progesterone (Channing et al, 1981). Such data indicate that FF inhibin in the normal cycle, like oestradiol, is a marker of follicular function and viability and is supported by results obtained with the RIA of plasma inhibin (McLachlan et al, 1986b). In sheep, inhibin levels vary widely between follicles, but show an increase in relation to follicular size (Tsonis et al, 1983). In gonadotrophin-treated human cycles, FF inhibin levels are much increased, but sex steroid concentrations are lower than those seen in normal cycles with differing profiles between clomiphene and human menopausal gonadotrophin (hMG) cycles (Channing et al, 1984b; Marrs et al, 1984). The significance of these changes is unclear as oocytes produced under each setting are capable of fertilization. As yet unanswered is the physiological role of FF inhibin in terms of a possible paracrine function within the ovary or as regards the release of inhibin into the circulation to modulate FSH release.

Inhibin circulates in peripheral plasma at low concentrations. De Paolo et al (1979b) detected inhibin bioactivity quantitatively in ovarian venous blood of rats at various times of the oestrous cycle and found its presence varied inversely with the peripheral FSH concentration. Lee et al (1981) used the pregnant mare serum gonadotrophin (PMSG)-primed immature female rat as a model for studying the in vivo control of inhibin production. Treatment resulted in a marked increase in plasma and ovarian inhibin levels as measured using a bioassay system of increased sensitivity (Lee et al, 1983). Peripheral FSH levels were lowered during PMSG treatment consistent with increased inhibin feedback upon pituitary FSH secretion (Lee et al, 1981). The trophic agent for enhanced inhibin production by the superovulating rat has been shown to be of pituitary origin (Tsukamoto et al, 1986). The effect is specific to FSH with a detectable increase in ovarian inhibin 6 hours after FSH administration (Lee et al, 1982). The mechanism of PMSG-induced inhibin production involves an increase in ovarian inhibin mRNA (Davis et al, 1986). Castration led to a rapid disappearance of inhibin from the circulation with a half-life of 30 minutes (Lee et al, 1982). Unilateral castration suggested that the remaining ovary undertook a compensatory increase in inhibin production to maintain FSH suppression. In agreement with the in vitro data, circulating inhibin levels were observed to fall rapidly following luteinizing doses of human chorionic gonadotrophin (hCG) (Carson and Lee, 1983). These data are strong evidence that, in vivo, inhibin is under the control of both FSH and LH, which are stimulatory and inhibitory respectively.

Circulating inhibin levels were first measured by radioimmunoassay in women undergoing ovarian hyperstimulation as part of an in vitro fertilization programme and were recently reported as showing a progressive increase during therapy (McLachlan et al, 1986b) (see also Chapter 7). Significant correlations were observed between plasma inhibin levels and plasma oestradiol and both the number of follicles detected on ultrasound and the number of oocytes collected at laparoscopy. Inhibin levels fell immediately following the endogenous LH surge or hCG administration. In some patients, discordant profiles of plasma inhibin and oestradiol were noted, with plasma inhibin tending to fall or plateau at a time when oestradiol levels continued to rise. In a subsequent study, women with a past history of failed conventional ovulation induction underwent ovarian suppression using an LHRH agonist followed later by the addition of exogenous gonadotrophin therapy (see Figure 2). Both oestradiol and inhibin showed an initial transient increase followed by a fall to undetectable levels during induction of a pseudomenopause with the LHRH agonist. A sharp and parallel increase in both hormones was seen during hMG therapy up until the time of ovulation induction with hCG. Overall, these studies confirmed in the human the animal data showing that inhibin circulates in plasma, is increased by its trophic agent FSH and is undetectable during withdrawal of gonadotrophin support. Evidence exists that oestradiol is primarily a theca cell product in the human (McNatty et al, 1979), whilst inhibin is a granulosa cell product and therefore the measurement of this protein in plasma may give a more direct assessment of follicular development and health. Whether it can be utilized as a clinically useful parameter is still under study.

INHIBIN PURIFICATION

The purification of inhibin has proved exceedingly difficult with the applica-

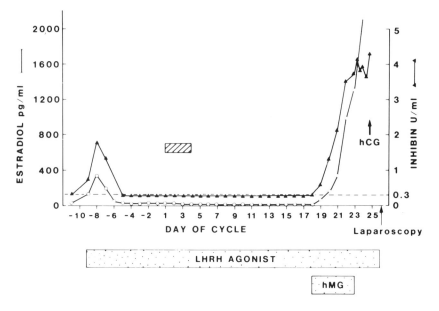

Figure 2. Plasma inhibin and oestradiol levels during ovarian suppression with the LHRH agonist buserelin (Suprafact, Hoechst AG) commenced in the late luteal phase. Note the transient rise in both hormones followed by the induction of a pseudomenopause (and menses ▨▨▨) with levels below assay limits of detection (dotted line). Subsequent exogenous gonadotrophin therapy is associated with a parallel rise of both hormones prior to hCG administration and oocyte recovery.

tion of a wide range of conventional purification techniques resulting in poor recoveries, an inability to achieve a homogeneous product and a wide range of reported molecular masses. It has now been shown that inhibin is a high molecular mass glycoprotein with prominent hydrophobic properties which presumably result in strong interactions with proteins and/or gel support systems leading to aberrant behaviour during chromatography. In addition, evidence has emerged that inhibin exists as multiple molecular mass forms in follicular fluid with different workers concentrating on one or two of these species. The failure of some authors to monitor the purification process with rigorously controlled PCC bioassay systems and the lack of an agreed inhibin standard have further impeded agreement. Fortunately, in recent years the advent of new isolation procedures, especially the use of reverse phase high-performance liquid chromatography (HPLC) (Dobos et al, 1983), has facilitated the purification of inhibin to homogeneity by several groups and has allowed partial sequence analysis and subsequent cloning and sequencing.

The starting materials used by various groups have included ovarian FF, rete testis fluid, testicular extract and seminal plasma. For reasons to be presented, inhibin from gonadal extracts should be viewed separately from 'inhibin-like' peptides in seminal plasma.

Follicular fluid inhibin

De Jong and Sharpe (1976) reported the presence of inhibin-like activity in bFF and subsequently FF has been recognised as the richest accessible source of inhibin for purification.

Bovine follicular fluid inhibin

A molecular mass of 60–70 kDa was proposed for bFF inhibin following partial purification (Jansen et al, 1981; Van Dijk et al, 1984). Inhibin was first purified to homogeneity by Robertson et al (1985) as a glycoprotein of 58 kDa consisting of two disulphide-linked subunits of apparent molecular masses 43 kDa and 15 kDa. Subsequently, a smaller 31 kDa form was reported (Robertson et al, 1986a) and proposed to result from the shortening of the 43 kDa subunit to a 20 kDa subunit (a concept later supported by structural analysis), whilst the 15 kDa subunit remained unchanged. The pure 31 kDa material had a median effective dose (ED_{50}) of 1 ng/ml in the PCC bioassay and was inactive following reduction to its subunits.

Multiple molecular mass forms of inhibin were also observed by Fukuda et al (1986) during their purification of a 32 kDa form of bFF inhibin with bioactivity also found in the 55 kDa and 96 kDa regions. Subsequent studies by that group using monoclonal antibodies to the subunits of inhibin have suggested that bFF contains inhibin bioactivity in the 32 kDa, 55 kDa, 65 kDa, 88 kDa, 108 kDa and 120 kDa regions (Miyamoto et al, 1986). This high degree of heterogeneity is thought to result from variable processing of the proforms of both subunits (see above).

The primary amino acid structure of the 43 kDa (termed A) and 15 kDa (termed B) subunits of bFF inhibin were subsequently established from the cloning and analysis of cDNA species derived from bovine granulosa cell mRNA (Forage et al, 1986). The A subunit is a protein of 300 amino acids with two potential N-glycosylation sites, two potential proteolytic processing sites and a preproregion of 60 amino acids. The B subunit arises from a separate gene, is a protein of 116 amino acids with no potential glycosylation points and has a large N-terminal extension of unknown function. These data support the proposition that the 31 kDa form is derived by proteolytic processing of the A subunit. The degradation of iodinated 58 kDa bFF inhibin to a 31 kDa form upon incubation with serum but not FF suggests that processing enzyme(s) are located in serum and makes it likely that inhibin circulates as the 31 kDa form (McLachlan et al, 1986a).

Porcine follicular fluid inhibin

pFF inhibin was first purified as a 32 kDa form and found to account for 70% of the total pFF bioactivity (Miyamoto et al, 1985). Bioactive higher molecular mass forms (55 kDa, 80–100 kDa) were also noted. Purified 32 kDa inhibin had properties similar to 31 kDa bovine inhibin in that it had similar biological activity in vitro, consisted of two subunits (20 kDa (A) and 15 kDa (B)) and was inactive following reduction. Charge heterogeneity of 32 kDa inhibin was observed on ion-exchange HPLC but no differences were observed in their N-terminal amino acid sequences. These charge differences are attributed to differences in glycosylation. These findings have been confirmed by others (Ling et al, 1985; Rivier et al, 1985). Two forms of 32 kDa inhibin bioactivity were isolated with differing bioactivities and different N-terminal amino acid sequences of the B subunit (termed inhibin B_A and B_B) (Ling et al, 1985).

The presence of two forms of pFF inhibin each sharing a common A subunit, but differing with respect to the B subunit, was confirmed when the amino acid sequences deduced from cDNA sequences for pFF inhibin were reported (Mason et al, 1985). The A subunit consisted of 132 amino acids (including a potential glycosylation site) separated from an extended N-terminal region by a potential dibasic processing site, similar to that observed with bovine inhibin. Evidence of greater molecular mass forms observed during purification could be explained by the incomplete processing of the A chain in an analogous way to bovine inhibin.

Neither of the two highly homologous B subunits corresponding to the two forms of pFF inhibin, B_A (116 residues) and B_B (115 residues), contained potential glycosylation sites. Both had nine cysteine residues in corresponding positions, and extended N-terminal proregions of unknown function containing potential cleavage and glycosylation sites. The combination of the A subunit with the B_A or B_B subunit resulted in the form of inhibin A or inhibin B respectively. As yet, no differing role in FSH regulation is apparent between the two proteins. The recently described homodimers of the B subunit will be discussed later.

Human follicular fluid inhibin

The purification of hFF inhibin has been even more difficult because of the low concentration of inhibin (1–5% of that in pFF or bFF). Inhibin has been partially purified from hFF using similar procedures to those used in the partial purification of bFF inhibin (van Dijk et al, 1985); nonetheless, hFF inhibin has not yet been purified to homogeneity.

The amino acid sequence of human inhibin has recently been reported, and was obtained utilizing mRNA extracted from a patient with polycystic ovary disease and a cDNA library produced and screened using fragments of porcine inhibin as hybridization probes (Mason et al, 1986) (see Figure 3). The A subunit showed a high degree (85%) of homology with the porcine and bovine subunits but included an additional potential N-glycosylation point. The B_A subunit was identical to the porcine and bovine B_A subunit and the B_B subunit differed by only one of 115 residues from that of the porcine B_B subunit confirming the existence of two inhibin forms differing in their B subunits. The structure of the A and B_A subunit have been confirmed using genomic DNA and bovine inhibin subunit probes (Stewart et al, 1986). Therefore, there is an unusually high degree of sequence conservation between human, bovine and porcine inhibin.

Immunological studies on follicular fluid inhibin

Polyclonal antisera raised to native inhibin of varying purity have been used

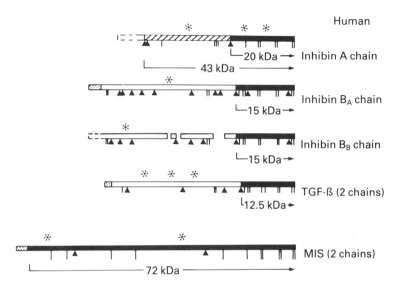

Figure 3. Schematic representation of the subunits of human inhibin, TGF-β, and MIS and their precursors. *, Asn-X-Ser-Thr; T̄, cysteine; ▲, two or more basic amino acids (Arg/Lys). Shaded/hatched regions represent the isolated or predicted forms of each subunit.

in attempts at immunopurification of inhibin (de Jong et al, 1983), in the bioneutralization of inhibin in vivo and in vitro (Channing et al, 1982; McLachlan et al, 1986a; van Dijk et al, 1986), and in the establishment of a radioimmunoassay (McLachlan et al, 1986a). The capacity of antisera raised against bovine inhibin to neutralize inhibin bioactivity derived from different species differs widely (McLachlan et al, 1986a; van Dijk et al, 1986). This suggests that the antigenic determinants responsible for bio-neutralization are similar but not identical between species. In addition, there is some evidence of sexual dimorphism of inhibin in terms of the ability of an antiserum to neutralize in vitro bioactivity (van Dijk et al, 1986). As the B subunits are virtually identical, these data further imply that the A subunit is responsible for the antigenic determinants responsible for bio-neutralization. Indeed, a synthetic six-amino-acid peptide derived from the porcine A subunit has been used to raise antibodies capable of in vitro neutralization of inhibin (Rivier et al, 1985).

Monoclonal antibodies to both subunits have recently been described allowing for effective immunopurification and a demonstration of six differing molecular mass species of bioactive inhibin in bFF (Miyamoto et al, 1986).

Seminal plasma

Franchimont et al (1975a) demonstrated the existence of inhibin-like material in bovine seminal plasma which was capable of specific dose-dependent suppression of circulating FSH in intact male rats. Subsequently, extensive work on the purification of inhibin-like activity in bovine and human seminal plasma (hSP) has been performed with the isolation of homogenous proteins with a wide range of molecular masses, mostly of less than 15 kDA. Despite considerable analysis of the structure of seminal plasma inhibin species, their position in physiology is still unclear.

A 94-amino-acid, non-glycosylated protein called 'β-inhibin' has been isolated from hSP (Seidah et al, 1984; Sheth et al, 1984) of which the 28 C-terminal amino acids were reported to contain the bioactive moiety (Arbatti et al, 1985). Evidence has accumulated that this is a prostatic peptide which is structurally identical to β globulin, a sperm-coating antigen (Johansson et al, 1984). A distinct 33-amino-acid peptide termed 'α-inhibin' (Ramasharma et al, 1984) was found to be a proteolytic degradation fragment of a 92-amino-acid peptide (Lilja and Jeppsson, 1985) which appears to be a seminal vesicular protein (Li et al, 1985).

The role, as a physiological regulator of FSH, of these alleged inhibin-like peptides is questionable not only because of their non-gonadal sites of production, but also because they are inactive in conventional inhibin bioassays (Yamashiro et al, 1984, Kohan et al, 1986) and, in the case of β-inhibin, its presence in semen, blood and urine of castrate men (Beksac et al, 1984).

Nonetheless, it seems likely that some gonadal inhibin is present in hSP following the studies of Scott and Burger (1980, 1981) who used a well characterized in vitro bioassay. Inhibin was absent from the semen of castrate and most azoospermic men, with an inverse correlation between serum FSH and seminal plasma inhibin. Nonetheless, low levels of inhibin activity were found in the semen of vasectomized men suggesting that some of the 'inhibin' activity present was of non-gonadal origin, or that it reached seminal plasma by an indirect route.

INHIBIN AND RELATED PEPTIDES

Within the inhibin molecule, structural homology exists between A and B subunits most clearly in relation to the position of cysteine residues (Mason et al, 1985; Forage et al, 1986). Primary structural homologies have been noted between the B subunits of inhibin, and the seemingly unrelated proteins of TGF-β and MIS. In addition to this remarkable discovery, the recent purification from pFF of two proteins consisting of dimers of the B subunit of inhibin with FSH-releasing properties or 'antiinhibin' activity indicates that inhibin and its related proteins represent an interesting and potentially important group from evolutionary, gene regulatory and physiological points of view.

Transforming growth factor-β

Transforming growth factors (TGFs) are mitogenic proteins which, by definition, induce anchorage-independent growth in mammalian cells (Massague, 1985). This induction process has been shown to be one of the best in vitro correlates of tumorigenicity in vivo (Roberts and Sporn, 1985). TGFs comprise two distinct forms, TGF-α (molecular mass approximately 6 kDa) which is structurally similar to epidermal growth factor (EGF) and competes for its receptor (Massague, 1983) and TGF-β which is composed of two identical disulphide-linked peptide chains with a combined molecular mass of approximately 25 kDa which does not compete for EGF receptors. TGF-β has been found widely in neoplastic and non-neoplastic tissues with platelets being a particularly rich source (Assoian et al, 1983). TGF-β may have stimulatory or inhibitory mitogenic or other effects depending upon the test system. The recent description of the amino acid sequence derived from the cDNA sequence for human TGF-β (Derynck et al, 1985) was followed by the observation of homology between TGF-β and A and B subunits of inhibin from all three species studied so far. Both inhibin and TGF-β are active as disulphide-linked dimeric structures with TGF-β being a homodimer.

Mullerian inhibitory substance

MIS is a Sertoli cell glycoprotein that causes regression of the Mullerian duct during development of the male foetus. The structures of bovine and human MIS have recently been derived using cloning techniques with human MIS consisting of a 535-amino-acid peptide (Cate et al, 1986). Significant homology was found between the C-terminal region of MIS and B_A and B_B subunits of inhibin and TGF-β. Furthermore, MIS is probably active as a disulphide-linked dimer.

Overall, these data are strong evidence for inhibin, TGF-β and MIS having a common ancestral origin. The striking structural homologies between the human inhibin subunits, TGF-β and MIS can be seen in Figure 3.

Inhibin B subunit dimers

The presence of specific FSH-stimulating activity (without an influence on LH) in fractions during the purification of pFF inhibin has been reported (Ying et al, 1986a). Two proteins with FSH-releasing activity have recently been purified to homogeneity from pFF (Ling et al, 1986; Vale et al, 1986). A 28 kDa peptide was found to be a dimer of the B_A subunit of inhibin, based on amino acid sequencing (Vale et al, 1986). In PCC it was a potent (ED_{50} = 25 pM) and specific releasing agent for FSH and was termed the FSH-releasing peptide (FRP) (Figure 4). No change was seen in LH and prolactin whilst basal and stimulated growth hormone and adrenocortico-trophic hormone (ACTH) release were impaired. FSH stimulation was not mediated by the LHRH receptor as judged by the slow onset (longer than 4 hours) of its effect, the failure of an LHRH antagonist to antagonize its biological effect and the observed increase in FSH cell content with longer term exposure (unlike the decrease seen with LHRH). Indeed, FRP and LHRH appear synergistic in enhancing FSH release. A 24 kDa material representing a $B_A B_B$ inhibin subunit dimer was termed 'activin' (as opposed

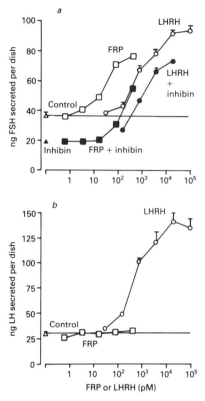

Figure 4. (a) Effects of FRP, porcine inhibin and LHRH on FSH secretion by rat anterior pituitary cells in primary culture. All substances were added simultaneously and incubation was continued for 72 h. Highly purified 32 kDa porcine inhibin was given at 40 pM. (b) Effects of LHRH and FRP on LH secretion by rat anterior pituitary cells in primary culture. For further details, see text. From Vale et al (1986).

to inhibin) and was also a potent FSH secretagogue active in picomolar concentrations (Ling et al, 1986).

Overall, these observations suggest that the gonad may secrete peptides derived from the same gene family which have opposing roles in FSH regulation (Figure 5). During coincubation, inhibin bioactivity was found to predominate over the FSH-releasing effect of both FRP and activin (Figure 4). In addition, there is far more inhibin in FF, leading to the overwhelmingly inhibitory nature of crude FF in terms of FSH secretion in vitro and in vivo and confirmed by the biological fact that FSH levels rise after castration. The coelution of inhibin and its B subunit dimers leads to the obscuration of the presence of the dimers during most chromatographic steps. Their combined presence in FF complicates the interpretation of pituitary cell inhibin bioassay systems as competition may exist leading to an incorrect assessment of either bioactivity. Very similar observations have also been made for TGF-β for which a potent FSH-releasing activity and a non-competitive inhibition by inhibin were reported (Ying et al, 1986a).

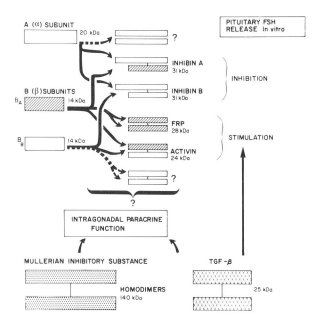

Figure 5. A schematic diagram of the interrelationship between inhibin subunits and related hormones and their biological activities.

POTENTIAL PHYSIOLOGICAL ROLE OF INHIBIN-RELATED PROTEINS

The complex relationships and functions of inhibin and its related proteins are outlined in Figure 5. The implication that inhibin A subunit dimers are important physiological regulators of FSH is highly speculative and they, unlike inhibin, have not yet been demonstrated in the circulation. It is tempting to speculate that the hypothalamus may contain inhibin B subunit dimers or related peptides that could act upon specific pituitary receptors to modulate FSH secretion.

Finally, an intraovarian paracrine role for inhibin, its B dimers and TGF-β remains a distinct possibility requiring further study. The enhancement of FSH-stimulated oestradiol production by TGF-β in rat granulosa cell culture gives initial support for a paracrine role of these proteins (Ying et al, 1986b). The clarification of the physiological role of each member of the inhibin-related protein group is currently one of the most exciting and challenging areas in reproductive endocrinology.

POTENTIAL ROLES FOR INHIBIN

In principle, the elucidation of any new step in the reproductive process provides an opportunity for fertility regulation. Since inhibin is postulated to play such a primary role in the regulation of FSH, manipulation of inhibin levels may provide a means of regulating fertility. Although it is clear from the evidence presented in this review that inhibin does circulate in plasma and is involved in FSH regulation, it is not clear to what extent inhibin is the only factor involved. Sex steroids clearly play a role in the pituitary release of gonadotrophins in both sexes and may complicate the clinical use of inhibin. Secondly, at an even more fundamental level, it is not clear what is the physiological role of FSH, particularly in the male. Some authors believe that the specific removal of FSH (for example by inhibin administration) is unlikely to be effective in producing azoospermia as limited spermatogenesis persists in the absence of FSH (Matsumoto et al, 1984; Nieschlag, 1986). There are, nonetheless, several observations cited in this review which could be exploited to regulate fertility either as a contraceptive or in the treatment of infertility.

Suppression of fertility following administration of impure inhibin preparations has been found in the sheep (Henderson et al, 1986) and in male primates (Moudgal et al, 1985). Further animal studies, particularly in primates, using pure inhibin preparations, are needed to examine its contraceptive possibilities. A potential advantage of inhibin would be its likely freedom from many of the side-effects associated with the steroid-based contraceptives.

In the promotion of fertility, two approaches have been examined in livestock. Active immunization with inhibin may lead to the formation of neutralizing antibodies and therefore presumably enhanced FSH secretion with accompanying increases in ovulation rates (Henderson et al, 1984; Cummins et al, 1986). It has also been found that short-term suppression of FSH with inhibin in sheep may be followed by rebound hypersecretion of FSH following cessation of treatment and subsequently increased ovulation rates (Wallace and McNeilly, 1985; Henderson et al, 1986). The applicability of such manoeuvres to the human is unknown.

Finally, a better understanding of the role of inhibin in normal reproduction will allow an assessment of its involvement in the pathophysiology of infertility. It may represent a valuable clinical marker of granulosa or Sertoli cell function and allow better diagnostic grouping of infertility and thereby facilitate the development of rational therapies.

SUMMARY

Inhibin is a gonadal glycoprotein produced by the granulosa and Sertoli cell under the influence of FSH and acts to specifically suppress pituitary FSH secretion. Recently, ovarian inhibin has been purified from several species and its amino acid sequence deduced using cloning techniques. Inhibin consists of two disulphide-linked heterologous subunits of which the smaller may exist in two different forms accounting for two different forms of inhibin in humans and pigs. Heterogeneity of inhibin also exists as a result of proteolytic processing of the molecule during its passage into the circulation. Significant homology exists between the subunits of inhibin and the dimeric peptides TGF-β and Mullerian inhibitory substance (MIS), suggesting they are all derived from a common ancestral gene. Furthermore, dimers of the smaller subunit of inhibin (FSH-releasing protein (FRP) or activin) have now been found in follicular fluid (FF) and, along with TGF-β, shown to be potent and specific stimulators of FSH secretion. These proteins may be involved in controlling FSH by another as yet unknown pathway and may prove to be the FSH-releasing factor, analogous to LHRH, which has been postulated to exist for some years.

Inhibin can no longer be simply considered as an isolated FSH-suppressing protein. The physiological significance and relationship between inhibin and its related proteins represent one of the most challenging and interesting areas in reproductive endocrinology. Further studies, particularly with the development and use of sensitive assays for both the FSH releasing hormone and inhibin will clarify their role in reproduction and their usefulness in monitoring or treating fertility.

REFERENCES

Arbatti NJ, Seidah NG, Rochemont J et al (1985) β$_2$-Inhibin contains the active core of human seminal plasma β-inhibin: synthesis and bioactivity. *FEBS Letters* **181:** 57–63.

Assoian RK, Komoriya A, Meyers CA, Miller DM & Sporn MB (1983) Transforming growth factor-β in human platelets. *Journal of Biological Chemistry* **258:** 7155–7160.

Au CL, Robertson DM & de Kretser DM (1983) In vitro bioassay of inhibin in testes of normal and cryptorchid rats. *Endocrinology* **112:** 239–244.

Au CL, Robertson DM & de Kretser DM (1984a) An in-vivo method for estimating inhibin production by adult rat testes. *Journal of Reproduction and Fertility* **71:** 259–265.

Au CL, Robertson DM & de Kretser DM (1984b) Relationship between testicular inhibin content and serum FSH concentrations in rats after bilateral efferent duct ligation. *Journal of Reproduction and Fertility* **72:** 351–356.

Au CL, Robertson DM & de Kretser DM (1985) Effects of hypophysectomy and subsequent FSH and testosterone treatment on inhibin production by adult rat testes. *Journal of Endocrinology* **105:** 1–6.

Au CL, Irby DC, Robertson DM & de Kretser DM (1986) Effects of testosterone on testicular inhibin and fluid production in intact and hypophysectomized adult rats. *Journal of Reproduction and Fertility* **76:** 257–266.

Baker HWG, Eddie LW, Higginson RE et al (1981) Assays of inhibin. In Franchimont P & Channing CP (eds) *Intragonadal Regulation of Reproduction*, pp 193–228. London: Academic Press.

Beksac MS, Khan SA, Eliasson R et al (1984) Evidence for the prostatic origin of immunoreactive inhibin-like material in human seminal plasma. **7:** 389–397.

Bramble RJ, Houghton AL, Eccles SS, Murray MAF & Jacobs HS (1975) Specific control of follicle stimulating hormone in the male: postulated site of action of inhibin. *Clinical Endocrinology* **4:** 443–449.

Carson RC & Lee VKW (1983) Inhibin content and production by antral, preovulatory, and luteinised rat ovarian follicles. *26th Annual Meeting of the Endocrine Society of Australia* (abstract).

Cate RL, Mattaliano RJ, Hession C et al (1986) Isolation of the bovine and human genes for Mullerian inhibiting substance and expression of the human gene in animal cells. *Cell* **45:** 685–698.

Channing CP, Gagliano P, Hoover DJ et al (1981) Relationship between human follicular fluid inhibin F activity and steroid content. *Journal of Clinical Endocrinology and Metabolism* **52:** 1193–1198.

Channing CP, Hoover DJ, Anderson LD & Tanabe K (1982) Control of follicular secretion of inhibin in vitro and in vivo. *Advances in the Biosciences* **34:** 41–55.

Channing CP, Tanabe K, Chacon M & Tildon JT (1984a) Stimulatory effects of follicle-stimulating hormone and luteinizing hormone upon secretion of progesterone and inhibin activity by cultured infant human ovarian granulosa cells. *Fertility and Sterility* **42:** 598–605.

Channing CP, Tanabe K, Seegar Jones G, Jones HW & Lebech P (1984b) Inhibin activity of preovulatory follicles of gonadotropin-treated and untreated women. *Fertility and Sterility* **42:** 243–247.

Chappel SC, Holt JA & Spies HG (1980) Inhibin: differences in bioactivity within human follicular fluid in the follicular and luteal stages of the menstrual cycle (40768). *Proceedings of the Society for Experimental Biology and Medicine* **163:** 310–314.

Chari S, Duraiswami S & Franchimont P (1976) A convenient and rapid bioassay for inhibin. *Hormone Research* **7:** 129–137.

Croze F & Franchimont P (1984) Biological determination of inhibin in rat ovarian-cell culture medium. *Journal of Reproduction and Fertility* **72:** 237–248.

Cummins LJ, O'Shea T, Al-Obaidi SAR, Bindon BM & Findlay JK (1986) Increase in ovulation rate following immunization of Merino ewes with a fraction of bovine follicular fluid containing inhibin activity. *Journal of Reproduction and Fertility* **77:** 365–372.

Davies RV, Main SJ & Setchell VP (1979) Inhibin in ram rete-testis fluid. *Journal of Reproduction and Fertility Supplement* **26:** 87–95.

Davis SR, Dench F, Nikolaidis I et al (1986) Inhibin A-subunit gene expression in the ovaries of immature female rats is stimulated by pregnant mare serum gonadotrophin. *Biochemical and Biophysical Research Communications* (in press).

Davoren JB & Hsueh AJW (1986) Growth hormone increases ovarian levels of immunoreactive somatomedin C/insulin-like growth factor I in vivo. *Endocrinology* **118:** 888–890.

de Jong FH & Sharpe RM (1976) Evidence for inhibin-like activity in bovine follicular fluid. *Nature* **263:** 71–72.

de Jong FH & Sharpe RM (1977) Gonadotrophins, testosterone and spermatogenesis in neonatally irradiated male rats: evidence for a role of the Sertoli cell in follicle-stimulating hormone feedback. *Journal of Endocrinology* **75:** 209–219.

de Jong FH, Smith SD & Van der Molen HJ (1979) Bioassay of inhibin-like activity using pituitary cells in vitro. *Journal of Endocrinology* **80:** 91–102.

de Jong FH, Janson EHJM, Steenbergen J, van Dijk S & van der Molen HJ (1983) In McCann SM & Dhindsa DS (eds) *Role of Peptides and Protein in Control of Reproduction*, pp 257–273. New York: Elsevier.

de Kretser DM, Burger HG, Fortune D et al (1972) Hormonal, histological and chromosomal studies in adult males with testicular disorders. *Journal of Clinical Endocrinology and Metabolism* **35:** 392–401.

de Paolo LV, Wise PM, Anderson LD, Barraclough CA & Channing CP (1979a) Suppression of the pituitary follicle-stimulating hormone secretion during proestrus and estrus in rats by porcine follicular fluid: possible site of action. *Endocrinology* **104L:** 402–408.

de Paolo LV, Shander D, Wise PM, Barraclough CA & Channing CP (1979b) Identification of inhibin-like activity in ovarian venous plasma of rats during the estrous cycle. *Endocrinology* **105:** 647–654.

Derynck R, Jarrett JA, Chen EY et al (1985) Human transforming growth factor-β complementary DNA sequence and expression in normal and transformed cells. *Nature* **316:** 701–705.

diZerega GS, Turner CK, Stouffer RL et al (1981) Suppression of follicle-stimulating hormone-dependent folliculogenesis during the primate ovarian cycle. *Journal of Clinical Endocrinology and Metabolism* **52:** 451–456.

Dobos M, Burger HG, Hearn MTW & Morgan FJ (1983) Isolation of inhibin from ovine follicular fluid using reversed-phase liquid chromatography. *Molecular and Cellular Endocrinology* **31:** 187–198.

Eddie LW, Baker HWG, Higginson RE & Hudson B (1979) A bioassay for inhibin using pituitary cell cultures. *Journal of Endocrinology* **81:** 49–56.

Erickson GF & Hsueh AJW (1978) Secretion of 'inhibin' by rat granulosa cells in vitro. *Endocrinology* **103:** 1960–1963.

Findlay JK, Robertson DM & Clarke IJ (1987) The influence of dose and route of administration of bovine follicular fluid and the suppressive effect of 31 kilodalton bovine inhibin (M_r

31,000) on plasma FSH concentration in ovariectomized ewes. *Journal of Reproduction and Fertility* (in press).

Franchimont P, Millet D, Vendrely E et al (1972) Relationship between spermatogenesis and serum gonadotropin levels in azoospermia and oligospermia. *Journal of Clinical Endocrinology and Metabolism* **34:** 1003–1008.

Franchimont P, Chari S, Hagelstein MT & Duraiswami S (1975a) Existence of a follicle-stimulating hormone inhibiting factor 'inhibin' in bull seminal plasma. *Nature* **257:** 402–404.

Franchimont P, Demoulin A & Bourguignon JP (1975b) Clinical use of LH-RH test as a diagnostic tool. *Hormone Research* **6:** 177–191.

Franchimont P, Verstraelen-Proyard J, Hazee-Hagelstein MT et al (1979) Inhibin: from concept to reality. *Vitamins and Hormones* **37:** 243–302.

Franchimont P, Hazee-Hagelstein MT, Charlet-Renard Ch & Jaspar JM (1986) Effect of mouse epidermal growth factor on DNA and protein synthesis, progesterone and inhibin production by porcine granulosa cells in culture. *Acta Endocrinologica* **111:** 122–127.

Forage RG, Ring JM, Brown RW et al (1986) Cloning and sequence analysis of cDNA species coding for the two subunits of inhibin from bovine follicular fluid. *Proceedings of the National Academy of Sciences (USA)* **83:** 3091–3095.

Fukuda M, Miyamoto K, Hasegawa Y et al (1986) Isolation of bovine follicular fluid inhibin of about 32 kDa. *Molecular and Cellular Endocrinology* **44:** 55–60.

Gomes WR, Hall RW, Jain SK & Boots LR (1973) Serum gonadotropin and testosterone levels during loss and recovery of spermatogenesis in rats. *Endocrinology* **93:** 801–809.

Henderson KM & Franchimont P (1981) Regulation of inhibin production by bovine ovarian cells in vitro. *Journal of Reproduction and Fertility* **63:** 1–12.

Henderson KM & Franchimont P (1983) Inhibin production by bovine ovarian tissues in vitro and its regulation by androgens. *Journal of Reproduction and Fertility* **67:** 291–298.

Henderson KM, Franchimont P, Lecomte-Yerna MJ, Hudson N & Ball K (1984) Increase in ovulation rate after active immunization of sheep with inhibin partially purified from bovine follicular fluid. *Journal of Endocrinology* **102:** 305–309.

Henderson KM, Prisk MD, Hudson N et al (1986) Use of bovine follicular fluid to increase ovulation rate or prevent ovulation in sheep. *Journal of Reproduction and Fertility* **76:** 623–635.

Hermans WP, van Leeuwen ECM, Debets MHM, Sander HJ & de Jong FH (1982) Estimation of inhibin-like activity in spent medium from rat ovarian granulosa cells during long-term culture. *Molecular and Cellular Endocrinology* **27:** 277–290.

Hoffman JC, Lorenzen JR, Weil T & Schwartz NB (1979) Selective suppression of the primary surge of follicle-stimulating hormone in the rat: further evidence for folliculostatin in porcine follicular fluid. *Endocrinology* **105:** 200–203.

Jansen EHJM, Steenbergen J, de Jong FH & van der Molen HJ (1981) The use of affinity matrices in the purification of inhibin from bovine follicular fluid. *Molecular and Cellular Endocrinology* **21:** 109–117.

Johansson J, Sheth A, Cederlund E & Jornvall H (1984) Analysis of an inhibin preparation reveals apparent identity between a peptide with inhibin-like activity and a sperm-coating antigen. *FEBS Letters* **176:** 21–26.

King RA & Witkop CJ (1976) Evidence for inhibin-like activity in bovine follicular fluid. *Nature* **263:** 71–72.

Kohan S, Froysa B, Cederlund E et al (1986) Peptides of postulated inhibin activity. *FEBS Letters* **199:** 242–248.

Lee VWK, McMaster J, Quigg H, Findlay J & Leversha L (1981) Ovarian and peripheral blood inhibin concentrations increase with gonadotropin treatment in immature rats. *Endocrinology* **108:** 2403–2405.

Lee VWK, McMaster J, Quigg H & Leversha L (1982) Ovarian and circulating inhibin levels in immature female rats treated with gonadotropin and after castration. *Endocrinology* **111:** 1849–1854.

Lee VWK, Quigg H, McMaster J, Burger HG & Leversha L (1983) A sensitive and rapid bioassay for inhibin based on inhibition of pituitary gonadotrophin secretion in vitro. *26th Annual Meeting of the Endocrine Society of Australia* (abstract).

Le Gac F & de Kretser DM (1982) Inhibin production by Sertoli cell cultures. *Molecular and Cellular Endocrinology* **28:** 487–498.

Le Lannou D, Chambon Y & Le Calve M (1979) Role of the epididymis in reabsorption of inhibin in rat. *Journal of Reproduction and Fertility* **26:** 117–121.

Li CH, Hammonds RG Jr, Ramasharma K & Chung D (1985) Human seminal inhibins: isolation, characterization, and structure. *Proceedings of the National Academy of Sciences (USA)* **82:** 4041–4044.

Lilja H & Jeppson J-O (1985) Amino acid sequence of the predominant basic protein in human seminal plasma. *FEBS Letters* **182:** 181–184.

Ling N, Ying S-Y, Ueno N et al (1985) Isolation and partial characterization of a M_r 32,000 protein with inhibin activity from porcine follicular fluid. *Proceedings of the National Academy of Sciences (USA)* **82:** 7217–7221.

Ling N, Ying S-Y, Ueno N et al (1986) Pituitary FSH is released by a heterodimer of the B-subunits from the two forms of inhibin. *Nature* **321:** 779–782.

Lumpkin MD, De Paolo LB & Negro-Vilar A (1984) Pulsatile release of follicle-stimulating hormone in ovariectomized rats is inhibited by porcine follicular fluid (inhibin). *Endocrinology* **114:** 201–206.

Mader ML, Channing CP & Schwartz NB (1977) Suppression of serum follicle stimulating hormone in intact and acutely ovariectomized rats by porcine follicular fluid. *Endocrinology* **101:** 1639–1642.

Marrs RP, Lobo R, Campeau JD et al (1984) Correlation of human follicular fluid inhibin activity with spontaneous and induced follicle maturation. *Journal of Clinical Endocrinology and Metabolism* **58:** 704–709.

Mason AJ, Hayflick JS, Ling N et al (1985) Complementary DNA sequences of ovarian follicular fluid inhibin show precursor structure and homology with transforming growth factor-β. *Nature* **318:** 639–643.

Mason AJ, Niall HD & Seeburg PH (1986) Structure of two human ovarian inhibins. *Biochemical and Biophysical Research Communications* **135:** 957–964.

Massague J (1983) Epidermal growth factor-like transforming growth factor. *Journal of Biological Chemistry* **258:** 13606.

Massague J (1985) Transforming growth factors. Isolation, characterization and interaction with cellular receptors. *Progress in Medical Virology* **32:** 142–158.

Matsumoto AM, Paulsen CA & Bremner WJ (1984) Stimulation of sperm production by human luteinizing hormone in gonadotropin-suppressed normal men. *Journal of Clinical Endocrinology and Metabolism* **55:** 882–887.

McCullagh (1932) Dual endocrine control of the testis. *Science* **76:** 19.

McLachlan RI, Robertson DM, Burger HG & de Kretser DM (1986a) The radioimmunoassay of bovine and human follicular fluid and serum inhibin. *Molecular and Cellular Endocrinology* **46:** 175–185.

McLachlan RI, Robertson DM, Healy DM, de Kretser DM & Burger HG (1986b) Plasma inhibin levels during gonadotropin-induced ovarian hyperstimulation for IVF: a new index of follicular function? *Lancet* **i:** 1233–1234.

McNatty KP, Makris A, de Grazia C, Osathanondh R & Ryan KJ (1979) The production of progesterone, androgens, and estrogens by granulosa cells, thecal tissue, and stromal tissue from human ovaries in vitro. *Journal of Clinical Endocrinology and Metabolism* **49:** 687–699.

Miller KF, Critser JK & Ginther OJ (1982) Inhibition and subsequent rebound of FSH secretion following treatment with bovine follicular fluid in the ewe. *Theriogenology* **18:** 45–53.

Miyamoto K, Hasegawa Y, Fukuda M et al (1985) Isolation of porcine follicular fluid inhibin of 32K daltons. *Biochemical and Biophysical Research Communications* **129:** 396–403.

Miyamoto K, Hasegawa Y, Fukuda M & Igarashi M (1986) Demonstration of high molecular weight forms of inhibin in bovine follicular fluid (bFF) by using monoclonal antibodies to bFF 32K inhibin. *Biochemical and Biophysical Research Communications* **136:** 1103–1109.

Moudgal MR, Murthy HMS, Murthy GS & Rao AJ (1985) In Sairam HR & Atkinson LE (eds) *Gonadal Proteins and Peptides and Their Biological Significance*, pp 21–37. Singapore: World Scientific Publishing.

Nieschlag E (1986) Reasons for abandoning immunization against FSH as an approach to male fertility regulation. In Zatuchni GI (ed.) *Male Contraception: Advances and Future Prospects*, pp 395–400. Philadelphia: Harper and Row.

Ramasharma K, Shashidara Murthy HM & Moudgal NR (1979) A rapid bioassay for measuring inhibin activity. *Biology of Reproduction* **20:** 831–835.

Ramasharma K, Sairam MR, Seidah NG et al (1984) Isolation, structure, and synthesis of a human seminal plasma peptide with inhibin-like activity. *Science* **223:** 1199–1201.

Reichert LE Jr & Abou-Issa H (1977) Studies on a low molecular weight testicular factor which inhibits binding of FSH to receptor. *Biology of Reproduction* **17:** 614–621.

Rivier J, Spiess J, McClintock R, Vaughan J & Vale W (1985) Purification and partial characterization of inhibin from porcine follicular fluid. *Biochemical and Biophysical Research Communications* **133:** 120–127.

Roberts AB & Sporn MB (1985) Transforming growth factors. *Cancer Surveys* **4:** 683–705.

Robertson DM, Au CL & de Kretser DM (1982) The use of ^{51}Cr for assessing cytotoxicity in an in vitro bioassay for inhibin. *Molecular and Cellular Endocrinology* **26:** 119–127.

Robertson DM, Foulds LM, Leversha L et al (1985) Isolation of inhibin from bovine follicular fluid. *Biochemical and Biophysical Research Communications* **126:** 220–226.

Robertson DM, de Vos FL, Foulds LM et al (1986a) Isolation of a 31 kDa form of inhibin from bovine follicular fluid. *Molecular and Cellular Endocrinology* **44:** 271–277.

Robertson DM, Giacometti MS & de Kretser DM (1986b) The effects of inhibin purified from bovine follicular fluid in several in vitro pituitary cell culture systems. *Molecular and Cellular Endocrinology* **46:** 29–36.

Schenken RS, Asch RH & Anderson WH (1984) Effect of porcine follicular fluid on the postcastration secretion of gonadotropins in rhesus monkeys. *Journal of Clinical Endocrinology and Metabolism* **59:** 436–440.

Schwartz NB & Channing CP (1977) Evidence for ovarian 'inhibin': suppression of the secondary rise in serum follicle stimulating hormone levels in proestrous rats by injection of porcine follicular fluid. *Proceedings of the National Academy of Sciences (USA)* **74:** 5721–5724.

Scott RS & Burger HG (1980) Inhibin is absent from azoospermic semen of infertile men. *Nature* **285:** 246–247.

Scott RS & Burger HG (1981) An inverse relationship exists between seminal plasma inhibin and serum follicle-stimulating hormone in man. *Journal of Clinical Endocrinology and Metabolism* **52:** 796–803.

Scott RS, Burger HG & Quigg H (1980) A simple and rapid in vitro bioassay for inhibin. *Endocrinology* **107:** 1536–1542.

Scott RS, Burger HG, Quigg H et al (1982) The specificity of inhibin bioassay using cultured pituitary cells. *Molecular and Cellular Endocrinology* **27:** 307–316.

Seethalakshmi L & Steinberger A (1983) Effect of cryptorchidism and orchidopexy on inhibin secretion by rat Sertoli cells. *Journal of Andrology* **4:** 131–135.

Seidah NG, Arbatti NJ, Rochemont J, Sheth AR & Chretien M (1984) Complete amino acid sequence of human seminal plasma β-inhibin. *FEBS Letters* **175:** 349–355.

Sheth AR, Arbatti N, Carlquist M & Jornvall H (1984) Characterization of a polypeptide from human seminal plasma with inhibin (inhibition of FSH secretion)-like activity. *FEBS Letters* **165:** 11–15.

Skinner MK & Fritz IB (1985) Testicular peritubular cells secrete a protein under androgen control that modulates Sertoli cell functions. *Proceedings of the National Academy of Sciences (USA)* **82:** 114–118.

Sluss PM & Reichert LE Jr (1984) Porcine follicular fluid contains several low molecular weight inhibitors of follicle-stimulating hormone binding to receptor. *Biology of Reproduction* **30:** 1091–1104.

Steinberger A (1981) Regulation of inhibin secretion in the testis. In Franchimont P & Channing CP (eds) *Intragonadal Regulation of Reproduction*, pp 283–298. London: Academic Press.

Steinberger A & Steinberger E (1976) Secretion of an FSH-inhibiting factor by cultured Sertoli cells. *Endocrinology* **99:** 918–921.

Stewart AG, Milborrow HM, Ring JM, Crowther CE & Forage RG (1986) Human inhibin genes: genomic characterization and sequencing. *FEBS Letters* (in press).

Stouffer RL & Hodgen GD (1980) Induction of luteal phase defects in rhesus monkeys by follicular fluid administration at the onset of the menstrual cycle. *Journal of Clinical Endocrinology and Metabolism* **51:** 669–671.

Tsonis CG, McNeilly AS & Baird DT (1986) Measurement of exogenous and endogenous inhibin in sheep serum using a new and extremely sensitive bioassay for inhibin based on inhibition of ovine pituitary FSH secretion in vitro. *Journal of Endocrinology* **110:** 341–352.

Tsonis CG, Quigg H, Lee VWK et al (1983) Inhibin in individual ovine follicles in relation to diameter and atresia. *Journal of Reproduction and Fertility* **67:** 83–90.

Tsukamoto I, Taya K, Watanabe G & Sasamoto S (1986) Inhibin activity and secretion of gonadotropin during the period of follicular maturation. *Life Sciences* (in press).

Uilenbroek JTJ, Tiller R, de Jong FH & Vels F (1978) Specific suppression of follicle-stimulating hormone secretion in gonadectomized male and female rats with intrasplenic ovarian transplants. *Endocrinology* **78:** 399–406.

Ultee-van Gessel AM, Leemborg FG, de Jong FH & van der Molen HJ (1986) In-vitro secretion of inhibin-like activity by Sertoli cells from normal and prenatally irradiated immature rats. *Journal of Endocrinology* **109:** 411–418.

Vale W, Rivier J, Vaughan J et al (1986) Purification and characterization of an FSH releasing protein from porcine ovarian follicular fluid. *Nature* **321:** 776–779.

van Dijk S, de Jong FH & van der Molen HJ (1984) Use of fast protein liquid chromatography in the purification of inhibin from bovine follicular fluid. *Biochemical and Biophysical Research Communications* **125:** 307–314.

van Dijk S, Steenbergen C, de Jong FH & van der Molen HJ (1985) Comparison between inhibin from human and bovine ovarian follicular fluid using fast protein liquid chromatography. *Molecular and Cellular Endocrinology* **42:** 245–251.

van Dijk S, Steenbergen C, de Jong FH & Gielen JTh (1986) Sexual dimorphism in immuno-neutralization of bioactivity of rat and ovine inhibin. *Journal of Endocrinology* (in press).

Van Thiel DH, Sherins RJ, Myers GH Jr & de Vita VT Jr (1972) Evidence for a specific seminiferous tubular factor affecting follicle-stimulating hormone secretion in man. *Journal of Clinical Investigation* **51:** 1009–1019.

Verhoeven G & Franchimont P (1983) Regulation of inhibin secretion of Sertoli cell-enriched cultures. *Acta Endocrinologica* **102:** 136–143.

Verjans HL & Eik-Nes KB (1976) Hypothalamic–pituitary–testicular system following testicular x-irradiation. *Acta Endocrinologica* **83:** 190–200.

Wallace JM & McNeilly AS (1985) Increase in ovulation rate after treatment of ewes with bovine follicular fluid in the luteal phase of the oestrous cycle. *Journal of Reproduction and Fertility* **73:** 505–515.

Welschen R, Hermans WP, Dullaart J & de Jong FH (1977) Effects of an inhibin-like factor present in bovine and porcine follicular fluid on gonadotrophin levels in ovariectomized rats. *Journal of Reproduction and Fertility* **50:** 129–131.

Yamashiro D, Li CH, Ramasharma K & Sairam MR (1984) Synthesis and biological activity of human inhibin-like peptide-(1–31). *Proceedings of the National Academy of Sciences (USA)* **81:** 5399–5402.

Ying S-Y, Becker A, Baird A et al (1986a) Beta transforming growth factor (TGF-β) is a potent stimulator of the basal secretion of follicle stimulating hormone (FSH) in a pituitary monolayer system. *Biochemical and Biophysical Research Communications* **135:** 950–956.

Ying S-Y, Becker A, Ling N, Ueno N & Guillemin R (1986b) Inhibin and beta type transforming growth factor (TGFβ) have opposite modulating effects on the follicle stimulating hormone (FSH)-induced aromatase activity of cultured rat granulosa cells. *Biochemical and Biophysical Research Communications* **136:** 969–975.

Zhiwen Z, Carson R, Herington A, Lee V & Burger H (1986) FSH and somatomedin-C stimulate inhibin production by rat granulosa cells in vitro. Submitted for publication.

6

Endocrine approaches to male fertility control

ULRICH A. KNUTH
EBERHARD NIESCHLAG

The ideal method for fertility regulation should be highly effective, free of toxic effects, reversible, rapid in onset and easily available. To be acceptable to both partners it should not interfere with spontaneous and pleasurable aspects of sexual intercourse.

In the female these requirements have been virtually achieved since oral contraceptives were introduced 25 years ago. In the male, however, a method with a similar profile of desired characteristics is still lacking. At present the condom, of all available male methods, still seems to fulfil the above requirements best. In a largely promiscuous society it offers the additional advantage of a certain protection against venereal diseases. Its use is obvious and guarantees the female that her partner is indeed using a contraceptive. In a more stable relationship, however, the use of condoms is frequently not acceptable to both partners. Since another potent, reversible male antifertility agent is not available, the woman is again forced to bear the contraceptive burden alone. Vasectomy may become an alternative when the family has been completed, but psychological factors and the desire to maintain potential fertility for unforeseen future events deter many men from this, in at least 50% of cases, irreversible step. Nevertheless, about 10% of all couples practising contraception in North America resort to vasectomy.

Since spermatogenesis is under hormonal control (see Chapter 4) the possibility of interfering with spermatogenesis via endocrinological mechanisms appears to be a reasonable target.

THE BASIC CONCEPT

In the female a delicate endocrine balance exists between negative and positive feedback mechanisms, which leads to the relatively rare events of ovulation. This balance can be disturbed easily, as clinical experience shows. Nature itself has provided an endocrine mechanism to interrupt ovulation during pregnancy. The same principle is the basic mechanism of oral contraceptives.

In contrast to the female gametogenesis in the male seems to be a more robust and vigorous event. Although ovulation occurs episodically about every four weeks, spermatogenesis is a long-term process with a developmental cycle of around 3 months for the single sperm and several million sperm being produced every day.

According to common knowledge, spermatogenesis is under the control of follicle stimulating hormone (FSH) and luteinizing hormone (LH), whose secretion is regulated by gonadal steroids and by peptides such as inhibin. Based on this negative feedback mechanism it should be possible to suppress gonadotrophin secretion by administration of appropriate substances and, as a consequence, block spermatogenesis.

The production of sperm and male hormones in the testes are so closely connected that it is difficult to suppress sperm production selectively without simultaneous suppression of androgen release. Since libido, potency, male behaviour and general metabolic processes (erythropoiesis, protein anabolism, bone metabolism) depend on a sufficient supply of testosterone, androgens must be substituted if the substance used for suppression of gonadotrophin secretion is not androgenic by itself. This leads to the general concept of endocrine male fertility regulation: combination of an anti-gonadotrophic substance with an androgen.

At first sight, testosterone and its esters combine these properties and appear to be the almost ideal agents for steroidal suppression of spermatogenesis. Testosterone administration inhibits hypophyseal LH secretion. The Leydig cells in close proximity to the testicular tubules are no longer stimulated and intratesticular androgen levels, required for regular spermatogenesis, decline. At the same time peripheral testosterone levels due to exogenous administration remain high enough to maintain libido and potency.

TESTOSTERONE

Injectable testosterone esters

The general validity of this basic concept was demonstrated in men more than three decades ago (Heller et al, 1950). Later more systematic studies were conducted by Reddy and Rao (1972), Mauss et al (1974) and finally a group of investigators supported by the National Institutes of Health (Patanelli, 1978). Several testosterone preparations were tested for their potential as male antifertility agents. With the exception of testosterone undecanoate all of these preparations have to be given parenterally.

Testosterone propionate

Complete azoospermia was seen in seven volunteers after 60 days of daily injection with 25 mg testosterone propionate (Reddy and Rao, 1972). Full recovery of sperm concentration was seen in all subjects after 5 months. Although effective in its basic concept, the necessity of daily injections prohibits widespread use of this regimen and consequently longer-acting testosterone esters were tested for male fertility control.

Testosterone enanthate

Mauss et al (1974) administered 250 mg testosterone enanthate (TE) to seven normal men weekly for 22 weeks. After 10 weeks, sperm counts were below 5×10^6/ml in all subjects; four of them revealed concentrations below 1×10^6/ml. In spite of the overall success one subject consequently showed an escape phenomenon with sperm counts above 10×10^6/ml while the treatment continued. Twenty-seven weeks after cessation of treatment, sperm counts had not returned to pretreatment values, although during the next 30 months seminal parameters of all seven men recovered completely (Mauss et al, 1978).

This study was followed by multicentre trials with TE in the USA (for summary see Patanelli, 1978). They were designed to identify the necessary frequency of TE injections required to attain and maintain azoospermia and to assess possible side-effects. Although 137 volunteers completed the trials, differences in duration and intervals of injection prohibit a concise summary. In general, results are similar to a study outlined in Figure 1 (Paulsen et al, 1978). Altogether studies showed that azoospermia or severe oligozoospermia with sperm counts below 5×10^6/ml could be achieved with weekly TE injections in a high number of men. However, when injections were given at intervals greater than 10–12 days, sperm counts increased in a larger number of volunteers even when the testosterone dose was doubled, indicating the relatively short half-life of the ester used.

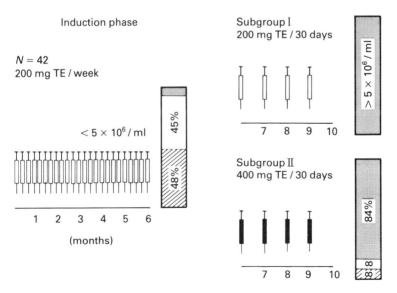

Figure 1. Design and results of a representative study using testosterone enanthate (TE) alone for male fertility regulation. Syringes indicate injections. The columns at the end of treatment periods indicate percentages of men with azoospermia (▨), severe oligozoospermia (□ = sperm counts below 5×10^6/ml) and proportion of volunteers where fertility may not be impaired (▦). Based on Paulsen et al (1978).

Other injectable testosterone esters

Although weekly intervals of TE injections offer an advantage over the daily administration of testosterone propionate, the frequency of injections required is still too high to render TE an acceptable general method for male fertility regulation. Since other available testosterone esters, such as testosterone cypionate and cyclohexanecarboxylate, possess pharmacological properties similar to those of TE (Schulte-Behrbühl and Nieschlag, 1980; Schürmeyer and Nieschlag, 1984) the possibility of more widely spaced injections of these esters is unlikely. Perhaps new testosterone esters currently under development by the World Health Organization (WHO) (Weinbauer et al, 1986) or testosterone microspheres as tested in feral mustangs (Kirkpatrick et al, 1982) may provide long-acting modalities suitable for fertility regulation.

Oral androgens

When the orally effective testosterone ester, testosterone undecanoate, became available for clinical use, it was reasonable to test this substance as a 'male pill'. To this end, seven normal volunteers received 240 mg testosterone undecanoate divided into three equal daily doses for 10–12 weeks (Nieschlag et al, 1978). This dose is two to three times above the dose required for substitution of hypogonadal patients. Nevertheless, only one of the seven subjects achieved azoospermia, whereas the others showed sperm counts still in a range compatible with fertility.

The reason for this failure of testosterone undecanoate to cause azoospermia is most probably caused by the particular pharmacokinetic property of this substance. Instead of a continuous, stable level of the androgen, short-lived serum testosterone peaks occur between 1 and 8 h after digestion of the capsules with unpredictable interindividual variation (Schürmeyer et al, 1983). Since gonadotrophin levels are not continuously suppressed, intermittent intratesticular stimulation of Leydig cells may be high enough to maintain spermatogenesis at a certain level.

In all clinical studies using testosterone esters no severe side-effects were noted. As a consequence of impaired spermatogenesis, testicular size decreased, but this was of no concern since most of the time the changes were not realized by the volunteers. Some men showed weight gain, acne, oily skin or slightly increased haemoglobin concentrations. Changes in sexual function were not reported.

ANTIANDROGENS

Animal studies and administration to sexual delinquents showed that the antiandrogen cyproterone acetate (CPA) suppressed spermatogenesis. This was not surprising since, owing to its strong gestagenic activity, CPA inhibits gonadotrophin secretion in addition to its antiandrogenic property. In clinical trials with 5–20 mg of CPA per day up to 16 weeks, sperm counts and sperm motility were drastically reduced (Fogh et al, 1979; Moltz et al, 1980; Wang and Yeung, 1980). However, testosterone levels in serum dropped and caused a decrease in libido and potency in some of the volunteers, so that clinical trials were not continued.

GESTAGENS PLUS TESTOSTERONE

The failure of testosterone esters alone injected at reasonable intervals to induce consistent azoospermia or severe oligozoospermia in volunteers led to the use of treatment schedules with a combination of different hormones.

Several steroid combinations were used in the past (Table 1). Progestin (progesterone)/testosterone (implanted as a testosterone pellet) and TE combinations received the widest attention. Multicentre trails were sponsored by WHO and the Population Council (for reference see Schearer, 1978; World Health Organization, 1972–1983). The best results were achieved with depot medroxyprogesterone acetate (DMPA) and TE supplementation. A representative study of this kind is shown in Figure 2 (Sanchez et al, 1979). DMPA and TE were injected monthly with a reduction of DMPA after 2 months. After 6 months of treatment 53% of participating volunteers had achieved azoospermia. An additional 33% showed severe oligozoospermia, whereas 14% did not respond as desired. The incidence of untoward side-effects was low. No effects on libido and potency were observed. A recent investigation of patients treated with DMPA for sexually offensive behaviour over long periods showed significant weight gain and increased blood pressure as well as an increased insulin response in the glucose tolerance test and indications of gall bladder dysfunction (Meyer

Table 1. Steroids and steroid combinations used in trials for male fertility regulation.

Supplement	Androgen								
	None	T implant	TP	TE	TC	TU	MT	T cream	19NT-HPP
None		*	*	*		*			*
Ethinyloestradiol							*		
Danazol				*					
CPA	*								
17-OH-Progesterone acetate				*			*		
17-OH-Progesterone capronate				*					
Megestrol acetate	*								
MPA				*				*	
DMPA		*	*	*	*			*	
Norethandrolone		*							
Norgestrienone		*							
Norgestrel		*		*					

T implant = pellets or testosterone-filled Silastic capsules; TP = testosterone propionate; TE = testosterone enanthate; TC = testosterone cypionate; TU = testosterone undecanoate; MT = methyltestosterone; 19NT-HPP = 19-nortestosterone hexyloxyphenylpropionate; DMPA = depot medroxyprogesterone acetate.

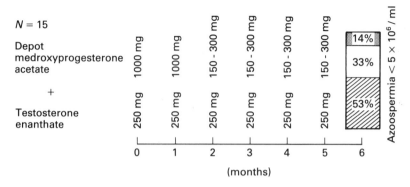

Figure 2. Design and results of a representative study using a combination of depot medroxy-progesterone acetate and testosterone enanthate for male fertility regulation. Doses refer to monthly i.m. injections. For further information see Figure 1. Based on Sanchez et al (1979).

et al, 1985). But in these cases DMPA was given without testosterone and the gestagen doses were higher than would probably be required for fertility regulation.

Oral gestagens plus testosterone cream

In order to develop a technique that could be self-administered, 20 mg medroxyprogesterone acetate were given orally plus 50–100 mg testosterone applied percutaneously via cream for one year (Soufir et al, 1983). Sperm counts in the six volunteers were suppressed to less than 5×10^6/ml but azoospermia was not reached. A further limitation of this approach was shown in another study when in five of 12 cases the wives of the treated men developed hirsutism due to testosterone transferred to their bodies by skin contact with their husbands (Delanoe et al, 1984).

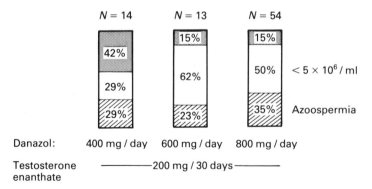

Figure 3. Results of a representative study using different doses of danazol and testosterone enanthate for male fertility regulation. Doses of danazol refer to daily oral administration. Testosterone enanthate was given additionally by injection once a month. Details on time course were not reported. For further information see Figure 1. Based on Leonard and Paulsen (1978).

DANAZOL PLUS TESTOSTERONE

Danazol, a derivative of ethinyltestosterone, when given orally, strongly inhibits LH and FSH secretion but is devoid of other significant oestrogenic or progestational activities. Various combinations of daily oral doses of danazol with monthly injections of 200 mg of TE were tested (Leonard and Paulsen, 1978). Details are given in Figure 3. Although the percentage of azoospermia or severe oligozoospermia rose with increasing doses of danazol, 15% of all participants showed sperm counts above 5×10^6/ml at the highest doses used.

19-NORTESTOSTERONE

Recently a search for an androgenic substance with a longer half-life, slow-release characteristics and strong antigonadotrophic activity was initiated. 19-Nortestosterone esters (19NT) were identified as potential candidates. These steroids have been on the market for more than 20 years without reports of serious side-effects. Binding studies with 19NT show a 54% higher affinity to the androgen receptor, compared with testosterone (Saartok et al, 1984). Reduction to dihydronortestosterone (DHNT) reduces this affinity, whereas the corresponding metabolism of testosterone to dihydrotestosterone (DHT) increases its binding affinity. When DHT is used as the 100% standard, binding affinity of 19NT is 30–40%, compared with 10–20% for testosterone and 12% for DHNT (Toth and Zarkar, 1982). This implies higher androgenic activity for 19NT in all target tissues without 5α-reductase activity such as muscle, haematopoietic stem cells, and possibly central brain areas (Mainwaring, 1977). In tissues with high 5α-reductase, however, 19NT, i.e. its metabolite DHNT, would exhibit only a fraction of the androgenic potency of comparable testosterone concentrations.

To study pharmacokinetic properties, a method for determination of 19NT in serum based on high-performance liquid chromatographic isolation and radioimmunological determination was developed (Belkien et al, 1985). Since two esters are commercially available, namely 19-nortestosterone hexyloxyphenylpropionate (19-NT-HPP, 19-nandrolonehexyloxyphenyl-propionate) (Anadur) and 19-nortestosteronedecanoate (Deca-Durabolin), pharmacokinetics of both substances were studied in six volunteers. Since Anadur was found to have a longer half-life than the decanoate ester (Figure 4), Anadur was used in a pilot study with five volunteers. Azoospermia was achieved in all participants after 12 weeks of injection (Schürmeyer et al, 1984a).

A follow-up study was conducted with a higher number of participants ($N = 12$) and a more elaborate design to test the effectiveness at injection intervals of 3 weeks (Knuth et al, 1985). Total time of treatment lasted 25 weeks succeeded by follow-up examinations for 17 additional weeks supplemented by a final test at week 52.

Differences in injection intervals during the second half of the treatment

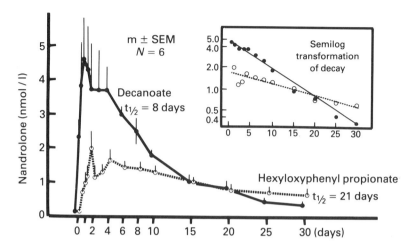

Figure 4. Serum concentration of 19-nortestosterone (nandrolone) in six volunteers after single injections of 50 mg of 19-nortestosterone decanoate or 19-nortestosterone hexyloxyphenyl-propionate. $t_{1/2}$ = half-life in days. Redrawn from Belkien et al (1985).

phase did not influence any of the measured parameters except 19NT serum levels themselves. Serum testosterone levels were completely suppressed, demonstrating the advantageous influence of the long half-life of the ester used. Gonadotrophin values in general were below detection levels.

Azoospermia occurred in two volunteers as early as 9 weeks after the first injection of 19NT-HPP with a rising frequency throughout the treatment period. Twenty-one days after the last injection, 27 weeks after the start of the treatment and theoretically the time point at which a maximal impact of treatment could be expected, six volunteers presented with azoospermia; a further two showed only single sperm in the sediment of the ejaculate and two had sperm counts below 5×10^6/ml. Only two of 12 men treated with 19NT-HPP revealed sperm counts in the normal range above 20×10^6/ml with unimpaired motility, representing a failure rate of 17%. One of them, however, had been azoospermic after 9 and 12 weeks of treatment with a recovery of sperm counts thereafter. Normalization in the other participants with sperm concentrations above 20×10^6/ml occurred as early as 15 weeks after the last injection and was complete in 11 of the 12 men after 28 weeks of follow up. The volunteer with sperm counts below 5×10^6/ml at week 52 presented with normal values 8 weeks later (Figure 5).

In spite of low testosterone concentrations no effect on libido or potency became apparent when weekly protocols on several parameters of sexual activity, desire and functions were evaluated. Complaints about impaired somatic functions or reduction of general well-being were not reported by any of the volunteers. Administration of 19NT-HPP did not affect liver enzymes, creatinine, uric acid, serum electrolytes or serum lipids. Haemoglobin, erythrocytes, haematocrit and mean corpuscular volume, however, were significantly elevated following 13 weeks of treatment when compared

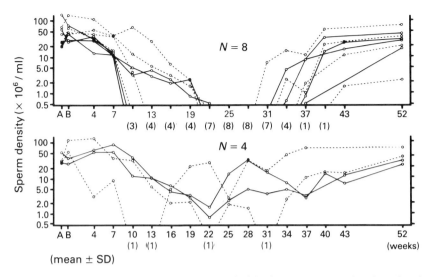

Figure 5. Individual sperm density in men treated with 19-nortestosterone hexyloxyphenyl-propionate. Shaded area represents treatment phase. Broken and solid lines indicate differences in injection intervals after 7 weeks (3 weeks versus weekly). Upper panel shows participants with azoospermia or few immotile sperm in the sediment at the end of the treatment phase. Number of azoospermic subjects at each time point is indicated by number in brackets. Lower panel displays sperm counts in men without constant suppression of spermatogenesis throughout the treatment. Please note logarithmic scale. From Knuth et al (1985), with permission.

to pretreatment values, although they did not leave the range considered normal by our standard values.

In comparison to the other clinical trials summarized in this chapter, 19NT as a single entity proved to be at least as effective as gestagen/TE combinations at longer injection intervals and more effective than luteinizing hormone releasing hormone (LHRH, gonadotrophin releasing hormone) analogue combinations (Figure 6). Whether uniform azoospermia can be achieved in combination with an additional antigonadotrophic substance awaits further clinical trials.

LHRH AGONISTIC ANALOGUES PLUS TESTOSTERONE

Following the synthesis of LHRH (Matsuo et al, 1971) it became clear that its gonadotrophin releasing activity depended on the mode of administration. When given physiologically, i.e. in a pulsatile pattern, it stimulated release of LH and FSH, whereas continuous administration led to a consequent decline in gonadotrophin levels (Belchetz et al, 1978). When long-acting LHRH analogues became available (for review see Karten and Rivier, 1986) this paradoxical effect could be achieved with single daily injections when given chronically (Happ et al, 1978).

In the rat, three sites and mechanisms of action have been identified to

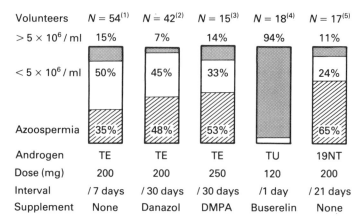

Figure 6. Comparison of success rate in representative experimental trials for male fertility regulation using different ways to suppress gonadotrophins. 'Androgen' indicates substance used to maintain virility: TE = testosterone enanthate, TU = testosterone undecanoate, 19NT = 19-nortestosterone hexyloxyphenylpropionate. 'Interval' describes the frequency of the androgen administration per multiple of days. 'Supplement' lists the antigonadotropic substance given in addition. Based on: (1) Paulsen et al, 1978; (2) Leonard and Paulsen, 1978; (3) Sanchez et al, 1979; (4) Schürmeyer et al, 1984b, and Michel et al, 1985; (5) Schürmeyer et al, 1984a, and Knuth et al, 1985.

explain this effect: (1) desensitization of the gonadotroph, (2) loss of gonadal receptors, and (3) changes in enzyme activity. In humans and non-human primates, however, no receptors for LHRH have been found in the testicular tissue (Clayton and Huhtaniemi, 1982) and a desensitizing effect of LHRH on testicular hormone production could not be detected (Mann et al, 1984; Schaison et al, 1984). A detailed review on the mechanism of action in the male has appeared recently (Bhasin and Swerdloff, 1986). These differences in basic physiological functions should caution against uncritical comparison between results from different species. Therefore in this review only data from human and non-human primate studies will be considered.

The first data on long-term effects of LHRH analogue administration to normal men were published in 1979 (Bergquist et al, 1979). D-Ser(Bu)^6,Pro^{9}Net-LHRH (buserelin) was injected at a dose of 5 µg-day subcutaneously (s.c.) for 17 weeks in four men. Although testosterone was not supplemented, an effect on sperm counts was not seen. Higher doses were tried when D-Trp^6,Pro^{9}Net-LHRH was given s.c. at a dose of 50 µg/day for up to 10 weeks in eight volunteers (Linde et al, 1981). No androgens were added and serum testosterone fell into the castrate range within a month. As a consequence five men became impotent after 6–7 weeks. Lowest sperm counts were seen after 14 weeks, when treatment had already been stopped. In six out of eight men the lowest sperm counts were below 6 × 10^6/ml. In two men values did not fall below 27.2 × 10^6 or 46 × 10^6/ml, respectively. Azoospermia was not achieved in any of the participants. Similar results without impotence were obtained when a similar regimen was used with addition of 100 mg of TE every other week for 20 weeks (Doelle et al, 1983). In contrast to the previous study, testosterone administration attenuated the decline in sperm counts to around 21 weeks. An increase in dose of D-Trp^6,Pro^{9}Net-LHRH to 100 μg/day or even 500 μg/day did not lead to azoospermia in all participating men (Rabin et al, 1984). A similar failure to achieve azoospermia was reported by Swerdloff's group (Bhasin et al, 1985a), when seven men were treated with 200 μg/day s.c. D-Nal(2)^6-LHRH for 16 weeks. Androgen supplementation was given every 2 weeks by an injection of 200 mg TE. An 83% decline in overall sperm counts was reported, but azoospermia did not occur in any participant.

Parallel experiments in non-human primates with daily s.c. injections showed similarly disappointing results. When treatment of rhesus monkeys was started with 4 μg/day of D-Ser(Bu)^6,Pro^{9}Net-LHRH followed after 8 weeks by an increase in dose to 10 μg twice a day for another 4 weeks, no decline in sperm counts could be elicited (Wickings et al, 1981). Similar results were reported by others (Resko et al, 1982; Sundaram et al, 1982). Neither the increase in dose of D-Ser(Bu)^6,Pro^{9}Net-LHRH to 100 μg/day for 10 weeks in four rhesus monkeys (Akhtar et al, 1982) nor extension of the treatment with 100 μg/day s.c. of (imBzl)-D-His^6-Pro^9-Net-LHRH to 40 weeks led to azoospermia (Sundaram et al, 1984). This was even more disappointing since no testosterone supplementation had been given in these studies.

Detailed analysis of hormone profiles during treatment demonstrated that the stimulatory effect of the analogue on LH and FSH secretion, although most pronounced during the first days of treatment, did not completely decline and remained constantly present at a reduced level. In rhesus monkeys Resko et al (1982) showed an increase of testosterone 3 h after each D-Ser(Bu)^6,Pro^{9}Net-LHRH injection with androgen levels above 30 ng/ml up to day 50 of treatment. Similar results were seen in our laboratory (Akhtar et al, 1982). To avoid intermittent LH and consequent testosterone peaks after single injections, studies with constant administration of LHRH analogues were initiated.

Trials with constant release formulations of D-Trp^6,Pro^{9}Net-LHRH and D-Ala^6-Pro^9-LHRH in the form of s.c. implanted pellets had already been performed in baboons (Vickery and McRae, 1980) but treatment had been too short to evaluate changes in sperm counts. To achieve a constant infusion of D-Ser(Bu)^6,Pro^{9}Net-LHRH (buserelin) in the free-moving animals osmotic mini-pumps were implanted in rhesus monkeys. Delivery rate was 2 μg/h. In four animals treated for 20 weeks, testosterone was supplemented after a decrease in sperm counts had already occurred (Ahktar et al, 1983a), whereas another group of three monkeys received testosterone supplementation by implanted Silastic capsules from the beginning of the study (Akhtar et al, 1983b). In the first group, in contrast to all previous studies, azoospermia was observed in all animals. Testosterone supplementation attenuated this effect in the other three monkeys. Sperm counts fell to a range between 1×10^6 and 5×10^6/ml, but azoospermia was not achieved. Continuous infusion by osmotic pumps implanted s.c. was reported by another group (Mann et al, 1984) but treatment of five rhesus

monkeys with Wy-40972 lasted only 8 weeks and no effect on sperm production was observed.

Based on monkey data and reported failures to achieve azoospermia in
normal men with daily analogue injections of LHRH, 11 men were treated
with continuous infusion of D-Ser(Bu)^6,Pro^{9}Net-LHRH (Schürmeyer et al,
1984b). Since osmotic pumps were not licensed to be implanted in the
human, they were attached to a s.c. catheter and carried close to the skin in a
small vial filled with 0.9% saline to provide the required osmotic pressure.
Seven men received on average 118 µg/day. A second group ($N = 4$) received
twice that dose (230 µg/day). Androgen supplementation with an orally
active testosterone ester (testosterone undecanoate, Andriol) was initiated
after 5 weeks of treatment. After 12 weeks of D-Ser(Bu)^6,Pro^{9}Net-LHRH
infusion at the low rate sperm counts were still above 40×10^6/ml, although
an additional decrease to around 20×10^6/ml was observed 4 weeks after the
end of infusion. With the higher dose, suppression was more pronounced,
but motile sperm were still present in the ejaculates. An increase in dose to
450 µg/day in another group of seven men had no effect on seminal
parameters, although testicular volume declined during the treatment
period of 12 weeks (Michel et al, 1985). In a preliminary report slightly
better results have been noted in a study with continuously administered
D-Nal(2)^6-LHRH at a dose of 400 µg/day and 200 mg TE every 14 days
(Swerdloff et al, 1985). After 16 weeks of treatment four men had sperm
counts below 10×10^6/ml and, in addition, one was azoospermic.

At present experiments with LHRH agonistic analogues have not yet led
to a practicable method for male fertility regulation. Even continuous
administration of LHRH analogues to avoid intermittent increase in LH,
although successful in monkeys, has not yet led to complete azoospermia in
men. Factors other than suppression of gonadotrophins could be responsible. A comparison in humans with intermittent and continuous administration of 20 µg or 200 µg nafarelin per day for a 28-day treatment period
showed no difference in LH and FSH level concentrations. The only advantage of the continuous administration was a better suppression of testosterone in some of the participants (Bhasin et al, 1985b). Furthermore, the
necessity to supplement testosterone appears to be counterproductive. New
forms of testosterone substitution avoiding high serum peaks may provide
better results.

In humans treated for 10 days with D-Nal(2)^6-LHRH 10 µg/day or
100 µg/day s.c., LH levels on day 10 were in the range of pretreatment values
after a previous increase (Heber et al, 1984). Others demonstrated that after
8 weeks of treatment with daily s.c. injections of 50 µg of D-Trp^6,Pro^{9}Net-
LHRH basal LH values were increased in one, unchanged in three and
decreased in three volunteers (Evans et al, 1984a). The responsiveness of
the Leydig cells to continuous LH infusion (1.3 IU/min for 48 h) was unimpaired. It has been shown that the comparatively high levels of immunoreactive LH in peripheral blood do not represent biological activity (Evans
et al, 1984b), a phenomenon which would explain the paradoxical decrease
in serum testosterone. However, at present we cannot exclude that LHRH
agonist treatment still allows some stimulation of intratesticular testo-

sterone production, which may maintain a certain level of spermatogenesis. Thus effects of LHRH analogues in combination with testosterone supplementation on spermatogenesis and testosterone production in young healthy volunteers seem to differ from results in older men treated for prostatic carcinoma with LHRH alone (Labrie et al, 1986).

LHRH ANTAGONISTIC ANALOGUES PLUS TESTOSTERONE

The problem of LH release and consequent stimulation of Leydig cells might be overcome by the use of LHRH antagonists. When these substances are administered, there is no initial increase in gonadotrophins, which may delay the onset of azoospermia, and no intermittent stimulation of LH release occurs. First studies in monkeys (*Macaca fascicularis*), however, showed that there were still animals in whom spermatogenesis was maintained in spite of antagonist treatment. In three of four animals azoospermia was reached after 7–9 weeks when 2 mg/day of the antagonist N-Ac-D-Nal(2)[1],D-pCl-Phe[2],D-Trp[3],D-hArg(Et$_2$)[6],D-Ala[10]-LHRH   (RS-68439) were given by osmotic minipump. The remaining animal had sperm counts below 5×10^6/ml (Weinbauer et al, 1984). Similar results were observed with a different substance (N-Ac-D-pCl-Phe[1,2],D-Trp[3],D-Arg[6],D-Ala[10]-LHRH; Org-30276) in five *Macaca fascicularis* monkeys (Akhtar et al, 1985) treated for 9 weeks with daily s.c. injections of 5 mg. Although three animals responded with azoospermia within 9 weeks the remaining two monkeys showed sustained spermatogenesis during another 8 weeks of treatment at an increased dose of 10 mg/day.

Antagonists appear to have a better potential for male fertility regulation than the agonists, although with available substances in humans approximately 1 g would be required per day! Before clinical trials can be initiated, toxicology of the compounds has to be fully assessed. Adverse reactions due to an apparent release of histamine were seen with tested material. With the available data one must conclude that, in comparison with medroxy-progesterone acetate/testosterone esters, the combination of LHRH analogues with available testosterone esters has so far proved to be less effective for male fertility regulation (Figure 6).

CONCLUSIONS

The failure of all treatment regimens to achieve uniform azoospermia in participating volunteers in spite of suppressed gonadotrophins could indicate that the starting hypothesis on the absolute requirement of FSH and LH for spermatogenesis in men or non-human primates is not correct. Data from studies using passive (Wickings and Nieschlag, 1983) and active immunization against FSH (Srinath et al, 1983) support these doubts. Rhesus monkeys were actively immunized against FSH. While booster immunization continued, they were followed for a period of four and a half years. Although suppression of spermatogenesis and reduction of sperm count in the ejaculate were observed, consistent azoospermia did not occur.

There are accumulating data from men and non-human primates that testosterone alone without LH may allow spermatogenesis to continue at a certain level, if testosterone concentrations within the testes are above a critical level (Marshall et al, 1983, 1984). This could mean that testosterone supplementation with presently available esters is detrimental to the goal of 100% azoospermia. Under physiological conditions intratesticular testosterone concentrations are up to 100 times higher than peripheral concentration. But there is very little information about what the minimal androgen requirements for spermatogenesis are. Studies with other androgen-dependent tissues show that due to a sigmoid dose–response curve a 95% reduction of serum testosterone causes only a 50–70% reduction of androgen activity (Labrie et al, 1985). Available testosterone preparations cause considerable fluctuations in serum levels with high levels after injection (Figure 7). These peaks may be sufficient to guarantee a certain proportion of receptor occupancy with maintenance or recovery of spermatogenesis. New testosterone preparations currently under development may contribute to overcome this problem.

Investigation of the available sex steroids and LHRH analogues have revealed the possibilities and limitations of hormonal fertility regulation in the male. It appears feasible to suppress spermatogenesis reversibly and without severe side-effects, but azoospermia cannot be achieved uniformly in all subjects. At present it is, however, generally accepted that azoospermia is the only criterion to ensure complete infertility in men. The presence of only a few sperm may be sufficient to induce pregnancy. Preg-

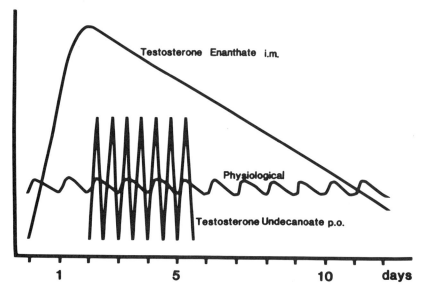

Figure 7. Schematic profiles of serum testosterone levels under physiological conditions after administration of a single testosterone enanthate injection, or oral testosterone undecanoate twice daily.

nancies have occurred in partners of men testing depot medroxyprogesterone acetate and testosterone at levels below 10×10^6 sperm per ml and even below 1×10^6 sperm per ml (Barfield et al, 1979). Therefore, the question prevails whether severe oligozoospermia combined with impaired morphology and decreased motility will be sufficient for male fertility regulation.

For some time it was hoped that assessment of the fertilizing capacity of human spermatozoa with hamster eggs in vitro might provide sufficient information to answer this question. In our first study with 19NT the hamster ova penetration test was used (Schürmeyer et al, 1984a). As long as sufficient sperm were available for testing, they were able to penetrate hamster ova, indicating that the remaining sperm under steroid suppression may be intact and fully functional sperm. However, recent studies have cast doubt on the potential value of the heterologous ovum penetration test for reliably predicting male fertility. Thus the open question can only be answered by clinical efficacy studies. Furthermore, the question whether 100% infertility is a must or whether severely reduced fertility would be acceptable at least to sectors of the world population requires discussion.

SUMMARY

As in the female, gametogenesis in the male is under the control of luteinizing hormone (LH) and follicle stimulating hormone (FSH). Their suppression should inhibit spermatogenesis. If a non-androgenic substance is used to suppress gonadotrophins, androgens must be supplemented to maintain virility, potency and metabolic processes. To avoid administration of several substances, testosterone and its esters were used to develop a male antifertility agent. Although azoospermia can be induced in a high proportion of men with administration of testosterone esters alone, this effect is not uniform. Even frequent injections with testosterone enanthate at weekly intervals fail to inhibit spermatogenesis in all participants. Combinations of gestagenic compounds with testosterone esters show a somewhat better effect, but again azoospermia is only achieved in around 50% of participants. LHRH analogues, although considered by many to offer a realistic potential for male fertility regulation, have not been proven to be successful for this purpose so far. Animal studies in monkeys and preliminary clinical trials demonstrate that agonistic analogues of LHRH have to be given continuously by pump or implant to achieve a pronounced effect on spermatogenesis. But even under these provisions, results in clinical trials have been worse than effects achieved with testosterone/gestagen combinations. Whether new antagonistic compounds offer a better potential awaits clinical trials. Studies in non-human primates demonstrate that testosterone by itself can maintain and initiate spermatogenesis. Based on these findings one could postulate an attenuating effect of high serum androgen levels after supplementation with available testosterone esters. Trials of alternative androgenic substances with slow-release characteristics and without high serum levels after single injections, like 19-nortestosterone hexyloxyphenylpropionate (19NT-HPP), tend to support this theory. With slow-release testosterone preparations under development by the WHO and more advanced delivery systems for LHRH analogues it is not unreasonable to speculate that an effective endocrine antifertility agent for the male will become available.

REFERENCES

Akhtar FB, Wickings EJ, Zaidi P & Nieschlag E (1982) Pituitary and testicular functions in sexually mature rhesus monkeys under high-dose LHRH-agonist treatment. *Acta Endocrinologica* **101**: 113–118.

Akhtar FB, Marshall GR, Wickings EJ & Nieschlag E (1983a) Reversible induction of azoospermia in rhesus monkeys by constant infusion of a GnRH agonist using osmotic minipumps. *Journal of Clinical Endocrinology and Metabolism* **56**: 534–540.

Akhtar FB, Marshall GR & Nieschlag E (1983b) Testosterone supplementation attenuates the antifertility effects of an LHRH agonist in male monkeys. *International Journal of Andrology* **6**: 461–468.

Akhtar FB, Weinbauer GF & Nieschlag E (1985) Acute and chronic effects of a gonadotrophin releasing hormone agonist on pituitary and testicular function in monkeys. *Journal of Endocrinology* **104**: 345–354.

Barfield A, Melo J & Coutinho E (1979) Pregnancies associated with sperm concentrations below 10 million/ml in clinical studies of a potential male contraceptive method, monthly depot medroxyprogesterone acetate and testosterone esters. *Contraception* **20**: 121–127.

Belchetz PE, Plant TM, Nakai Y, Keogh EJ & Knobil E (1978) Hypophyseal responses to continuous and intermittent delivery of hypothalamic gonadotropin-releasing hormone. *Science* **202**: 631–633.

Belkien L, Schürmeyer T, Hano R, Gunnarsson PO & Nieschlag E (1985) Pharmacokinetics of 19-nortestosterone esters in normal men. *Journal of Steroid Biochemistry* **22**: 623–629.

Bergquist C, Nillius SJ, Bergh T, Skarin G & Wide L (1979) Inhibitory effects on gonado-trophin secretion and gonadal function in men during chronic treatment with a potent stimulatory luteinizing hormone-releasing hormone analogue. *Acta Endocrinologica* **91**: 601–608.

Bhasin S & Swerdloff RS (1986) Mechanisms of gonadotropin-releasing hormone agonist action in the human male. *Endocrine Reviews* **7**: 106–114.

Bhasin S, Heber D, Steiner BS, Handelsman DJ & Swerdloff RS (1985a) Hormonal effects of gonadotropin-releasing hormone (GnRH) agonist in the human male. III. Effects of long term combined treatment with GnRH agonist and androgen. *Journal of Clinical Endocrinology and Metabolism* **60**: 998–1003.

Bhasin S, Steiner B & Swerdloff RS (1985b) Does constant infusion of gonadotropin-releasing hormone agonist lead to greater suppression of gonadal function in man than its intermittent administration? *Fertility and Sterility* **44**: 96–101.

Clayton RN & Huhtaniemi IT (1982) Absence of gonadotropin-releasing hormone receptors in human gonadal tissue. *Nature* **299**: 56–59.

Delanoe D, Fougeyrollas B, Meyer L & Thonneau P (1984) Androgenisation of female partners of men on medroxyprogesterone acetate/percutaneous testosterone contra-ception. *Lancet* **i**: 276.

Doelle GC, Alexander AN & Evans RM (1983) Combined treatment with an LHRH agonist and testosterone in man: reversible oligospermia without impotence. *Journal of Andrology* **4**: 298–302.

Evans RM, Doelle GC, Alexander AN, Uderman HD & Rabin D (1984a) Gonadotropin and steroid secretory pattern during chronic treatment with a luteinizing hormone releasing hormone analog in men. *Journal of Clinical Endocrinology and Metabolism* **58**: 862–867.

Evans RM, Doelle GC, Lindner J & Bradley V (1984b) A luteinizing hormone-releasing hormone agonist decreases biological activity and modifies chromatographic behavior of luteinizing hormone in man. *Journal of Clinical Investigation* **73**: 262–266.

Fogh M, Corcker CS, Hunter WM et al (1979) The effects of low doses of cyproterone acetate on some functions of the reproductive system in normal men. *Acta Endocrinologica* **91:** 545–552.

Happ J, Scholz P, Weber T et al (1978) Gonadotropin secretion in eugonadotropic human males and postmenopausal females under long-term application of a potent analog of gonadotropin-releasing hormone. *Fertility and Sterility* **30:** 674–678.

Heber D, Bhasin S, Steiner B & Swerdloff RS (1984) The stimulatory and down-regulatory effects of a gonadotropin-releasing hormone agonist in man. *Journal of Clinical Endocrinology and Metabolism* **58:** 1084–1088.

Heller CG, Nelson WO & Hall IC (1950) Improvement in spermatogenesis following depression of human testes with testosterone. *Fertility and Sterility* **1:** 415–422.

Karten MJ & Rivier JE (1986) Gonadotropin-releasing hormone analog design. Structure–function studies toward the development of agonists and antagonists: rationale and perspectives. *Endocrine Reviews* **7:** 44–66.

Kirkpatrick J, Turner JW & Perkins (1982) Reversible chemical fertility control in feral horses. *Equine Veterinary Sciences* **22:** 114–118.

Knuth UA, Behre H, Belkien L, Bents H & Nieschlag E (1985) Clinical trial of 19-nortestosterone-hexoxyphenylpropionate (Anadur) for male fertility regulation. *Fertility and Sterility* **44:** 814–821.

Labrie F, Dupont A & Belanger A (1985) Complete androgen blockade for the treatment of prostate cancer. In De Vita VT Jr, Hellman S, Rosenberg SA (eds) *Important Advances in Oncology*, p 193. Philadelphia: JB Lippincott.

Labrie F, Dupont A, Belanger A et al (1986) Treatment of prostate cancer with gonadotropin releasing hormone agonist. *Endocrine Reviews* **7:** 67–74.

Leonard JM & Paulsen CA (1978) Contraceptive development studies for males: oral and parenteral steroid hormone administration. In Patanelli DJ (ed.) *Hormonal Control of Male Fertility*, pp 223–238. Bethesda: Department of Health, Education and Welfare, National Institutes of Health.

Linde R, Doelle GC, Alexander N et al (1981) Reversible inhibition of testicular steroidogenesis and spermatogenesis by a potent gonadotropin-releasing hormone agonist in normal men. *New England Journal of Medicine* **305:** 663–667.

Mainwaring WIP (1977) *The Mechanism of Action of Androgens*. New York: Springer.

Mann DR, Gould KG & Collins DC (1984) Influence of continuous gonadotropin-releasing hormone (GnRH) agonist treatment on luteinizing hormone and testosterone secretion, the response to GnRH, and the testicular response to human chorionic gonadotropin in male rhesus monkeys. *Journal of Clinical Endocrinology and Metabolism* **58:** 262–267.

Marshall GR, Wickings EJ, Lüdecke DK & Nieschlag E (1983) Stimulation of spermatogenesis in stalk-sectioned rhesus monkeys by testosterone alone. *Journal of Clinical Endocrinology and Metabolism* **57:** 152–159.

Marshall GR, Wickings EJ & Nieschlag E (1984) Testosterone can initiate spermatogenesis in an immature nonhuman primate (*Macaca fascicularis*). *Endocrinology* **114:** 2228–2233.

Matsuo H, Baba Y, Nair RM, Arimura A & Schaly AV (1971) Structure of the porcine LH- and FSH-releasing hormone I. The proposed amino acid sequence. *Biochemical and Biophysical Research Communications* **43:** 1334–1339.

Mauss J, Börsch G, Richter E & Bormacher K (1974) Investigations on the use of testosterone oenanthate as male contraceptive agent. *Contraception* **10:** 281–289.

Mauss J, Börsch G, Richter E & Bormacher K (1978) Demonstration of the reversibility of spermatozoa suppression by testosterone oenanthate. *Andrologia* **10:** 149–153.

Meyer WJ III, Walker PA, Emory LE & Smith ER (1985) Physical, metabolic, and hormonal effects on men of long-term therapy with medroxyprogesterone acetate. *Fertility and Sterility* **43:** 102–109.

Michel E, Bents H, Akhtar FB, Hönigl W, Knuth UA, Sandow J & Nieschlag E (1985) Failure of high-dose sustained release luteinizing-releasing hormone agonist (buserelin) plus oral testosterone to suppress male fertility. *Clinical Endocrinology* **23:** 663–675.

Moltz L, Römmler A, Post A, Schwartz U & Hammerstein J (1980) Medium dose cyproterone acetate (CPA): effects on hormone secretion and on spermatogenesis in men. *Contraception* **21:** 393–413.

Nieschlag E, Hoogen H, Bölk M, Schuster H & Wickings EJ (1978) Clinical trial with testosterone undecanoate for male fertility control. *Contraception* **18:** 607–614.

Patanelli DJ (ed.) (1978) *Hormonal Control of Male Fertility.* Bethesda: Department of Health, Education and Welfare, National Institutes of Health.

Paulsen CA, Leonard JM, Burgess EC & Ospina LF (1978) Male contraceptive development: re-examination of testosterone enanthate as an effective single entity agent. In Patanelli DJ (ed.) *Hormonal Control of Male Fertility*, pp 17–35. Bethesda: Department of Health, Education and Welfare, National Institutes of Health.

Rabin D, Evans RM, Alexander AN et al (1984) Heterogeneity of sperm density profiles following 20-week therapy with high dose LHRH analog plus testosterone. *Journal of Andrology* 5: 176–180.

Reddy PRK & Rao JM (1972) Reversible antifertility action of testosterone propionate in human males. *Contraception* 5: 295–301.

Resko JA, Belanger A & Labrie F (1982) Effects of chronic treatment with a potent luteinizing hormone releasing hormone agonist on serum luteinizing hormone and steroid levels in the male rhesus monkey. *Biology of Reproduction* 26: 378–384.

Saartok T, Dahlberg E & Gustafsson J-A (1984) Relative binding affinity of anabolic-androgenic steroids: comparison of the binding to the androgen receptors in skeletal muscle and in prostate, as well as to sex hormone-binding globulin. *Endocrinology* 114: 2100–2106.

Sanchez FA, Brache V & Leon P, Faundes A (1979) Inhibition of spermatogenesis with monthly injections of medroxyprogesterone acetate and low dose testosterone enanthate. *International Journal of Andrology* 2: 136–149.

Schaison G, Brailly S, Vuagnat P, Bouchard P & Milgrom E (1984) Absence of a direct inhibitory effect of the gonadotropin-releasing hormone (GnRH) agonist D-Ser (TBU)6, des-Gly-NH$_2$10 GnRH ethylamide (buserelin) on testicular steroidogenesis in men. *Journal of Clinical Endocrinology and Metabolism* 58: 885–888.

Schearer SB (1978) The use of progestins and androgens as a male contraceptive. *International Journal of Andrology* (supplement 2): 680–711.

Schulte-Beerbühl M & Nieschlag E (1980) Comparison of testosterone, DHT, LH and FSH in serum after injection of testosterone enanthate or testosterone cypionate. *Fertility and Sterility* 33: 201–203.

Schürmeyer T & Nieschlag E (1984) Comparative pharmacokinetics of testosterone enanthate and testosterone cyclohexanecarboxylate as assessed by serum and saliva testosterone in normal men. *International Journal of Andrology* 7: 181–187.

Schürmeyer T, Wickings EJ, Freischem CW & Nieschlag E (1983) Saliva and serum testosterone following oral testosterone undecanoate administration in normal and hypo-gonadal men. *Acta Endocrinologica* 102: 456–462.

Schürmeyer T, Knuth UA, Belkien L & Nieschlag E (1984a) Reversible azoospermia induced by the anabolic steroid 19-nortestosterone. *Lancet* i: 417–420.

Schürmeyer T, Knuth UA, Freischem CW et al (1984b) Suppression of pituitary and testicular function in normal men by constant gonadotropin-releasing hormone agonist infusion. *Journal of Clinical Endocrinology and Metabolism* 59: 19–28.

Soufir J-C, Jouannet P, Marson J & Soumah A (1983) Reversible inhibition of sperm production and gonadotropin secretion in men following combined oral medroxypro-gesterone acetate and percutaneous testosterone treatment. *Acta Endocrinologica* 102: 625–632.

Srinath BR, Wickings EJ, Witting C & Nieschlag E (1983) Active immunization with follicle stimulating hormone for fertility control: a 4½-year study in male rhesus monkeys. *Fertility and Sterility* 40: 110–117.

Sundaram K, Connell KG, Bardin CW, Samojlik E, Schally AV (1982) Inhibition of pituitary testicular function with D-Trp6-LHRH in rhesus monkeys. *Endocrinology* 110: 1308–1314.

Sundaram K, Thau RB, Goldstein M et al (1984) Effect of an LHRH agonist on pituitary and testicular function in rhesus monkeys. *Journal of Reproduction and Fertility* 72: 365–371.

Swerdloff RS, Handelsman DJ & Bhasin S (1985) Hormonal effects of GnRH agonist in the human male: an approach to male contraception using combined androgen and GnRH agonist treatment. *Journal of Steroid Biochemistry* 23: 855–861.

Toth M & Zarkar T (1982) Relative binding affinities of testosterone, 19-nortestosterone and their 5-alpha-reduced derivatives to the androgen receptor and other androgen-binding proteins: a suggested role of 5-alpha-reductive steroid metabolism in the dissociation of 'myotropic' and 'androgenic' activities of 19-nortestosterone. *Journal of Steroid Biochemistry* **17**: 653–660.

Vickery BH & McRae GI (1980) Effects of continuous treatment of male baboons with superagonists of luteinizing-releasing hormone. *International Journal of Fertility* **25**: 179–184.

Wang C & Yeung KK (1980) Use of low-dosage oral cyproterone acetate as a male contraceptive. *Contraception* **21**: 245–269.

Weinbauer GF, Surmann FJ, Akhtar FB et al (1984) Reversible inhibition of testicular function by a gonadotropin hormone-releasing hormone antagonist in monkeys (*Macaca fascicularis*). *Fertility and Sterility* **42**: 906–914.

Weinbauer GF, Marshall GR & Nieschlag E (1986) New injectable testosterone ester maintains serum testosterone of castrated monkeys in the normal range for four months. *Acta Endocrinologica* (in press).

Wickings EJ, Zaidi P & Nieschlag E (1981) Effects of chronic, high-dose LHRH-agonist treatment on pituitary and testicular functions in rhesus monkeys. *Journal of Andrology* **2**: 72–79.

Wickings EJ & Nieschlag E (1983) Immunological approach to male fertility control. In Diczfalusy E & Benagiano P (eds) *Comprehensive Endocrinology: Endocrine Mechanisms in Fertility Regulation*, pp 249–259. New York: Raven Press.

World Health Organization (WHO) (1972–1983) Special Programme of Research Development and Research Training in Human Reproduction, Annual Reports (1972–1983). Geneva: World Health Organization.

7

Contributions of in vitro fertilization to knowledge of the reproductive endocrinology of the menstrual cycle

D. L. HEALY
L. MORROW
M. JONES
M. BESANKO
P. A. W. ROGERS

S. OKAMATO
A. THOMAS
V. McLACHLAN
F. MARTINEZ

The birth of the first baby following in vitro fertilization (IVF) in 1978 will remain a milestone in reproductive medicine. Edwards and Steptoe aspirated a single oocyte in a spontaneous ovarian cycle for this index IVF pregnancy. Thereafter, it was thought critical that the natural ovarian cycle be used for IVF treatment: no attempt was made to employ drugs or hormones in an attempt to induce multiple follicular and oocyte development. Then Trounson and associates reported in 1981 that IVF pregnancies could result in women following the use of clomiphene citrate (CC) and human chorionic gonadotrophin (hCG) to induce multiple follicular development in endocrine-normal patients.

In our opinion, these two IVF reports have provided a great stimulus within the past decade to clinical studies of the ovarian and menstrual cycle. In particular, they have presented endocrinologists with the challenge of administering ovulation induction agents to patients who are infertile, not from chronic anovulation, but from tubal disease and who normally undergo spontaneous ovulation. Furthermore, the phenomenon of IVF stimulated the use of real-time ultrasound to examine the ovaries biophysically for the first time and to bring a new dimension to knowledge of ovarian function and structure. In this chapter, we attempt to examine the impetus which IVF has given to clinical ovarian physiology in seven sections: (1) the primate ovarian and menstrual cycles; (2) follicular phase contributions; (3) endocrine events about oocyte aspiration; (4) luteal phase contributions; (5) lessons from abandoned IVF treatment cycles; (6) contributions from artificial menstrual cycles; and (7) summary.

THE PRIMATE OVARIAN AND MENSTRUAL CYCLE

A primordial ovarian follicle in the human measures 0.05 mm in diameter

(Baker, 1963). Typically, on day 1 of the menstrual cycle, the smallest antral follicle in women is approximately 4 mm in diameter and contains one million granulosa cells. Just prior to ovulation, the human follicle is 20–25 mm in diameter and contains 50 million granulosa cells (McNatty et al, 1979). Understanding of the hormonal mechanisms controlling this remarkable 50-fold growth, which occurs within a fortnight, has come from a number of studies in non-human primates.

A definition of terms may help understanding of these mechanisms. A primordial follicle contains an oocyte surrounded by a single layer of spindle-shaped cells. A primary follicle is surrounded by one or more layers of recognizable granulosa cells, but no fluid-filled antrum is seen. A secondary follicle contains a variable volume of antral fluid which increases markedly as the Graafian follicle approaches ovulation (Ross and Van de Wiele, 1981). Follicle recruitment is a process whereby a follicle begins to mature in a milieu of sufficient gonadotrophic stimulation to permit progress towards ovulation (Hodgen, 1982). Recruited follicles correspond histologically to small antral follicles. Recruitment normally occurs during days 1–4 of the primate ovarian cycle (Figure 1). Selection is the process by which typically a single follicle is chosen. Ultimately, the selected follicle alone can avoid atresia and is competent to achieve timely ovulation. Selection normally occurs during days 5–8 of the normal ovarian cycle. Dominance is the means by which the selected or dominant follicle, or its successor, the corpus luteum, maintains its eminence bilaterally over all other follicles (Goodman et al, 1977). This process dictates the course of events in the hypothalamus, pituitary and ovaries both temporally and spatially for the duration of that menstrual cycle. Normally, dominance of the preovulatory follicle occupies days 8–12 of the primate ovarian cycle, whereas the corpus luteum reigns from about days 16 to 24. Demise of the corpus luteum in the non-fertile menstrual cycle ends the authority of this antecedent dominant structure.

A key issue to understanding the regulation of follicle growth is to learn what determines whether a follicle remains at rest, develops and ovulates or becomes atretic. Of the cohort of follicles recruited in each ovarian cycle in the higher primates, normally only one escapes atresia and achieves ovulation of an oocyte competent to produce a normal pregnancy. Folliculogenesis, then, is the integration of three processes of the follicle: rest or latency, growth culminating in ovulation, or, more often, atresia.

Taken by itself, follicular size is not a reliable guide to follicle and oocyte viability. The dominant follicle is identifiable by day 7 of the ovarian cycle on the basis of fluoresceinated hCG binding to thecal tissue (diZerega and Hodgen, 1980). At this time, several equally large antral follicles are present bilaterally in the ovaries, but none shows this unique pattern of thecal fluorescence; all but the authentic dominant follicle are destined for atresia.

Healthy follicles have other characteristics that distinguish them. Firstly, optimal numbers of granulosa cells in human follicles of 4, 8 and 20 mm diameter are 2×10^6, 5×10^6 and 50×10^6 respectively (McNatty and Baird, 1978). Secondly, viable follicles usually contain measurable follicle stimulating hormone (FSH) levels in follicular fluid (>1.3 mIU/ml; McNatty and

Sawers, 1975). Thirdly, the preovulatory follicle in women typically contains oestradiol (E_2) concentrations which reach 2–3 µg/ml, as well as comparatively low androgen values (Hillier et al, 1980). In contrast to the dominant follicle, other large antral follicles destined to be atretic contain relatively few granulosa cells, scarcely any intrafollicular FSH, lower E_2 concentrations and higher androgen and progesterone (P) levels (Vrailly et al, 1981).

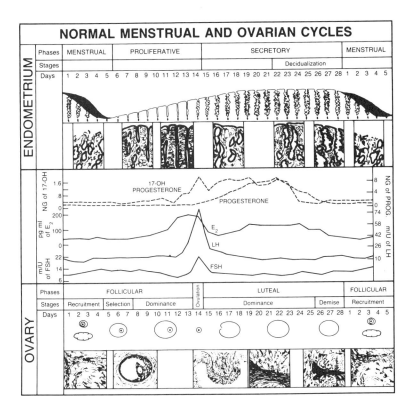

Figure 1. Schematic representation of the relationship between the menstrual cycle and endometrium with the ovarian cycle and ovary. From Healy & Hodgen (1981), with permission.

IVF has enabled access to the follicular fluid of immediately preovulatory follicles. Carson et al (1982) demonstrated that pregnancy-potent oocytes retrieved from follicles during IVF therapy came from a follicular milieu with the highest concentrations of E_2, low concentrations of androgens, but with a high androstenedione to testosterone ratio and low P concentrations. Secondary and tertiary follicles, which are still capable of yielding an oocyte at IVF egg collection, but are not pregnancy-potent, had lower concentrations of follicular E_2 and higher levels of intrafollicular P and testosterone.

FOLLICULAR PHASE CONTRIBUTIONS

Oestradiol

Following the initial report of multiple follicular development and pregnancy using CC and hCG in patients entered in an in vitro fertilization and embryo transfer (IVF–ET) programme (Trounson et al, 1981) a number of stimulation regimens were described for such subjects. These included CC alone (Wood et al, 1981; Trounson and Leeton, 1982; Fishel et al, 1984), human menopausal gonadotrophin (hMG) (Jones et al, 1982; Laufer et al, 1983), CC plus hMG (Trounson, 1983), purified FSH (Jones et al, 1984a; Bernardus et al, 1985), pulsatile luteinizing hormone releasing hormone (LHRH) (Liu et al, 1983), and LHRH agonists followed by hMG (Porter et al, 1984; Fleming et al, 1985). Monitoring of ovarian stimulation during these treatments was usually by a combination of plasma E_2 measurement and ovarian follicular ultrasound morphometry. At the present time, many IVF groups use a combination of CC and hMG for ovarian stimulation.

In the clinical management of IVF patients, we believe an important question is: What is a desirable plasma E_2 concentration for each day of an IVF treatment cycle? Previous studies reporting plasma E_2 concentrations during IVF ovarian stimulation contained results which limited their clinical usefulness. These included reports analysing cycles arising from more than one type of stimulation regimen (Jones et al, 1984b), IVF cycles that were non-conceptual as well as conceptual (Quigley et al, 1984a,b), IVF cycles which were analysed in a retrospective fashion from a reference day chosen, usually as the day of hCG administration, rather than prospectively (Lopata, 1983), and use of inappropriate parametric statistics to analyse E_2 levels without prior logarithmic transformation (Vargyas et al, 1982; Dlugi et al, 1984, 1985). Our approach has been to use the patient's previous six menstrual cycle lengths to predict the most likely day of the expected midcycle LH surge as reported by McIntosh et al (1980). Their method, developed from analysing apparently endocrine-normal women receiving artificial insemination, derived linear regression equations to predict the day of the LH surge and its 95% confidence limits. At Monash University, we have typically commenced IVF ovarian stimulation 10 days before this anticipated LH surge.

We recently analysed a consecutive series of 102 IVF conception cycles stimulated by a standard regimen of CC and hMG in order to determine the follicular phase plasma E_2 profiles in such patients and to derive clinically useful predictors of satisfactory E_2 values during IVF ovarian stimulation (Okamoto et al, 1986a).

In our IVF programme, CC, 100 mg/day for 5 days, was begun 10 days before the calculated midpoint of the cycle. hMG, 150 IU/day, was started 1 day later and continued until the plasma E_2 was 500–1000 pg/ml and steadily rising. The duration and daily dosage of hMG treatment was often adjusted between 0 and 150 IU/day depending on the patient's individual response as judged by E_2 and ovarian ultrasound determinations. Endocrine results were reviewed at a clinical IVF meeting each afternoon where the next day's stimulation was decided. The timing of the blood sampling, hCG injection, oocyte collection technique and other IVF–ET methods were described previously (Downing, 1984; McBain and Trounson, 1984). In brief, when 0800 h plasma E_2 concentrations were approximately 1000 pg/ml, patients were admitted to hospital and blood taken at 0800, 1400 and 2100 h for plasma E_2, LH and P determinations. Treatment continued until plasma E_2 concentrations reached approximately 500 pg/ml per 18 mm follicle and provided plasma P concentrations remained below 2 ng/ml. If a surge in plasma LH had not occurred, within 36 h of the predicted day of the LH surge, 5000 IU of hCG was administered and the operating theatre booked 28–36 h later for oocyte aspiration.

Figure 2 displays plasma E_2 concentrations from 102 consecutive IVF conception cycles after standard CC–hMG stimulation. The percentile envelopes thus generated demonstrate the range of E_2 values associated with an IVF pregnancy. Nineteen patients who conceived had at least one plasma E_2 below the 5th percentile, whereas 15 individuals had at least one

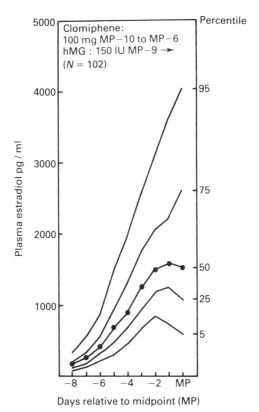

Figure 2. Plasma E_2 concentrations in 102 consecutive IVF conception cycles using 100 mg CC for 5 days beginning 10 days before the calculated midpoint of the cycle and 150 IU hMG, commencing the day following CC. Percentiles are given on the right of the figure. The dotted line indicates median E_2 concentrations on each day.

plasma E_2 above the 95th percentile. Seven subjects had two E_2 values and five subjects had three E_2 values on consecutive days below the 5th percentile. Eight patients had two consecutive daily E_2 values above the 95th percentile whereas six individuals had three consecutive E_2 concentrations above this level.

In an important contribution, Jones et al (1982) classified the serum E_2 concentrations in 175 IVF cycles (33 pregnancies) stimulated by hMG treatment, on the basis of the shape of the E_2 response around the time of discontinuing hMG injections. Pregnancy rates varied from 27% for the most 'favourable' A pattern to zero per cent for D- or E-shaped E_2 response patterns. To our knowledge, this was the first report to suggest a method which enabled the clinician to cancel IVF treatment cycles which were unlikely to result in pregnancy. More recently, however, Diamond et al (1985) analysed 151 IVF–hMG cycles using these criteria, but found no significant differences in fertilization, cleavage or pregnancy rates between these types of E_2 response patterns. Only seven pregnancies occurred in their study. In our series of 102 consecutive IVF pregnancies, conception often occurred despite 'unfavourable' E_2 response patterns (Table 1). Cancellation of all cycles showing these types of E_2 response patterns would have lost almost one-third of our IVF pregnancies. Although we used CC–hMG rather than hMG alone, it indicates that the precise shape of the plasma E_2 response pattern is not clinically useful as a predictor of the likelihood of an IVF pregnancy.

Table 1. Distribution of the shape of the plasma E_2 profiles in 102 IVF conception cycles following a standard regimen of CC and hMG.

Plasma E_2 pattern*	Percentage of conception cycles
A + G	70.6
B + C	13.7
D + E	15.7

* Patterns as described in Jones et al (1982): A and G patterns showed increasing E_2 values until hCG injection; B and C patterns showed increasing E_2 values during hMG injection but not later; D and E patterns showed decreasing E_2 values while hMG was being administered.

It is inevitable that derivation of a normal plasma E_2 range is retrospective in that the knowledge that a particular IVF treatment cycle resulted in pregnancy is known. Such information is, of course, not known to the clinician managing a patient during an IVF superovulation treatment cycle, who is faced with an individual who is not yet pregnant. We suggest that the 5–95 percentile envelope best describes the desirable plasma E_2 concentrations during IVF superovulation. Five and six patients respectively had plasma E_2 concentrations below the 5th percentile and above the 95th percentile of this range for at least three consecutive days. Although in one sense it is arbitrary in choosing between a 5–95 and 0–100 percentile envelope for a treatment range, accepting a non-parametric tolerance interval (γ) of 0.90 allows the probability of including 96% of observations between the sample extremes (Dixon and Massey, 1983). Moreover, over 1000 IVF conception treatment cycles would have to be analysed to be statistically confident of satisfactorily describing a 1–99 percentile plasma E_2 range.

A clinical plasma E_2 range for IVF therapy has a number of advantages. Firstly, it allows both the clinician as well as the IVF patient to determine objectively whether the plasma E_2 response is proceeding satisfactorily. Secondly, it provides an objective definition of an adequate plasma E_2 concentration on each day of IVF treatment rather than an arbitrary definition of a 'low responder' close to the day of anticipated oocyte retrieval (Garcia et al, 1983; Mantzavinos et al, 1983). Low (< 5th percentile) E_2 values on one or two consecutive days allow the clinician to increase the amount of gonadotrophin injected in order to reach satisfactory folliculogenesis. Thirdly, our E_2 range allows the clinician to cancel an IVF treatment cycle at an early stage rather than after several days of expensive but disappointing treatment. Fourthly, this clinical E_2 range defines IVF hyperstimulation as plasma E_2 concentrations higher than the 95th percentile on each day of our routine CC–hMG regimen (Figure 2).

In conclusion, we believe that such an analysis of plasma E_2 concentrations following a single regimen of ovarian stimulation in a large number of IVF conception cycles is clinically useful. The envelope describing the 5–95 percentiles of plasma E_2 values seems a valid marker of satisfactory folliculogenesis.

Inhibin

It has long been postulated that the gonads produce a non-steroidal factor (inhibin) which is secreted in response to FSH stimulation and inhibits pituitary FSH secretion (McCullagh, 1932; Baker et al, 1976). Recently, inhibin from bovine (Robertson et al, 1985; Forage et al, 1986) and porcine (Ling et al, 1985; Mason et al, 1985; Miyamoto et al, 1985; Rivier et al, 1985) follicular fluid has been purified, cloned and sequenced. In cattle, inhibin exists as a glycoprotein of molecular mass 58 kDa (consisting of subunits of 43 kDa and 15 kDa) and is processed to a 31 kDa form (consisting of 20 kDa and 15 kDa subunits) which is also bioactive (Robertson et al, 1986). A similar subunit structure for 32 kDa porcine follicular fluid inhibin has been shown.

To date, it has been difficult to define the physiological role of inhibin in the regulation of the human pituitary–ovarian axis because no suitably specific and sensitive assay system has been available. Recently, plasma inhibin concentrations have been measured in women during IVF ovarian hyperstimulation using a radioimmunoassay.

In brief, this assay utilized an antiserum raised to purified 58 kDa inhibin which has been shown to neutralize the inhibin bioactivity in bovine and human follicular fluid and that of purified 31 kDa and 58 kDa inhibin in an in vitro bioassay (Scott et al, 1980). This antiserum bound iodinated 31 kDa bovine inhibin and was used in the establishment of a discontinuous, second antibody radioimmunoassay (RIA) system. Serial dilution of human plasma yielded parallel dose–response lines to a purified 31 kDa inhibin standard of defined bioactivity which was used as an interim standard as the appropriate standard for human inhibin has not been established (McLachlan et al, 1986a). The subunits of inhibin obtained following reduction and alkylation of the native hormone showed <0.5% cross-reaction in the RIA. Assay sensitivity was 0.5 U/ml (1.3 ng/ml) and the interassay coefficient of variation was 9.3%.

Plasma was obtained from 26 unselected women undergoing ovulation induction in the Monash University IVF programme. Briefly, CC 100–150 mg daily and hMG 75–225 IU daily were administered between days 4 and 12 of a treatment menstrual cycle as previously described. Follicular number and development were assessed by the progressive increase in plasma oestradiol and by ovarian ultrasound (Aloka LS SSD 270 electronic sector scanner, 3.5 mHz transducer, sensitivity 8 mm, Tokyo). Human chorionic gonadotrophin 5000 IU was administered in 15 cases to induce ovulation in the absence of an endogenous LH surge. The latter was seen in eight subjects whilst treatment was discontinued in three subjects because of poor follicular development. Plasma from two normal women during spontaneous menstrual cycles was obtained from early in the follicular phase until the time of ovulation. Plasma E_2, LH and FSH were measured by RIA.

During gonadotrophin administration, plasma inhibin rose progressively and in parallel with plasma E_2 (McLachlan et al, 1986b; Figure 3). Peak

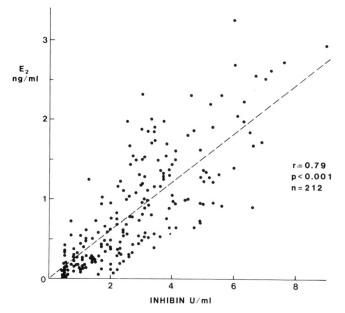

Figure 3. The relationship between plasma inhibin and E_2 levels during gonadotrophin administration to induce superovulation for IVF. From McLachlan et al (1986b), with permission.

inhibin concentrations were significantly correlated with the number of follicles detected on ultrasound (Figure 4). The number of oocytes recovered at laparoscopy also significantly correlated with both the peak plasma inhibin ($r = 0.45$, $P < 0.05$, $N = 21$) and peak plasma E_2 concentrations ($r = 0.48$, $P < 0.05$, $N = 21$). Data are shown for individual patients representative of the groups in whom hCG was administered (Figure 5A) and in whom a spontaneous LH surge occurred (Figure 5B). In four cases (Figure 5C), a dissociation between plasma inhibin and E_2 profiles was observed with inhibin reaching a plateau or falling whilst plasma E_2 either reached a peak 1–2 days later or continued to increase. In the two normal women having spontaneous menstrual cycles, inhibin immunoactivity was below the limit of assay detection (< 0.5 U/ml) prior to day 13 then rising to concentrations up to 1.8 U/ml in the periovulatory period.

The stimulation of inhibin by exogenous gonadotrophins during ovarian hyperstimulation supports the trophic role of FSH in ovarian inhibin production. This evidence confirms in women the extensive animal data both in vivo and in vitro that inhibin is a follicular product under FSH control with granulosa cells being the likely site of production (Erickson and Hsueh, 1978; Lee et al, 1982).

The close correspondence between plasma inhibin and E_2 concentrations supports the broad concept they are both monitoring follicular growth. This view is supported by the significant correlation of peak plasma inhibin concentrations with both the number of follicles on ultrasound and the

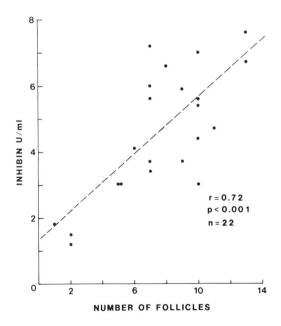

Figure 4. The relationship between peak inhibin levels and numbers of follicles detected ultrasonically prior to oocyte aspiration for IVF. From McLachlan et al (1986b), with permission.

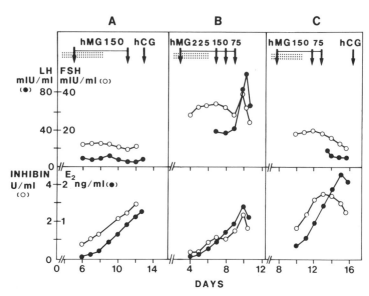

Figure 5. Circulating levels of inhibin, E_2, FSH and LH in three women undergoing ovarian hyperstimulation. A: Pattern typical of a cycle in which hCG was administered to induce ovulation. B: Pattern typical of a cycle with a spontaneous LH surge. Note the rise and fall in inhibin and E_2 levels. C: Example of dissociation between plasma inhibin and E_2 levels. Note the fall in inhibin whilst E_2 continues to rise. Treatment consisted of CC 100 mg daily (shaded area) and hMG at the dose specified, with arrows indicating the day of dosage alteration. From McLachlan et al (1986b), with permission.

number of oocytes recovered at laparoscopy. Plasma E_2, although an established parameter of follicular development, is predominantly a theca cell product in the human (McNatty et al, 1979). However in vitro studies (Erickson and Hsueh, 1978) have demonstrated that inhibin is a granulosa cell product and thus the levels measured in human plasma represent a circulating protein marker of granulosa cell function. Inhibin levels are observed to fall after the midcycle LH and E_2 surge, at which time luteinization of the follicle begins. This is again consistent with the experimental observations in the rat where hCG administration leads to a fall in circulating inhibin concentrations (Lee, 1983).

The four subjects who demonstrated dissociation between plasma inhibin and E_2 profiles late in the induction process are of particular interest as these data suggest a differential regulation of these two parameters of follicular growth. Inhibin could be considered a more direct index of follicular development and its assessment may become of therapeutic importance in the procedure and timing of ovulation induction and oocyte collection for IVF. For instance, the plateau and decline of inhibin prior to E_2 may suggest that the follicle has reached maturity prior to the oestradiol peak.

In view of the confounding effect of hMG therapy upon the measurement of plasma FSH, no correlation of plasma inhibin and FSH is as yet apparent. The measurement of inhibin in spontaneous cycles has shown detectable levels only in the periovulatory period. A more thorough examination of the relationship between plasma inhibin and FSH throughout the IVF cycles will assess the predictive value of plasma inhibin as an index of follicular function and oocyte health.

Luteinizing hormone

It has recently been suggested that the follicular phase concentrations of LH can predict fertilization rates and the likelihood of pregnancy in patients on IVF therapy. Stanger and Yovich (1985) reported that the fertilization rate of mature oocytes was reduced in patients whose basal serum LH was greater than 1 standard deviation above the mean LH concentration a few days before egg collection. Howles et al (1986) used urinary LH levels in monitoring IVF patients and also suggested that those who are destined not to become pregnant had significantly higher LH levels on the two days prior to egg collection. The methodological difficulties with these contributions include the uncertainty of the correlation between urinary LH and bioactive serum LH affecting the ovary, the use of correct statistical methods for data interpretation and the absence of a normal range against which to compare IVF LH levels. A final difficulty is the fact that 10–15% of seemingly mature oocytes with a dispersed oocyte–cumulus complex have chromosomal abnormalities (Plachot et al, 1986).

Despite these caveats, the predictive value of serum LH may be clinically significant and of importance, not only in IVF treatment, but also in basic and clinical knowledge of the reproductive endocrinology of the menstrual cycle. Serum LH concentrations could be used diagnostically in the management of patients with chronic anovulation receiving ovarian stimulants, or in IVF patients undergoing superovulation. Furthermore, the availability of purified FSH may allow FSH to be injected without concomitant LH, so reducing circulating LH concentrations and leading to improved oocyte health.

Data from the Monash University IVF Programme show that LH concentrations in a series of 97 consecutive cycles induced with CC 100 mg/day and hMG 150 IU/day show a significant fall two and three days before the calculated midpoint of these IVF cycles. Serum LH concentrations from a series of 75 spontaneous cycles do not show this fall in circulating LH levels in the late follicular phase. Further work is needed to show if this changed pattern of LH concentrations during IVF treatment predicts pregnancy (Okamoto et al, 1986b).

Oocyte number

The use of ovarian stimulants to induce codominant folliculogenesis has enabled the reproductive endocrinologist to produce more than one fertilizable oocyte per cycle in endocrine-normal women. The availability of embryo freezing/cryobiology facilities, and the imminent availability of oocyte freezing techniques will provide methods to freeze excess oocytes or embryos if a large number (say 20–30) of fertilizable oocytes could be obtained in a single IVF treatment.

To address the question of whether the induction of a large number of fertilizable oocytes is indeed an advantage to an individual patient, and whether such treatment will improve the chances of pregnancy, we have retrospectively analysed our data over 662 consecutive IVF treatment cycles (Howlett et al, 1986). Forty-five of 662 IVF patients had more than seven oocytes recovered at laparoscopy. The pregnancy rate per laparoscopy and embryo transfer of these patients was twice that of the control group (pregnancy rate per laparoscopy = 31% versus 15%, $P<0.01$; pregnancy rate per embryo transfer = 34% versus 18%, $P<0.02$). This increased pregnancy rate occurred despite there being no difference between the mean number of embryos transferred in either patient group. The median number of embryos transferred in each group was three and this produced a similar incidence of multiple pregnancy, although there was a trend towards fewer abortions in those patients who had seven oocytes or more recovered at laparoscopy. Not surprisingly, the plasma E_2 concentrations were significantly higher in the follicular phase of patients yielding more than seven oocytes than in the control group of IVF patients.

These results confirm the clinical benefit of using ovarian stimulants in order to obtain a large number of fertilizable oocytes, either at IVF or gamete intrafallopian transfer (Asch, 1986). Such results also suggest that gonadotrophin ovulation induction in patients with idiopathic infertility may improve in vivo conception and pregnancy rate by the release of more than one fertilizable oocyte. However, clinical trials of such methods for patients with long-standing idiopathic infertility have not been reported.

ENDOCRINE EVENTS ABOUT OOCYTE ASPIRATION

Progesterone (P)

During the normal menstrual cycle in primates, an increase in P production can be detected in venous blood from the ovary bearing the dominant follicle as early as 48 h before spontaneous ovulation (diZerega et al, 1980). Twelve to 24 h before spontaneous ovulation in humans, a small but significant rise in P can be detected in peripheral plasma (Moghissi et al, 1972). The rise in P has been shown to begin within a few hours of the spontaneous LH surge (Hoff et al, 1983). After ovulation, P levels rise sharply and adequate P secretion is required, not only to convert the endometrium from proliferative to secretory, but also to suppress endogenous gonadotrophin release and to regulate new follicular growth just before the next menstrual cycle (diZerega et al, 1981; Fritz and Speroff, 1982).

During cycles stimulated with CC–hMG, high levels of P occur and these show marked diurnal fluctuations around the time of the LH surge (Trounson and Calabrese, 1984). Coincident with the plasma LH surge, P levels show a sharp and sustained rise parallel to the increase in LH concentrations.

When follicles are aspirated at IVF procedures, up to 20% of the total population of granulosa cells are removed (Kreitmann and Hodgen, 1981). The most severe disruption of P production in the subsequent luteal phase of the IVF cycle is likely to occur in natural ovulatory cycles with a single follicle. The use of ovarian stimulants to induce multiple follicular maturation in IVF therapy ameliorates the threat of luteal deficiency through the collective secretion of more than one corpus luteum. In IVF cycles stimulated with CC–hMG, there is little evidence of shortening of the luteal phase despite multiple follicular aspiration (Kerin et al, 1984).

Taylor et al (1986) have studied the nature of the acute changes that occur in serum P values immediately before, during and after laparoscopic oocyte retrieval. Circulating P levels fell to 20% of their initial concentration within 2 h of the induction of anaesthesia for IVF oocyte collection. The decrease in P levels was not related to the number of follicles aspirated. The mean circulating P values showed an increase above this nadir within 4 h of the induction of anaesthesia, and by 24 h P levels were increasing above pre-anaesthetic concentrations.

It was of interest in this study that the four patients who became pregnant were those with the highest circulating P concentrations just before anaesthesia and during the 2 h sampling period after initiation of anaesthesia. With one exception in this group of 20 subjects, all patients who failed to conceive were below the range of P levels recorded for the pregnant patients. Further studies are needed to establish whether preovulatory P concentrations do indeed have value predictive of oocyte fertilization and pregnancy, both for IVF therapy as well as for the natural ovarian/menstrual cycle.

Prolactin

The induction of anaesthesia is known to elevate serum prolactin concentrations significantly (Healy and Burger, 1977). In a small study, patients were randomly allocated to placebo or 2.5 mg of bromocriptine 12 and 2 h before the induction of anaesthesia for oocyte collection (Taylor et al, 1986). Such treatment prevented the marked elevation in prolactin during oocyte recovery and also appeared to inhibit P secretion, but neither P levels nor pregnancy were related to prolactin concentrations. These negative results are of significance since higher follicular fluid prolactin concentrations have been suggested as a marker of oocyte fertilizing capacity and pregnancy potential (Laufer et al, 1984).

LUTEAL PHASE CONTRIBUTIONS

In contrast to the follicular phase and midcycle, study of the luteal phase resulting from IVF treatment has provided little new insight into the reproductive endocrinology of the ovarian/menstrual cycle. Several publications have appeared reporting E_2 and P concentrations after oocyte collection and the concentrations of E_2, P and the E_2/P ratio have all been suggested as predictive of IVF pregnancy (Gidley-Baird et al, 1986). Most of these studies have involved relatively small numbers of patients receiving different stimulation regimens and often receiving hCG or exogenous progesterone supplements. Moreover, the presence of multiple corpora lutea after IVF oocyte collection makes it impossible to assess the secretory function of a single corpus luteum at that time. Several large studies have indicated that ovulation induction using hMG alone is associated with a short luteal phase (Jones et al, 1984b), but that the length of the luteal phase is normal in patients receiving CC–hMG treatment (Kerin et al, 1984).

The appearance of hCG in peripheral plasma in IVF conception cycles is often delayed compared with either spontaneous cycles or pregnancy induced with gonadotrophic hormones alone (Englert et al, 1984). An international collaborative study of the detection of hCG in pregnancies achieved by IVF showed that after hCG was detected in peripheral plasma, hCG concentrations rose exponentially with a doubling time of approximately 1.3 days, consistent with spontaneous conception (Lenton et al, 1982; Confino et al, 1986). This international study analysed 300 IVF pregnancies obtained by 15 IVF centres. In comparison to the β hCG curve for ongoing singleton pregnancies, hCG concentrations in pregnancies destined for spontaneous abortion or for ectopic pregnancies showed statistically lower hCG concentrations. In this study, 37% of all IVF pregnancies resulted in pregnancy wastage.

At Monash University, we have analysed 110 consecutive IVF pregnancies and reviewed the value of a single plasma hCG concentration 14 days after oocyte collection (Okamoto et al, 1986c). This large study from a single institution confirms the finding of lower hCG concentrations in ectopic pregnancy and indicates that, in our hands, hCG concentrations below the 25th percentile for ongoing singleton IVF pregnancies represents a high predictive value (27%) for ectopic pregnancies. Such data are not available for the prediction of ectopic pregnancy in spontaneous conceptions or following artificial insemination and it is possible that IVF results here may make a further contribution to clinical reproductive medicine.

LESSONS FROM ABANDONED IVF TREATMENT CYCLES

Somewhere between 10 and 30% of patients who commence IVF superovulation treatment are discharged before an attempt at oocyte collection is made (Jones, 1985). Reasons for abandoning IVF treatment will vary from one IVF centre to the other and include not only biological factors, such as low plasma E_2 concentrations, but also organizational factors such as the presence of a spontaneous LH rise in patients attending clinics where out of hours oocyte collection is not possible. Table 2 shows in a consecutive series of 75 IVF cycles which were regarded as unsatisfactory, that inadequate E_2 concentrations was the reason for discharging the patients from treatment in two-thirds of cases.

There are three clinical choices when faced with a patient with unsatisfactory stimulation. The couple can be discharged from further attempts at IVF treatment. Option two is to have the superovulation regimen repeated in a few months' time in the hope of some spontaneous improvement. Option three is to assess a spontaneous menstrual cycle and to endeavour to

Table 2. Classification of abandoned IVF cycles ($N = 75$).

Serum E_2 < 5th percentile	48
Decreasing serum E_2 despite hMG	6
Serum P > 2 ng/ml	8
Serum LH > 35 U/l	7
Organization and other reasons	6

devise more appropriate stimulation in the next IVF attempt. In our hands, mere repetition of the same superovulation regimen results in satisfactory folliculogenesis in only approximately 10% of patients. As it is not clear why all women with regular spontaneous menstrual cycles do not respond to IVF superovulation treatment, we have investigated 41 consecutive patients in this category at least 3 months after their IVF attempt. A weekly blood sample was taken from day 1 of a spontaneous menstrual cycle and assayed for FSH, LH, prolactin, E_2 and P concentrations and compared with normal ranges for regular spontaneous menstrual cycles. Twenty-two of these 41 cycles showed abnormal endocrine profiles.

Premature follicle selection was apparent in six of these 22 abnormal cycles. In these patients, although progesterone concentrations were apparently satisfactory in the midluteal phase, progesterone levels were also markedly elevated as early as day 15 of the spontaneous cycle. This suggests that ovulation in these patients occurred as early as day 10 or 11 and that follicle selection probably also occurred several days before the usual time of days 5–8. If this hypothesis is true, commencement of ovarian stimulants at an earlier time should rescue at least some follicles from atresia and prevent repetition of the IVF failure. In our experience, commencement of super-ovulation treatment on day 1 of the menstrual cycle in patients with apparent premature follicle selection has been satisfactory in the induction of multiple codominant follicles in the second IVF treatment cycle.

Occult ovarian failure has been noticed in five of the 22 patients with abnormal endocrine profiles in our studies. In this condition, analysis of the spontaneous menstrual cycle demonstrates that, although progesterone levels in the luteal phase are in a satisfactory range, plasma FSH and LH concentrations in the follicular phase of this spontaneous cycle are markedly elevated into the menopausal range. We believe this condition represents an early stage of the premature ovarian failure syndrome (Board et al, 1979). In our experience alteration in the day of onset of IVF treatment has not benefited these patients.

We have treated 19 patients with previous failed IVP therapy with the LHRH agonist buserelin, 600 μg per day intranasally (6 × 100 μg) in an attempt to suppress endogenous gonadotrophin secretion and to enable simpler gonadotrophin control of the folliculogenic process in the next IVF cycle (Fleming et al, 1985). Buserelin was commenced in either the mid-luteal or early follicular phases following reports in non-human primates that luteal phase commencement more rapidly induced a hypogonado-trophic state (Fraser and Sandow, 1985). Commencement of buserelin treatment on day 21 of the menstrual cycle required only 8 days until E_2

concentrations remained below 50 pg/ml for at least three consecutive days whilst, in contrast, commencement of buserelin treatment on day 1 of menses required 18 days of treatment before a hypo-oestrogenic state was induced. In three patients with occult ovarian failure studied in this way, no folliculogenesis occurred with combined buserelin–hMG treatment up to a daily dose of 825 IU per day. By contrast, buserelin–hMG treatment in other types of failed superovulation yielded a total of 114 oocytes in 16 patients. This resulted in a median yield of seven oocytes per patient, ranging from two to 13 oocytes. One hundred and six of these oocytes appeared to have a mature oocyte–cumulus complex and 89 were fertilized (85%), allowing 13 patients to have embryo transfer of three embryos. Three pregnancies resulted.

This early study suggests that, in appropriately selected IVF patients, use of an LHRH agonist to induce hypogonadotrophism is of benefit in a subsequent IVF attempt. The most simple hypothesis for this improvement is the removal of endogenous gonadotrophins from competing with administered gonadotrophins upon the ovaries. It is not yet clear whether use of an LHRH agonist in typical IVF patients will also lead to codominant folliculogenesis and yield a larger number of oocytes than would be produced with conventional IVF treatment.

CONTRIBUTIONS FROM ARTIFICIAL MENSTRUAL CYCLES

Lutjen et al (1984) have reported a steroid replacement regimen for women with premature ovarian failure or ovarian agenesis which achieves plasma concentrations and profiles of E_2 and P within the normal range of the menstrual cycle. This regimen induces development of a normal secretory phase endometrium. With this regimen, plasma concentrations of LH were within the normal range by the end of the first cycle of treatment with endogenous steroids. However, plasma FSH remained above the normal range, even during the third treatment cycle (Lutjen et al, 1986). These data are consistent with the necessity of a gonadal feedback factor such as inhibin for maintaining FSH concentrations in the normal range. A radioimmunoassay for inhibin in human plasma has been applied to such patients and no measurable inhibin was identified. Although the majority of these patients had a surge of LH at midcycle, only three of eight individuals had concomitant FSH surges, supporting a role for progesterone in facilitating the midcycle FSH rise.

SUMMARY

The administration of ovarian stimulants to endocrine-normal women in IVF programmes gives the clinical endocrinologist an opportunity to modify natural folliculogenesis. Use of antioestrogens and/or gonadotrophins at the correct time has demonstrated that follicular atresia can be prevented and that multiple pregnancy-potent haploid ova can be obtained.

Scrutiny of spontaneous menstrual cycles in patients who show unsatisfactory IVF responses has identified two new syndromes, premature follicle selection and occult ovarian failure, in these patients. The incidence of these disorders in fertile women is still unclear. Early results suggest that endocrine manipulations may overcome premature follicle selection and induce codominant folliculogenesis.

Inhibin is a recently characterized ovarian protein which is increased in peripheral blood during IVF treatment. Results from IVF cycles suggest that plasma inhibin may be a new index of follicular function. Other potential indices of ovarian function, such as the luteal protein relaxin, may also develop from the application of basic research to IVF and advance knowledge of the human ovarian and menstrual cycles.

REFERENCES

Asch RH, Balmaceda JP, Ellsworth LR & Wong PG (1986) Preliminary experiences with gamete intra-Fallopian transfer (GIFT). *Fertility and Sterility* **45**: 366–372.

Baker TG (1963) A quantitative and cytological study of germ cells in human ovaries. *Proceedings of the Royal Society of London* **158**: 417–433.

Baker HWG, Bremner WH, Burger HG et al (1976) Testicular control of follicle-stimulating hormone secretion. *Recent Progress in Hormone Research* **32**: 429–476.

Bernardus RE, Jones GS, Acosta AA et al (1985) The significance of the ratio in follicle-stimulating hormone and luteinizing hormone induction of multiple follicular growth. *Fertility and Sterility* **43**: 373–379.

Board JA, Redwine FO, Moncure CW, Frable WJ & Taylor JR (1979) Identification of differing etiologies of clinically diagnosed premature menopause. *American Journal of Obstetrics and Gynecology* **134**: 936–943.

Carson RS, Trounson AO & Findlay JK (1982) Successful fertilization of human oocytes in vitro: concentrations of oestradiol 17β, progesterone and androstenedione in antral fluid of donor follicles. *Journal of Clinical Endocrinology and Metabolism* **55**: 798–800.

Confino E, Demir RH, Friberg J & Gleicher M (1986) The predictive value of HCG beta subunit levels in pregnancies achieved by in vitro fertilization and embryo transfer: an international collaborative study. *Fertility and Sterility* **45**: 526–531.

Diamond MP, Webster BW, Garner HC et al (1985) Selection of superior stimulation protocols for follicular development in a program for in vitro fertilization. *Fertility and Sterility* **43**: 251–255.

Dixon WJ & Massey FJ Jr (1983) *Introduction to Statistical Analysis*, p 401. New York: McGraw-Hill.

diZerega GS & Hodgen GD (1980) Fluorescence localization of luteinizing hormone-human chorionic gonadotropin uptake in the primate ovary. II. Changing distribution during selection of the dominant follicle. *Journal of Clinical Endocrinology and Metabolism* **51**: 903–907.

diZerega GS, Marut EL, Turner CK & Hodgen GD (1980) Asymmetrical ovarian function during recruitment and selection of the dominant follicle in the menstrual cycle of the Rhesus monkey. *Journal of Clinical Endocrinology and Metabolism* **51**: 698–703.

diZerega GS, Lynch A & Hodgen GD (1981) The initiation of asymmetrical ovarian oestradiol secretion in the primate ovary after luteectomy. *Endocrinology* **108**: 1233–1239.

Dlugi AM, Laufer N, DeCherny AH et al (1984) The periovulatory and luteal phase of conception cycles following in vitro fertilization and embryo transfer. *Fertility and Sterility* **41**: 530–537.

Dlugi AM, Laufer N, Botero-Ruiz W et al (1985) Altered follicular development in clomiphene citrate versus human menopausal fertilization. *Fertility and Sterility* **43**: 40–46.

Downing B (1984) Oocyte pick-up. In Wood C & Trounson A (eds) *Clinical In Vitro Fertilization*, p 67. New York: Springer-Verlag.

Englert Y, Roger M, Belaisch-Allart J et al (1984) Delayed appearance of plasmatic chorionic gonadotropin in pregnancies after in vitro fertilization and embryo transfer. *Fertility and Sterility* **42:** 835–840.

Erickson GF & Hsueh AJW (1978) Secretion of 'inhibin' by rat granulosa cells in vitro. *Endocrinology* **103:** 1960–1963.

Fishel SB, Edward RG & Purdy JM (1984) Analysis of infertile patients treated consecutively by in vitro fertilization at Bourn Hall. *Fertility and Sterility* **42:** 191–193.

Fleming R, Haxton MJ, Hamilton MPR et al (1985) Successful treatment of infertile women with oligomenorrhoea using a combination of an LHRH agonist and exogenous gonadotropins. *British Journal of Obstetrics and Gynaecology* **92:** 369–372.

Forage RG, Ring JM, Brown RW et al (1986) Cloning and sequence analysis of cDNA species coding for the two subunits of inhibin from bovine follicular fluid. *Proceedings of the National Academy of Sciences (USA)* **83:** 3091–3095.

Fraser HM & Sandow J (1985) Suppression of follicular maturation by infusion of a luteinizing hormone-releasing hormone agonist started during the late luteal phase in the stumptailed macaque monkey. *Journal of Clinical Endocrinology and Metabolism* **60:** 579–584.

Fritz MA & Speroff L (1982) The endocrinology of the menstrual cycle: the interaction of folliculogenesis and neuroendocrine mechanisms. *Fertility and Sterility* **38:** 509–513.

Garcia JE, Jones GS, Acosta AA & Wright G Jr (1983) Human menopausal gonadotropin/ human chorionic gonadotropin follicular maturation for oocyte aspiration: phase I, 1981. *Fertility and Sterility* **39:** 167–171.

Gidley-Baird AA, O'Neill C, Sinosich MJ et al (1986) Failure of implantation in human in vitro fertilization and embryo transfer patients: the effects of altered progesterone/estrogen ratios in humans and mice. *Fertility and Sterility* **45:** 69–74.

Goodman AL, Nixon WE, Johnson DK & Hodgen GD (1977) Regulation of folliculogenesis in the cycling Rhesus monkey: selection of the dominant follicle. *Endocrinology* **100:** 155–161.

Healy DL & Burger HG (1977) Human prolactin. *Australian and New Zealand Journal of Obstetrics and Gynaecology* **17:** 61–78.

Healy DL & Hodgen GD (1981) *Obstetrical and Gynecological Survey* **34:** 341.

Hillier SG, van den Voogaard ANJ, Reichert LE & van Hall EV (1980) Intraovarian sex steroid hormone interaction and the regulation of follicular maturation: aromatization of androgens by human granulosa cells in vitro. *Journal of Clinical Endocrinology and Metabolism* **50:** 640–647.

Hodgen GD (1982) The dominant ovarian follicle. *Fertility and Sterility* **38:** 281–300.

Hoff JD, Quigley ME & Yen SSC (1983) Hormonal dynamics at midcycle: a re-evaluation. *Journal of Clinical Endocrinology and Metabolism* **57:** 792–796.

Howlett DT, Okamoto S, Trounson AO & Healy DL (1986) Retrieving seven or more oocytes double IVF pregnancy rates. Submitted for publication.

Howles CM, McNamee MC, Edwards RG & Pickering JD (1986) Early embryo mortality and failure of implantation during IVF: endocrine correlates. *European Society of Human Reproduction and Embryology, Second Meeting*, Brussels, Belgium, June 22–25. Abstract 66.

Jones GS (1985) Use of purified gonadotrophins for ovarian stimulation in IVF. In Wood C & Trounson A (eds) *New Clinical Issues in In Vitro Fertilization*, pp 775–784. London: Saunders.

Jones HW Jr, Jones GS, Andrews MC et al (1982) The program for in vitro fertilization at Norfolk. *Fertility and Sterility* **38:** 14–21.

Jones GS, Garcia JE & Rosenwaks Z (1984a) The role of pituitary gonadotropins in follicular stimulation and oocyte maturation in the human. *Journal of Clinical Endocrinology and Metabolism* **59:** 178–180.

Jones HW Jr, McDowell JS, Acosta AA et al (1984b) Three years of in vitro fertilization at Norfolk. *Fertility and Sterility* **42:** 826–833.

Kerin JFT, Warnes GM, Quinn P et al (1984) The effect of clomid-induced superovulation on human follicular and luteal function for extracorporeal fertilization and embryo transfer. *Clinical Reproduction and Fertility* **2:** 129–135.

Kreitmann O & Hodgen GD (1981) Induced corpus luteum dysfunction after aspiration of the preovulatory follicle in monkeys. *Fertility and Sterility* **35:** 671–675.

Laufer N, DeCherney AH, Haseltine FP et al (1983) The use of high-dose human menopausal gonadotropin in an in vitro fertilization program. *Fertility and Sterility* **40**: 734–737.

Laufer N, Botero-Ruiz W, deCherney AH et al (1984) Gonadotropin and prolactin levels in follicular fluid of human ova successfully fertilized in vitro. *Journal of Clinical Endocrinology and Metabolism* **58**: 430–437.

Lee VW (1983) PMSG treated immature female rat. A model system for studying control of inhibin secretion. In Greenwald GS & Terranova PF (eds) *Factors Regulating Ovarian Function.* New York: Raven Press.

Lee VW, McMaster J, Quigg H & Leversha L (1982) Ovarian and circulating inhibin levels in immature female rats treated with gonadotropin and after castration. *Endocrinology* **111**: 1849–1854.

Lenton BA, Neal, LM & Sulaiman R (1982) Plasma concentrations of human chorionic gonadotropin from the time of implantation until the second week of pregnancy. *Fertility and Sterility* **37**: 773–780.

Ling N, Ying S-Y, Ueno N et al (1985) Isolation and partial characterization of a M_r 32000 protein with inhibin activity from porcine follicular fluid. *Proceedings of the National Academy of Sciences (USA)* **82**: 7217–7221.

Liu JH, Durfee RD, Muse K & Yen SSC (1983) Induction of multiple ovulation by pulsatile administration of gonadotropin-releasing hormone. *Fertility and Sterility* **40**: 18–23.

Lopata A (1983) Concepts in human in vitro fertilization and embryo transfer. *Fertility and Sterility* **40**: 289–293.

Lutjen P, Trounson A, Leeton J et al (1984) The establishment and maintenance of pregnancy using in vitro fertilization and embryo donation in a patient with primary ovarian failure. *Nature* **307**: 174–176.

Lutjen PJ, Findlay JK, Trounson AO, Leeton JF & Chan LK (1986) The effect on plasma gonadotropin of cyclic steroid replacement in women with premature ovarian failure. *Journal of Clinical Endocrinology and Metabolism* **62**: 419–424.

Mantzavinos T, Garcia JE & Jones HW (1983) Ultrasound measurement of ovarian follicular stimulated by human gonadotropins for oocyte recovery and in vitro fertilization. *Fertility and Sterility* **40**: 461–465.

Mason AJ, Hayflick JS, Ling N et al (1985) Complementary DNA sequences of ovarian follicular fluid inhibin show precursor structure and homology with transforming growth factor β. *Nature* **318**: 659–663.

McBain JC, Trounson A (1984) Patient management–treatment cycle. In Wood C & Trounson A (eds) *Clinical In Vitro Fertilization*, p 49. New York: Springer-Verlag.

McCullagh DR (1932) Dual endocrine activity of testis. *Science* **76**: 19–20.

McIntosh JEA, Matthews CD, Crocker JM, Broom TJ & Cox LW (1980) Predicting the luteinizing hormone surge: relationship between the duration of the follicular and luteal phases and the length of the human menstrual cycle. *Fertility and Sterility* **34**: 125–130.

McLachlan RI, Robertson DM, Burger HG & De Kretser DM (1986a) The radioimmunoassay of bovine and human follicular fluid and serum inhibin. *Molecular and Cellular Endocrinology* **46**: 175–185.

McLachlan RI, Robertson DM, Healy DL, De Kretser DM & Burger HG (1986b) Plasma inhibin levels during gonadotrophin-induced ovarian hyperstimulation for IVF: a new index of follicular function? *Lancet* **i**: 1233–1234.

McNatty KP & Baird DT (1978) Relationship between follicle stimulating hormone, androstenedione and oestradiol in human follicular fluid. *Journal of Endocrinology* **76**: 527–531.

McNatty KP & Sawers RS (1975) The relationship between the endocrine environment within the Graafian follicle and the subsequent rate of progesterone secretion by human granulosa cells in vitro. *Journal of Endocrinology* **66**: 391–400.

McNatty KP, Makris A, de Grazia C, Osathanondh R & Ryan KJ (1979) The production of progesterone androgens and oestrogens by granulosa cells, thecal tissue and stromal tissue from human ovaries in vitro. *Journal of Clinical Endocrinology and Metabolism* **49**: 687–699.

Miyamoto K, Hasegawa Y, Fukuda M et al (1985) Isolation of porcine follicular fluid inhibin of 32K daltons. *Biochemical and Biophysical Research Communications* **129**: 396–403.

Moghissi KF, Syner FN & Evans TN (1972) A composite picture of the menstrual cycle. *American Journal of Obstetrics and Gynecology* **114**: 405–411.

Okamoto S, Healy DL, Howlett DT et al (1986a) An analysis of plasma estradiol concentrations during clomiphene citrate (CC)–human menopausal gonadotropin (HMG) stimulation in an in vitro fertilization–embryo transfer (IVF–ET) program. *Journal of Clinical Endocrinology and Metabolism* **63**: 736–740.

Okamoto S, Thomas, A, McLaughlin V, Morrow L & Healy DL (198b) Do serum LH concentrations really predict IVF fertilization rates and pregnancy? Submitted for publication.

Okamoto S, Morrow L & Healy DL (1986c) Predictive value of serum HCG concentrations in IVF pregnancies. Submitted for publication.

Plachot M, Junca AM, Mandelbau J et al (1986) Cytogenetical analysis of human oocytes and embryos in an IVF programme. *European Society of Human Reproduction and Embryology, Second Meeting*, Brussels, Belgium, June 20–25. Abstract 69.

Porter RN, Smith W, Lenton BA, Neal, LM & Sulaiman R (1984) Plasma concentrations of human chorionic gonadotropin from the time of implantation until the second week of pregnancy. *Fertility and Sterility* **37**: 773–780.

Quigley M, Berkowitz AS, Gilbert SA & Wolf DP (1984a) Clomiphene citrate in an in vitro fertilization program: hormonal comparisons between 50- and 150-mg daily dosage. *Fertility and Sterility* **41**: 809–816.

Quigley MM, Schmidt CL, Beauchamp PJ et al (1984b) Enhanced follicular recruitment in an in vitro fertilization program: clomiphene alone versus a clomiphene/human menopausal gonadotropin combination. *Fertility and Sterility* **42**: 25–31.

Rivier J, Spiess J, McClintock R, Vaughan J & Vale W (1985) Purification and partial purification of inhibin from porcine follicular fluid. *Biochemical and Biophysical Research Communications* **133**: 120–127.

Robertson DM, Foulds LM, Leversha L et al (1985) Isolation of inhibin from bovine follicular fluid. *Biochemical and Biophysical Research Communications* **126**: 220–226.

Robertson DM, de Vos FL, Foulds LM et al (1986) Isolation of a 31 kD form of inhibin from bovine follicular fluid. *Molecular and Cellular Endocrinology* **44**: 271–277.

Ross GT & Van de Wiele RL (1981) The ovary. In Williams R (ed.) *Textbook of Endocrinology*, 6th edn, pp 355–399. Philadelphia: Saunders.

Scott RS, Burger HG & Quigg H (1980) A simple and rapid in vitro bioassay for inhibin. *Endocrinology* **107**: 1536–1542.

Stanger JD & Yovich JL (1985) Reduced in vitro fertilization of human oocytes from patients with raised basal luteinising hormone levels during the follicular phase. *British Journal of Obstetrics and Gynaecology* **92**: 385–393.

Taylor TJ, Trounson A, Besanko M, Burger HG & Stockdale J (1986) Plasma progesterone and prolactin changes in superovulated women before, during and immediately after laparoscopy for in vitro fertilization and their relation to pregnancy. *Fertility and Sterility* **45**: 680–686.

Trounson AO (1983) In vitro fertilization at Monash University, Melbourne, Australia. In Crosignani PG & Rubin BL (eds) *In Vitro Fertilization and Embryo Transfer*, p 315. New York: Academic Press.

Trounson AO & Calabrese R (1984) Changes in plasma progesterone concentrations around the time of the luteinizing hormone surge in women superovulation for in vitro fertilization. *Journal of Clinical Endocrinology and Metabolism* **59**: 1075–1079.

Trounson AO & Leeton JF (1982) The endocrinology of clomiphene stimulation. In Edwards RG & Purdy JM (eds) *Human Conception In Vitro*, p 51. New York: Academic Press.

Trounson AO, Leeton, JF, Wood C, Webb J & Wood J (1981) Pregnancies in humans by fertilization in vitro and embryo in the control of ovulatory cycles. *Science* **212**: 681–684.

Vargyas JM, Marrs RP, Kletzky OA & Mishell DR (1982) Correlation of ultrasonic measurement of ovarian follicle size and serum estradiol levels in ovulatory patients following clomiphene citrate for in vitro fertilization. *American Journal of Obstetrics and Gynecology* **144**: 569–574.

Vrailly S, Gougeon A, Milgrom E, Vonsel-Helmreich O & Papiernik E (1981) Androgens and progestins in the human ovarian follicle: differences in the evolution of preovulatory, healthy non-ovulatory and atretic follicles. *Journal of Clinical Endocrinology and Metabolism* **53**: 128–134.

Wood C, Trounson A, Leeton JF et al (1981) A clinical assessment of nine pregnancies obtained by in vitro fertilization and embryo transfer. *Fertility and Sterility* **35**: 502–507.

8

Pathophysiological relationships between the biological and immunological activities of luteinizing hormone

MARIA L. DUFAU
JOHANNES D. VELDHUIS

Over the last few years there has been a growing realization of the potential value of highly sensitive bioassays for the measurement of protein hormone concentrations in blood. The establishment of radioimmunoassays (RIAs) of sufficient specificity and sensitivity to measure virtually all known peptide and protein hormones in body fluids has been accompanied by the recognition that in some cases the immunoactive hormone concentration does not precisely reflect the content of biologically active hormone in the circulation. This is of particular importance for glycoprotein hormones, since there is now good evidence for the essential role of the carbohydrate residues of hormones such as luteinizing hormone (LH), human chorionic gonadotrophin (hCG), follicle stimulating hormone (FSH) and thyroid stimulating hormone (TSH) in the expression of bioactivity at the target cell level as well as on metabolic clearance. The need for more exact estimates of serum hormone bioactivity has begun to be answered by the use of highly sensitive target cells (e.g. cells acutely dispersed or in short-term culture, from gonads, adrenal and other end organs, or tumour cells from established cultures) for bioassay of their respective trophic hormones. This approach has been particularly successful in the case of dispersed Leydig cells for the assay of plasma concentrations of LH and hCG in human and animal species.

THE LH BIOASSAY

The LH bioassay is based on the acute dose-related testosterone response of testicular interstitial cells to gonadotrophin in vitro (Dufau et al, 1971a, 1972). Testosterone responses of dispersed rat (Dufau et al 1974, 1976a) interstitial cells and mouse (Van Damme et al, 1974) to unknown samples are compared with the responses evoked by standard hormones. Potencies are derived in terms of the standard used. The assay termed RICT (rat interstitial cell testosterone) described by Dufau et al (1974, 1976a) has been

applied to the measurement of pituitary and serum LH and LH-like gonadotrophins in man, rhesus monkey, rat, shrew, sheep, rabbit, mink, reptiles,
turtles and various exotic animals.

The RICT assay is five to 10 times more sensitive than RIA for LH
measurement in humans and is of comparable sensitivity for measurement
of circulating rat LH (Dufau et al, 1974, 1976a; Solano et al, 1979). This has
permitted the measurement of LH in one-hundredth of a millilitre of human
male and female serum and has allowed multiple and frequent sampling for
the measurement of bioactive LH profiles in adults and children during
physiological and diagnostic studies and during therapy to suppress gonadotrophin secretion.

The in vitro LH bioassay can be performed in laboratories throughout the
world, and can be expected to give similar results when a uniform standard is
employed. This is an improvement over certain aspects of RIAs which are
subject to the individual characteristics of each antibody employed for
assay. The high sensitivity of the RICT assay permits measurement of levels
of bioactive LH in unextracted serum from birth to puberty with good
precision. This also offers advantages over RIA on those frequent occasions
when the RIA levels are only slightly above the lower limit of sensitivity of
the assay.

CHEMISTRY AND STRUCTURE–FUNCTION STUDIES

Since the carbohydrate moieties of LH and hCG play a predominant role in
the molecular mechanism of gonadotrophin action at the target cell, we will
review briefly some aspects of the chemistry of gonadotrophins. The glycoprotein hormones LH, hCG, FSH and TSH are composed of two poly-
peptide subunits (α and β) that are associated through non-covalent interactions. The intact hormone (α and β combined) is required for expression
of receptor binding and biological activity, but individual subunits are
devoid of biological activity. The α subunits within a species possess nearly
the same amino acid sequence with some heterogeneity at their N-termini.
The β subunits are of different structures conferring the hormonal specificity
for interaction with respective receptors only in association with the α
subunit. The carbohydrate moieties constitute about 16% of the weight of
the LH molecule with two asparagine N-linked oligosaccharide groups on
the α subunit and one in the β subunit. The β subunit of hCG contains two
N-linked oligosaccharides and four additional oligosaccharide chains O-
linked to serine (Kessler et al, 1979). The branched carbohydrate chain is
formed by mannose, galactose, fucose, glucosamine and galactosamine with
a predominance of terminal sialic acid in hCG (20 residues per molecule
compared with 1 or 2 in human LH) or fucose and galactose in LH. Some LH
branches also contain one residue of N-acetylgalactosamine and N-acetyl-
glucosamine covalently linked to a sulphate group (Parsons and Pierce,
1980). The oligosaccharide content and structure including the sialic acid
appear to be responsible for the charge microheterogeneity which is
reflected in the differences of isoelectric point (pI) observed for hCG of 3–5,

(Nwokoro et al, 1981), and that for LH of 7.8–9.8. In the case of LH, six isoforms are resolved on isoelectrofocusing polyacrylamide gels of rat pituitary extracts, within the indicated range of pIs resulting from differences in carbohydrate structure (Dufau et al, 1982) (see Table 1 and also page 167). A similarly defined pattern for rat pituitary LH has been reported using isoelectric focusing column separation of pituitary LH (Wakabayashi, 1977; Hattori, 1983), whereas microelectrofocusing in sucrose gradients showed a less clear resolution of pI isoforms of LH in rat pituitary extracts. Using the isoelectrofocusing column procedure for characterization of human serum LH, a heterogeneous profile of LH activity was found in both pituitary and plasma samples, with a larger proportion present in the pH range of 6.5–10 (Robertson et al, 1977, 1982). An additional isoform (pI 9.8) of high biological activity was reported in recent chromatofocusing studies (Keel and Grotjan, 1985). Isoforms of higher pI species could result from higher terminal acetylhexosamine content. The bioactive/immunoactive ratio (B : I ratio) of LH isohormones decreases with decreasing pI values (Dufau et al, 1982; Keel and Grotjan, 1985). Removal of the terminal sialic acid residue significantly reduces the half-life of the circulating hormone. This is particularly marked in the case of hCG, for which the plasma half-life falls from 55 min to 1 min in the rat (Van Hall et al, 1971; Tsuruhara et al, 1972b). Also the content of sialic acid explains the

Table 1. Summary of LH immunoactivity (I) and bioactivity (B) (ng/ml) and B : I ratios of LH components resolved by isoelectrofocusing (IEF) of pituitary extracts from control and orchiectomized animals.

Peak fraction from IEF components	I	B	B : I	Fraction number	I	B	B : I
	Control				5 Days		
I	16.0	40.0	2.5	I	26.0	36.5	1.4
II	31.5	55.0	1.7	II	40.0	71.7	1.8
III	33.0	40.0	1.2	III	36.0	52.7	1.5
IV	13.0	13.0	1.0	IV	17.0	18.2	1.1
V	11.0	8.5	0.77	V	13.0	11.0	0.84
VI	13.5	8.5	0.62	VI	8.0	5.0	0.62
	20 Days				45 Days		
I	55.0	54.0	0.98	I	155.0	140.3	0.90
II	97.5	83.5	0.85	II	192.0	142.7	0.74
III	77.5	72.5	0.93	III	170.0	65.4	0.38
IV	40.0	21.5	0.53	IV	185.0	52.0	0.28
V	35.0	20.5	0.58	V	150.0	49.5	0.33
VI	22.5	10.0	0.44	VI	110.0	36.0	0.32
	60 Days						
I	42.5	54.0	1.27				
II	67.5	97.7	1.45				
III	87.5	128.5	1.46				
IV	55.0	61.5	1.10				
V	34.0	32.3	0.94				
VI	30.0	19.5	0.65				

pIs of components: I (9.44); II (9.20); III (9.02); IV (8.76); V (8.64); VI (8.46). From Dufau et al (1982).

differences in the half-life for hCG (12 h) and LH (15–40 min) in man. The latter findings were derived from early studies using in vivo bioassays where the marked reduction of biological activity observed by these assays mainly reflected rapid clearance of the hormone from the circulation. The in vitro assay, which is unaffected by in vivo clearance, has permitted evaluation of the effects of deglycosylation on the intrinsic biological activity of pituitary and circulating glycoprotein hormones.

Early studies using the Leydig cell assay demonstrated that desialylation of human LH and hCG, with consequent marked changes in their isoelectric points, caused a 50% loss of bioactivity (Dufau et al, 1971b). Enzymically deglycosylated hCG and LH bind to Leydig cell and ovarian LH receptors with a higher affinity than the intact hormones (Tsuruhara et al, 1972b). However such hormone–receptor complexes are apparently deficient in their ability to couple with adenylate cyclase in the cell membrane with consequent reduction in cyclic adenosine monophosphate (cAMP) production and steroidogenesis (Catt et al, 1974; Moyle et al, 1975). The additional removal of galactose by treatment of asialo-hCG with β-galactosidase had no further effect on the receptor binding properties of the modified hormone (Tsuruhara et al, 1972a). However, the steroidogenic activity of asialoagalacto-hormone was reduced to about 15% of that of the native hormone (Dufau et al, 1971b). The ability of the modified glycoproteins to stimulate cAMP in the testis was also substantially reduced, particularly for the asialoagalacto-preparation (Catt et al, 1974).

These findings demonstrated that the two terminal amino sugar residues do not participate in the process of hormone recognition and interaction with specific plasma membrane receptors in the testis and ovary. The decrease in potency of the deglycosylated hormones, accompanied by their retention of receptor binding activity, suggested that such derivatives could act as competitive antagonists of the native hormone under appropriate in vitro conditions. Furthermore chemical deglycosylation of LH (Sairam and Schiller, 1979; Sairam and Fleshner, 1981), and hCG (Chen et al, 1982; Manjunath and Sairam, 1982), with anhydrous hydrogen fluoride or trifluoromethane sulphonic acid (Kalyan and Bahl, 1981), was able to remove 76–87% sialic acid, galactose, mannose and fucose, 52% of N-acetylglucosamine and 14% of N-acetyl-D-galactosamine (with cleavage occurring at the mannose residues of the asparagine-linked moiety and the galactose residues of the serine-linked moiety). Structure–function studies demonstrated an increase in binding of the modified hormone by testicular and ovarian LH receptors with an accompanying marked decrease in the ability to stimulate cAMP and testosterone production. In addition, the preparation antagonized the actions of the native hormone in vitro.

More recent studies have demonstrated a dominant role of sugar residues of the α subunit in the transduction of the hormonal signal (Sairam and Barghavi, 1985). Such results are consistent with the earlier demonstration of preferential masking of the receptor by α subunit immunoreactive sites (Milius et al, 1983). Also, during cross-linking of intact hCG labelled in the α or β subunit to pure LH receptor, only the α subunit readily cross-linked to the receptor (Kusuda and Dufau, 1986). Taken together these observations indicate that the α subunit possesses for the most part the recognition sites for interaction with the receptor and the oligosaccharide chain for signal transduction, while the β subunit's predominant role would be to confer the necessary specific conformational changes on the α subunit for interaction with the corresponding recognition site, in this case the LH receptor.

LH BIOACTIVITY AND BIOIMMUNORATIOS

The in vitro LH bioassay permits accurate measurement of LH and hCG in the human under all physiological circumstances. In addition to the absolute measurement of intrinsic biological activity of the circulating hormone, the evaluation of B:I ratios can provide a useful sensitive index of qualitative changes of the LH molecule. Biochemical changes in secreted LH, such as degree of glycosylation and possible sulphation, could modify the B:I ratio and reflect significant pathophysiological regulatory events in the brain/hypothalamic/pituitary system (see below, Figure 3 and page 167).

The plasma levels of bioactive LH in men and postmenopausal women have been generally higher than those measured by RIA, although the two values are frequently closer in cycling women (Dufau et al, 1976a,b). In men and postmenopausal women, B:I ratios are usually 3–5 (Dufau et al, 1976a, 1977a, 1983), whereas those in normal women at all stages of the cycle are closer to unity (Dufau et al, 1976b; Veldhuis et al, 1984). The ratios indicated were derived from plasma LH assays with potencies expressed in terms of the urinary standard, human menopausal gonadotrophin (2nd International Reference Preparation (hMG)). The absolute values of the ratios are subject to changes according to the standard used; however, the differences observed between groups should not be significantly affected provided the same antibody is used. Furthermore, the above differences are observed whether B:I ratio values are derived from single samples from groups with large numbers of subjects (Dufau et al, 1976a,b, 1977a) or, as more recently, from multiple, frequent sampling (each 10–15 min over 6–8 h) in a series of six to eight subjects per group (Dufau et al, 1983; Veldhuis et al, 1983, 1984).

The intermittent nature of gonadotrophin secretion that was originally defined by RIA was subsequently analyzed by RICT assay initially in men and postmenopausal women to assess whether bioactive LH exibits similar pulsatility. As was observed earlier for individual samples, in the more recent study, bioactive LH values were considerably higher than immuno-active levels throughout the profiles analyzed (41.4 ± 15.1 and 450 ± 243 mIU/ml by RICT assay versus 10.2 ± 2.3 and 83 ± 35 by RIA for males (Figure 1) and postmenopausal females respectively, with corresponding B:I ratios of 3.95 ± 0.97 and 5.4 ± 1.3). Furthermore the total area under the bioactive LH secretion profile was four-fold higher than that defined by the immunoactive hormone profile and the absolute amplitude of the bio-active LH peaks was increased 0.5- to 11-fold over the immunoactive values. Although the majority of the LH peaks were coincident by bioassay and RIA, dissociation occurred in about 25% of the total LH peaks. A small

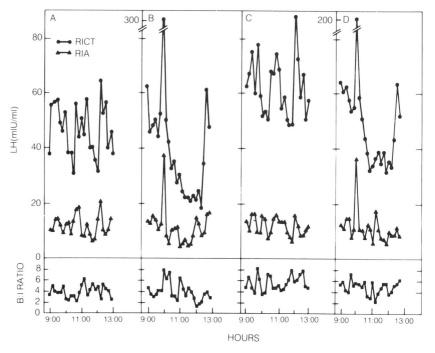

Figure 1. Bioactive (●—●) and immunoactive (▲–▲) patterns of serum LH in four young men from whom blood samples were drawn every 10 min. LH values are expressed in terms of the 2nd International Reference Preparation (hMG). B : I ratio profiles were derived from the data shown in the upper panel. From Dufau et al (1983), with permission.

proportion of bioactive LH peaks (13%) were not detected by RIA. A larger proportion of immunoactive LH peaks were devoid of increases in biological activity. This dissociation was more marked in postmenopausal women (45%) than in men (23%). Such disparities could be explained by the differences in sensitivity of the two assays, and/or pituitary secretion of LH molecules that are devoid of biological activity but are recognized by the antibody, and that may or may not be capable of binding the receptor but are unable to stimulate the target cell (i.e. subunit or deglycosylated hormone).

There are several important differences between the patterns of bioactive LH in men and postmenopausal women (Dufau et al, 1983). The pulses of biologically active LH occurred less frequently in postmenopausal women with a periodicity of 190 ± 122 min (compared with 76 ± 35 min in men), and although substantial concentrations of hormone are released, the fractional increase over the baseline was relatively small (3.5-fold lower than in men). In the male, a consistently more distinct pattern of bioactive LH pulses is observed. In a few subjects who displayed low frequency of LH release, secretion occurred in a surge-like fashion, with pulses that reached levels up to 300 mIU/ml (Figure 1; Subjects B and D). Also, such LH peaks were short-lived with an initial estimated half-life of 5–10 min. In contrast, in the majority of subjects pulses were more frequent and reached levels up to 60–90 mIU/ml with usually a relatively longer apparent initial half-life of 15–30 min. It is clear from this study that because of the marked differences observed between absolute values within pulses and during the interpulse intervals and also between the profiles of different subjects, evaluation of single samples is of limited use. Rather, multiple frequent sampling is preferable to assess physiological status or for diagnostic purposes. Alternatively, for convenience and to reduce assay costs, estimation of pooled multiple samples collected over the 3 hours (every 10 min) provides a useful integrated value.

A finding of major importance is the observed significant increases in the B : I ratios within pulses over interpulse B : I ratios in 98% of the pulses in men (Figure 1, lower panel) and 83% in postmenopausal women. This observation indicates that the LH secreted in pulses (intrapulse) is of higher biological activity than the basal (interpulse) levels and could reflect the release of a compartmentalized LH pool induced by the endogenous LH releasing hormone (LHRH) signal. Such increases were not evident in previous studies of men and postmenopausal women in response to exogenous LHRH using either a single large bolus of LHRH (100 µg subcutaneously) or continuous infusion with low doses of LHRH (2 µg/min), (Dufau et al, 1976b, 1977a; Beitins et al, 1977, 1980). This could be explained in the former case by an increased secretion from all pituitary pools yielding an integrated B : I value instead of selective increases from the highly bioactive pool, and in the latter by a lack of definition of a small early pool (presumably of high bioactivity) and considerably mixing with the late pool of reduced bioactivity. Demonstration of such compartments, which mimicked the increase in B : I ratio observed within the pulse by endogenous LHRH, has been recently obtained by exogenous low doses of LHRH (10 µg intravenous) administered in pulse-like fashion (Veldhuis and Dufau, 1986; Figure 2). Thus, the physiological mode of episodic LH secretion is such that it avoids gonadal desensitization that could occur if similar concentrations of highly bioactive hormone were secreted in a constant manner.

Of interest are the recent findings demonstrating that chronic treatment with D-Trp[6]Pro N-ethylamide, a highly potent LHRH agonist (LHRHA), markedly reduced the biological activity of circulating LH in men (Evans et al, 1984; Swerdloff et al, 1985). After a period of initial stimulation, subsequent pituitary responses to LHRH are blunted and spontaneous LH pulsations abolished, a finding that indicated pituitary desensitization.

Although mean 12-hour radioimmunoactive LH levels were unchanged from pretreatment values (Evans et al, 1984), plasma testosterone values declined to 200 ng/dl or < 50 ng/dl, after treatment with LHRHA for 12 days (Evans et al, 1984) or 16–18 weeks (Swerdloff et al, 1985) respectively. Since the Leydig cell responded normally to exogenous gonadotrophin, despite low testosterone values, the above findings indicated that the abnormality caused by LHRHA treatment is due to secretion of LH of reduced biological activity. RICT assay showed marked reduction of the biological activity of circulating LH with a consequent fall in B : I ratios. Furthermore, characterization of the serum immunoreactive LH (12-day study) by Sephadex

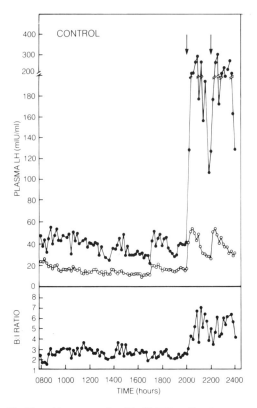

Figure 2. Bioactive (●—●) and immunoactive (○—○) LH profile of a young male subject during basal 10 min sampling (0800–2000) with pulsations induced by endogenous LHRH pulses. Administration of low-dose bolus intravenous LHRH (10 μg) at 2 h intervals elicited magnified LH pulses enriched in biological activity with B:I ratios of 6–8. From Veldhuis and Dufau (1986), with permission.

chromatography, revealed a retarded elution profile during short treatment with LHRHA (Evans et al, 1984), whereas no changes in the gel filtration profiles on a polyacrylamide agarose column (Ultrogel, AcA54) or high performance liquid chromatography (Bio Sil TSK-125) were observed in the long-term study. Chromatofocusing of urinary LH, however, revealed a significant shift in the isoelectric point of the predominant LH species to a more acid range suggesting a change in the carbohydrate side-chain. The blunted pituitary responses and disappearance of spontaneous LH pulsations most likely result from marked homologous down-regulation of LHRH receptors (Clayton and Catt, 1981). Presumably the marked reduction of LHRH receptors, possibly coupled to pituitary desensitization, would be responsible for production of only basal levels of gonadotrophin of reduced biological activity. This type of pharmacological dysfunction could serve as a model to unravel the complex pathophysiological mechanisms of altered gonadotrophin secretion observed in patients with central or hypothalamic disorders with reductions in LH pulse frequency or amplitude and consequently of B : I ratio (see also page 167).

In cycling women, biologically active LH is also secreted in discrete pulsations preferentially enriched in bioactive hormone. At each of the three stages of the menstrual cycle, B : I LH ratios within LH pulses were significantly increased (Veldhuis et al, 1984). The mean pulse and interpulse B : I ratios exceeded unity (2.42) but were significantly lower than those defined in normal men (3.95) and postmenopausal women (5.4). The mean B : I LH ratio increased in the late follicular phase (Dufau et al, 1977a; Veldhuis et al, 1984). Furthermore, only at this stage of the cycle did bolus injection of LHRH cause a significant increase in the B : I ratio (Dufau et al, 1977a,b). Since the observed increases in B : I ratio could be induced by a large dose of exogenous LHRH, it is likely that the highly bioactive LH pool is considerably expanded at this stage of the cycle, allowing its expression despite dilution by LH secreted from less bioactive pools. Although the exact endocrine factors that influence variations in the biopotency of circulating LH in women are not fully understood, acute oestrogen increases may significantly modify bioactive LH release through positive feedback effects in the hypothalamus. The increased B : I LH ratios in the late follicular phase are consistent with observations in the preovulatory stage of the menstrual cycle and oestrous cycle of the monkey and rat (Dufau et al, 1977b; Solano et al, 1980b; Marut et al, 1981). In the rat the significant increase of LH B : I ratio at pro-oestrus is abolished by gonadectomy, even though an LH peak of similar radioimmunoactive magnitude occurs at the same time as in the control (Dufau et al, 1982).

In cycling women, individual peaks of bioactive and immunoactive LH are significantly discrepant, as they are for men and postmenopausal women. The majority of the discordance is accounted for by immunoactive LH pulses, 30% of which occur without a significant rise in bioactivity. Conversely 14% of bioactive LH pulses occur without a demonstrable immunoactive LH peak. Since a significant discordance exists between immunoactive and bioactive LH pulsations in all groups of normal subjects studied, it is clear that estimates of circulating concentrations of biologically active LH rather than immunoactive LH alone are necessary to characterize fully pathological and physiological patterns of LH secretion.

The sequence involved in the control of gonadotrophin secretion is initiated presumably by an endogenous hypothalamic rhythm generator ('gonadostat' or 'pulse generator') which controls the frequency of LHRH pulses that are responsible for the corresponding LH pulses observed in plasma (Figure 3). Modulation of LHRH secretion is exerted through opioid neurons as well as other peptidergic and catecholaminergic neurons which originate in the hypothalamic and diencephalic regions of the brain. Their axonal projections interconnect with LHRH neurons in or near the preoptic tuberal region of the hypothalamus and either enhance or slow the frequency of LH pulses by corresponding alterations in LHRH outflow. Opioids acutely slow LHRH pulses at this level directly through interactions with LHRH neurons or indirectly by modifying the output of other cells (i.e. noradrenergic fibres). In addition, a direct paracrine effect of opioids on the gonadotroph has been postulated (Blank et al, 1985). The latter could contribute to the chronic inhibition of gonadotrophin secretion, e.g. in heroin addicts and or in hypogonadism associated with strenuous prolonged exercise. Steroids also modify LHRH secretion at several levels. For example, oestrogen replacement reinstates opioid suppression of LH secretion in orchidectomized patients with testicular feminization (Veldhuis et al, 1985a).

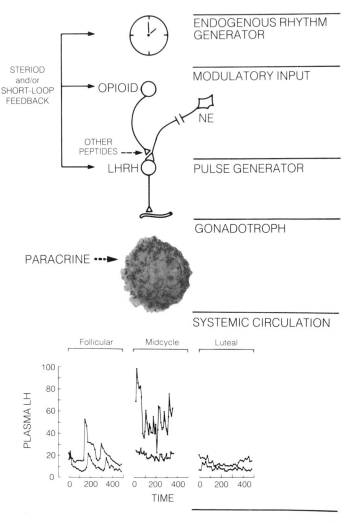

Figure 3. Neuronal pathways and modulatory circuits involved in the control of gonadotropin secretion (modified by Blank et al (1985) after Kalra SP (1985)). The panel below shows bioactive (higher level profiles) and immunoactive (lower level profiles) LH profiles in the early follicular phase (follicular); late follicular phase (near mid-cycle); and luteal phase. Increases in the B:I LH ratio and frequency of pulses in relation to stage of the menstrual cycle are demonstrated.

LHRH is released from nerve terminals in the median eminence of the hypothalamus in a pulsatile fashion to reach the pituitary through the portal vein system. LHRH binds to specific high-affinity receptors on the gonado-troph and activates the secretory mechanism leading to LH release. The physiological variations in LH secretion that occur during the menstrual cycle are accompanied by significant changes in the periodicity of LH pulses and reflect the operation of distinct neuroendocrine modulatory mechan-isms (Figure 3, below). Bioactive pulses of LH increase from 0.5 pulse/h in the early follicular phase to 1 pulse/h in the late follicular phase, and during the luteal phase there is a significant reduction in the frequency of bioactive LH pulses to 0.3 pulse/h (Veldhuis et al, 1984). The enhancement of ovarian function prior to ovulation might be attributed to this increase in LH frequency, since such frequency modulation is an important physiological mechanism for regulating the blood concentration of LH available to the ovary prior to ovulation. The long-term changes in LH periodicity during the menstrual cycle could reflect among other mechanisms changes in hypothalamic opioid tone. This is consistent with the observation that when the endogenous LHRH signal in men is amplified by opiate-receptor blockade following oral administration of the long-acting opioid antagonist naltrexone, LH is released in more frequent and augmented pulses of high biological activity with a significant increase in androgen production (Veldhuis et al, 1983) (Figure 4). Thus, in addition to increases in the B:I ratio, the changes in the amplitude and frequency of LH pulses may

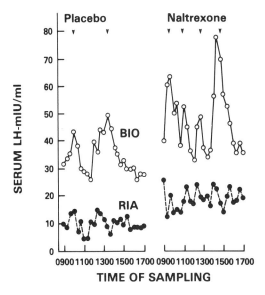

Figure 4. Increased frequency and amplitude of bioactive LH pulses during oral treatment with the long-acting opiate-receptor antagonist naltrexone. A representative profile is given of LH bioactivity and immunoactivity determined in a normal man after placebo or naltrexone administration. Arrows over the upper curve are used to designate significant bioactive LH pulses. From Veldhuis et al (1983), with permission.

effectively enhance stimulation of gonadal steroidogenesis.

The consistent and significant differences in B:I ratios between pre-menopausal women and normal male or postmenopausal women could be due to a number of factors: differences in secretion rate, metabolic clearance, and the effects of gonadal steroids upon the nature as well as the secretion rates of pituitary gonadotrophins. Increased LH endogenous pro-duction in normal males has been suggested by earlier studies showing greater urinary excretion of LH in men than in cycling women. In two reports, urine from normal men was found to contain considerably higher quantities of biologically active LH than urine of adult women during the follicular or luteal phases (Loraine and Brown, 1956; McArthur et al, 1958). The urinary excretion of LH in normal males was found to overlap with values of the lower range of postmenopausal women (McArthur et al, 1958). In addition a higher blood LH production rate of immunoactive LH was demonstrated in males than in cycling women (Pepperell et al, 1975). Moreover, more recent studies have demonstrated that previous estimates of LH blood production rates from immunoassay data (Kohler et al, 1968; Yen et al, 1968; Marshall et al, 1973; Pepperell et al, 1975; Raiti et al, 1975) markedly underestimated the quantity of biologically active hormone secreted in man (Veldhuis et al, 1986). The estimated blood production rate for bioactive LH in normal men, derived from steady-state metabolic clearance rates in hypogonadotrophic patients at physiological plasma con-centrations of immunoactive and bioactive LH, is about three-fold higher than for LH immunoactivity (1937 IU/24h compared with 589 IU/24h). Such values are in accord with the plasma LH B:I ratio of 4 in normal men. In contrast, the metabolic clearance rate for LH bioactivity was only 33% less than that for immunoactivity. These results indicate that the markedly higher endogenous production rates of bioactive compared to immuno-active LH activity, rather than changes in metabolic clearance, represent the predominant factor responsible for the high plasma B:I ratio that is characteristic of plasma LH in normal men under physiological conditions.

Another factor which could influence the B:I ratio in normal subjects is the action of gonadal steroids upon the nature, as well as on the secretion rate, of pituitary gonadotrophins. This is indicated by the higher B:I ratios that are observed in plasma LH of subjects with relatively low oestrogen secretion. Like men and postmenopausal women, patients with Turner's syndrome have higher B:I ratios than cycling women (Dufau et al, 1976a). These increased values can be reduced to the normal cycling values by prolonged oestrogen replacement therapy, while minimally affecting im-munoactive LH concentrations (Lucky et al, 1979) (Figure 5). In more recent studies, infusion of oestradiol-17β to seven normal men (oestradiol infused continuously for 3½ days) decreased mean plasma bioactive LH concentrations and diminished the B:I LH ratio. Conversely, the anti-oestrogen tamoxifen increased bioactive LH pulse frequency, bioactive LH pulse amplitude and plasma B:I ratios. These results clearly indicate that oestradiol modulates the biological activity and pulsatile secretion of LH (Veldhuis and Dufau, 1986). Furthermore, evaluation of LH during epi-sodes of vasomotor flushing in perimenopausal women showed significant

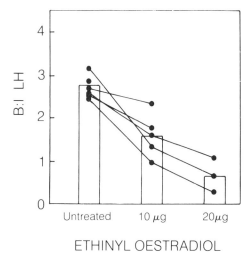

ETHINYL OESTRADIOL

Figure 5. Serum B:I LH ratios in girls with gonadal dysgenesis prior to and after chronic treatment with low doses of oestrogen. B:I ratios were significantly higher prior to the treatment with ethinyloestradiol (2.76 ± 0.14) than after 3 months of treatment (1.54 ± 0.14). From Lucky et al (1979), with permission.

increases in the B:I ratio. Conjugated oestrogen plus depomedroxy-progesterone treatment significantly ameliorated the vasomotor symptoms and caused marked reduction of LH B:I ratio to the premenopausal range, with no change in the radioimmunoactive LH level (Chang et al, 1984). Thus, in these circumstances, as in other cases described here, bioactive LH and B:I ratios correlate better than radioimmunoactive LH with the physiological status.

At variance with the effects of chronic oestrogen treatment, acute oestrogen exposure can increase LH bioactivity and B:I ratios as observed during LHRH stimulation in the late follicular phase, near midcycle in normal cycling women (Dufau et al, 1976a,b). Furthermore, an increase in the plasma B:I ratio was observed at the time of the midcycle LH peak in the monkey, and at the rat oestrous surge, concomitant with a decrease in the B:I ratio of pituitary LH (Dufau et al, 1977b; Solano et al, 1980b). Furthermore, castration at a time prior to the maximal increase in oestrogen prevented the preovulatory rise in B:I ratio (Dufau et al, 1982). These studies suggest that the acute rise in oestrogen could be responsible for the release of LH with high bioactivity from the pituitary into the circulation at the time of the surge. There is also evidence that oestrogen and other sex steroids can influence the B:I ratio in the gonadotroph cell per se. Previous studies have indicated that oestrogen can influence the incorporation of [^{3}H]glucosamine as well as [^{14}C]alanine into pituitary LH in vitro (Liu and Jackson, 1977), and it is likely that sex steroids could affect terminal glycosylation and hence the bioactivity of LH (see also under 'Chemistry and structure–function studies' above). In addition, androgen-dependent changes in the properties and B:I ratio of pituitary FSH (Bogdanove et al,

1974) and a decrease in the molecular radius of pituitary FSH have been described after orchiectomy in the rat. Qualitative variations in circulating LH detected by altered B:I ratios are also found in patients undergoing certain physiological changes. The plasma LH of prepubertal boys has a B:I ratio close to unity, and exhibits an increased ratio after the onset of testicular androgen secretion with the initiation of rapid gonadotrophic increments. In the cited studies the changes in ratio reflected predominantly a change in bioactive LH (Reiter et al, 1978, 1984; Lucky et al, 1980a). In contrast, Warner et al (1983) reported that older men with prostate cancer had significantly lower B:I ratios than healthy young men. This early report indicated the potential importance of changes in B:I ratio with age and sickness. In a follow-up of the latter study, lower B:I ratios were found in older, apparently healthy men compared to young men (2.52 ± 0.33 compared with 4.10 ± 0.24). These resulted from modest changes in LH immunoactivity and larger alterations in LH bioactivity that were associated with lower mean testosterone levels. Regression analysis showed that the

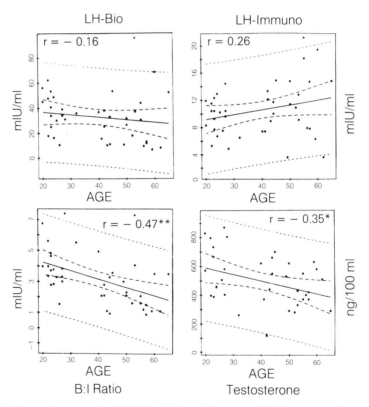

Figure 6. Regression analysis of LH bioactivity and immunoactivity (upper panel), and B:I ratios and testosterone production (lower panel) in healthy men of several ages. The dotted lines indicate the standard deviation and the dashed lines the standard error of the regression line. The decrements in B:I ratio and plasma testosterone were highly correlated with age. From Warner et al (1985), with permission.

reductions in B : I ratio and plasma testosterone were highly correlated with age (Warner et al, 1985) (Figure 6). Furthermore, the same study described a more pronounced reduction in B : I ratio as a function of sickness in men of similar age. Systemically ill men over the age of 40 had lower ratios than age-matched healthy men (1.05 ± 0.08 compared with 2.52 ± 0.33). In this case the changes in B : I ratio reflected solely reduction in the bioactive LH (36.7 ± 3.3 mIU/ml compared with 11.7 ± 1.1 mIU/ml) with no significant changes in radioimmunoactivity (11.4 ± 1.0 mIU/ml compared with 11.8 mIU/ml). These findings indicate that the qualitative nature of LH varies as a function of ageing and illness in men. Also of interest in the study by Warner et al (1983) is that three out of nine castrate men had normal LH levels by RICT (but not by RIA). This may reflect the lowered B : I ratios that occur after castration (Solano et al, 1979, 1980a; Dufau et al, 1982).

An effect of low testosterone on the B : I ratio is suggested by investigations in the rodent. The LH B : I ratio in male rats (1.2) was significantly higher than that in pituitary extracts (0.97). This minor but significant difference reflects the presence in the circulation of highly bioactive LH presumably released from a selective pool (basic isoforms) residing in a population of granules with considerable mixing with less bioactive pools.

The B : I ratio of stored and secreted LH is significantly decreased 5–25 days after castration (by 50%) and restored to control levels thereafter. The decrease in the B : I ratio of LH in castrated males was not due to increased subunit production and was prevented by administration of testosterone propionate or dihydrotestosterone beginning at the time of castration (Solano et al, 1980a). After castration the pituitary exhibited a higher B : I ratio than the circulating hormone, though both were decreased compared to ratios in intact animals. This explained the marked B : I ratio reduction of basic LH isoforms which in intact animals have the highest B : I ratios. It was also deduced from these studies that the chemical or structural changes in the LH molecule responsible for the reduction of the B : I ratio that occur in the rat during castration do not affect the charge of the molecule (Dufau et al, 1982) (Table 1).

The demonstration of a decrease in the LH B : I ratio after castration (Dufau et al, 1982), the previous observation of higher ratios in men than in premenopausal women (Dufau et al, 1976a) and the changes in B : I ratio observed in puberty and ageing suggest that androgens modulate the biological activities of both stored and circulating LH.

Bioactive LH measurements in pathological states

The RICT assay has been applied to the measurement of biologically active serum LH in several groups of hypogonadal patients (Table 2). The most interesting results were observed in the groups of patients with dysgenic gonads (young patients with Klinefelter's syndrome) or germinal aplasia, either idiopathic or due to drug therapy. In the former, bioactive serum LH values were as high as those observed during LHRH stimulation, when only a moderate rise in radioimmunoactive LH was noted. In particular, two of four patients in this group showed a significant elevation of the B : I ratio

Table 2. Bioactive LH measurements in pathological states.

Code	Patient diagnosis	Age	Testosterone (ng/100 ml)	FSH (mIU/ml)	LH mIU/ml		
					RICT bioassay	RIA	LH B:I ratio
A	Klinefelter's syndrome	22	350	30	201.8	26.8	7.52
B	Klinefelter's syndrome	19	600	105	160.5	40.7	3.93
C	Klinefelter's syndrome	22	332	37	240.0	39.0	6.15
D	Klinefelter's syndrome (mosaicism)	23	275	52	66.5	22.0	3.02
11	Germinal cell aplasia (spontaneous)	25	400	50	115.57	41.8	2.76
12	Germinal cell aplasia (spontaneous)	29	275	45	13.19	14.5	0.91
100	Germinal cell aplasia (chemotherapy)	23	350	32	15.5	14.0	1.11
101	Germinal cell aplasia	25	530	50	80.5	15.4	5.22
102	Germinal cell aplasia (chemotherapy)	32	—	40	64.0	40.0	1.6
103	Germinal cell aplasia (chemotherapy)	24	—	52	46.2	27.9	1.65
201	Chromophobe adenoma	50	—	<2	0	<2	—
202	Hand–Schüller–Christian disease	18	112	8.0	6.2	6.2	1.0
203	Panhypopituitarism	27	30	7.0	0	3.0	—
204	Fertile eunuch syndrome	24	180	11.0	0	4.0	—
205	Fertile eunuch syndrome	20	<50	15.0	8.6	12.0	0.72
301	Kallmann's syndrome	19	<50	<2	0	<2	—
302	Kallmann's syndrome	25	<50	<2	0	<2	—
A*	Kallmann's syndrome	22	<50	<2	0	2.9	—
B*	Kallmann's syndrome	39	<50	<2	0	2.3	—
C*	Kallmann's syndrome	33	<50	<2	11.6	9.2	1.26
D*	Hypopituitarism (suprasellar tumour)	21	<50	<2	0	8.9	—
E*	Kallmann's syndrome	29	<50	<2	0	3.8	—
F*	Kallmann's syndrome	21	<50	<2	0	3.8	—
G*	Panhypopituitarism	19	177	<2	5.3	4.4	1.2
Normal values†		21–40	250–1200 mean 580 ± 49	4–25	36.7 ± 49 (SEM)	9.4 ± 0.63	4.10 ± 0.2

Code: A–302 from Dufau et al (1977a).
  * from Veldhuis et al (1986).
† Normal values from Dufau et al (1983).

compared to normal subjects. In the germinal aplasia group, bioactive LH values were increased in several patients. Such elevated levels of bioactive LH in both groups of patients occurred in some cases when radioimmuno-active serum LH was normal or only slightly increased.

In patients with hypogonadotrophic hypogonadism, bioactive LH levels were undetectable in eight out of nine subjects (Table 2) and in all seven patients of a previous study (Dufau et al, 1976a). In contrast low values of radioimmunoassayable LH were always found in these samples.

The abnormal nature of LH secreted with low levels of bioactive LH and consequently low LH pulse amplitude and low B:I ratio may be aetiologi-cally relevant in patients with impotence and normal immunoreactive pituitary hormones, LH periodicity, and low–normal testosterone levels. The increased B:I ratio during exogenous bolus LHRH administration, 100 µg, (Figure 7) or clomiphene therapy (which is believed to enhance endogenous LHRH release) in a patient with this type of disorder, and known to have a pituitary stone (calcification) suggests a functional relation-

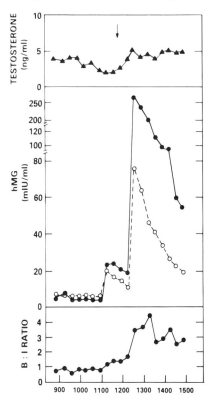

Figure 7. Bioactive and immunoactive LH profiles during basal collections and after a single dose of LHRH (100 µg) subcutaneously in a male patient with a complaint of impotence. After exogenous LHRH (arrow), marked increases were observed in bioactive LH with correspond-ing increases in the B:I ratio and testosterone production. From Plourde et al (1985), with permission.

ship between pituitary LHRH exposure and the potency of secreted LH (Plourde et al, 1985). The results of this study also suggest an association between the low LH B:I ratio and the anatomical disruption of the hypothalamic–pituitary portal system by the pituitary stone which prevented adequate exposure to endogenous LHRH. Normal men do not have a significant change in their B:I ratios after stimulation with a large bolus dose (100 μg) of LHRH (Dufau et al, 1977a; Beitins et al, 1977) suggesting that the LH secreted is derived from several pools presumably with mixing of small pools of highly bioactive LH with large pools of lower activity (also see page 159). In this interesting case report, it seems that a high biological LH pool was present that was not releasable by the low-amplitude endogenous LHRH pulses but was effectively released by a large, pharmacological LHRH stimulus. More recently, qualitative abnormalities of secreted LH characterized by a low B:I ratio (1.0 ± 0.1 standard deviations compared with 4.5 ± 0.4 standard deviations) with low–normal testosterone levels and normal radioimmunoactive LH were observed in seven of a group of 12 male patients age 24–50 with complaint of impotence for 4–5 months. It is conceivable that the defect of LH bioactivity in this group of patients is derived from a central dysfunction, psychogenic in nature, altering the frequency and or amplitude of LHRH release (Fabbri et al, 1986).

There are at least two cases reported of patients with a hypogonadal condition arising through a genetic defect which was expressed in the formation of anomalous LH that was immunologically active but devoid of biological activity (Axelrod et al, 1979; Gattucio et al, 1980). There was evidence in each patient's history of familial infertility and of parental consanguinity. Both cases were initially identified through the production of large amounts of radioimmunoactive LH, exaggerated LH increases in response to LHRH (Figure 8, right) and diminished testosterone levels

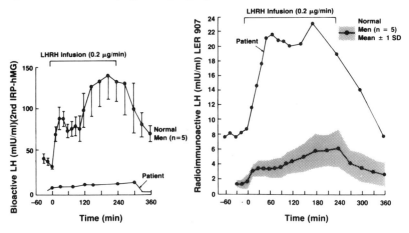

Figure 8. Effect of LHRH infusion on immunoactive LH (left) in a 33-year-old hypogonadal man with biologically inactive LH. The LH responses of five normal men to the LHRH infusion are shown in the shaded area. Measurement of LH bioactivity (right) in the serum of the patient in control samples and after LHRH infusion of 0.2 μg/min LHRH compared with the profile of five normal men (mean ± SD). From Beitins et al (1977, 1981), with permission.

unable to support spermatogenesis after the spermatid stage of development. The testis retained its functional integrity and capability to recognize the exogenous hormone (hCG), but was unable to recognize the endogenous gonadotrophic stimulus. Further studies of the patient described by Axelrod et al (1979) demonstrated that the in vitro bioactivity of LH in serum and urine, measured by RICT assay, was low in comparison with values found in normal men (Beitins et al, 1981) (Figure 8, left). Furthermore, circulating subunits were not present in excess, and the immunological LH had a molecular weight comparable to that of authentic LH. Also of interest was that the biological activity of the patient's serum and urinary LH increased by about 100%, but was still below the normal (20% of normal levels), during testosterone treatment. Moreover, serum testosterone and oestradiol concentrations rose further during LHRH infusion when testosterone was administered but not in the untreated state. Thus, the in vivo gonadal responses to LH correlated with the in vitro measurement by RICT assay of the LH molecule.

The endocrine consequences of reversible endogenous oestrogen excess on the pituitary–gonadal axis in man were analysed in a detailed study of a patient with an oestrogen-producing adrenal tumour (Veldhuis et al, 1985b). In this case, hypogonadism was attributable to a selective reduction in bioactive LH and a low B : I ratio and altered Leydig cell function. The LH reduction could result from oestradiol action at the hypothalamic level to reduce LHRH secretion, and from direct effects on pituitary processing of LH.

After initial observations indicating the value of measurements of bioactive LH content in blood in the assessment of sexual maturation, the analysis of bioactive LH parameters was evaluated as an additional discriminator in abnormal pubertal states. Rich et al (1982) have investigated the pituitary reserve of bioactive LH during normal and hypogonadotrophic states. Bioactive and immunoactive LH both correlated with the maturation achieved by hypogonadotrophic males and discriminated equally well between teenagers with delayed puberty and those with gonadotrophin deficiency once testosterone levels exceeded 30 ng/dl (testosterone levels which occur in late prepuberty, very early puberty or adrenarche (Rich et al, 1982)). Furthermore, the pituitary bioactive LH reserve is greater during midpuberty than before or after this time. In contrast to most of the pubertal or adult controls, many of the patients with pituitary deficiencies had lower bioactive and immunoactive LH levels at 4 h than at 1 h after LHRH treatment. Thus the level of LH after 4-hour treatment has been considered an indicator of normality by both assay criteria (Rich et al, 1982). Bioactive LH was found to be a useful test to discriminate true precocious puberty from premature thelarche and adrenarche (Rich et al, 1982). Although the immunoactive LH levels were three times higher in girls with true precocious puberty than in the other two groups, there was considerable overlap. However, the bioactive LH levels were 16 times higher in girls with isosexual precocity than in the other groups and there was no overlap.

The value of the in vitro LH bioassay has been clearly demonstrated in two separate areas. First, this assay provides valid cross-species comparisons to be performed between intrinsic biological activities of a wide variety of human and animal gonadotrophins, and permits assay of circulating levels in a large number of animal species. The latter feature has allowed the investigation of modulatory influences on LH bioactivity that are relevant to human pathophysiology. Second, and most importantly, the in vitro bioassay permits the most sensitive measurements of circulating LH in human serum under all physiopathological circumstances. Evaluation of bioactive parameters (absolute circulating bioactive level and B : I ratio) has demonstrated that LH secreted during pulses is of significantly higher biological activity than that measured between pulses. Such increases seem to reflect the release of a compartmentalized gonadotrophin pool of high biological activity. The findings of significant discordance between immunoactive and bioactive LH pulsations in males, cycling females and postmenopausal women indicate that estimates of bioactive LH are necessary to fully characterize LH profiles. Increases in frequency observed in normal men during therapy with naltrexone (a long-acting opiate antagonist) were accompanied by significant increases in testosterone production. Similarly, modulation of the frequency of bioactive pulses occurs during the late follicular phase of the menstrual cycle. Thus, the change in frequency appears to be an important mechanism for regulating the blood concentration of LH available to the gonads and provides the basis for optimal treatment during the use of LHRH for induction of ovulation.

The measured bioactive parameters are indicative of the production rate of the hormone under the concerted modulatory influences of gonadal steroids, and the periodicity and amplitude of the LHRH stimulus. Alterations of these parameters may explain a number of gonadal endocrine abnormalities which are poorly defined by conventional radioimmunoassay.

REFERENCES

Axelrod L, Neer RM & Kliman B (1979) Hypogonadism in a male with immunologically active, biologically inactive luteinizing hormone: an exception to a venerable rule. *Journal of Clinical Endocrinology and Metabolism* 48: 279–287.

Beitins EZ, Dufau ML, O'Loughlin K, Catt KJ & McArthur J (1977) Analysis of biological and immunological activities in the two pools of LH released during constant infusion of LHRH in men. *Journal of Clinical Endocrinology and Metabolism* 45: 605–608.

Beitins IZ, Dufau ML, O'Laughlin K et al (1980) Biological and immunological activities of serum LH in normal women during LH-RH infusion and in Turner's syndrome during estrogen treatment. In Belling CG & Wentz AC (eds) *LH-Releasing Hormone*, pp 135–155. New York: Masson.

Beitins IZ, Axelrod L, Ostrea T, Little R & Badger TM (1981) Hypogonadism in a male with an immunologically active, biologically inactive luteinizing hormone: characterization of the abnormal hormone. *Journal of Clinical Endocrinology and Metabolism* 52: 1143–1149.

Blank MS, Fabbri A, Catt KJ & Dufau ML (1985) Direct inhibition of gonadotroph function by opiates. *Transactions of the Association of American Physicians* XCVII: 1–9.

Bogdanove EM, Campbell GT & Peckman WD (1984) FSH pleomorphism in the rat–regulation by gonadal steroids. *Endocrine Research Communications* 1: 87–99.

Catt KJ, Tsuruhara T, Mendelson C, Ketelslegers JM & Dufau ML (1974) Gonadotropin binding and activation of interstitial cells of the testis. In Means AR (ed.) *Hormone Binding and Target Cell Activation in the Testis*, pp 1–30. New York: Plenum Press.

Chang SP, Soupe D, Kletzky DA & Lobo RA (1984) Differences in the ratio of bioactive to immunoreactive serum luteinizing hormone during vasomotor flushes and hormonal therapy in postmenopausal women. *Journal of Clinical Endocrinology and Metabolism* **58**: 925–928.

Chen H-C, Shimohigashi Y, Dufau ML & Catt KJ (1982) Characterization and biological properties of chemically deglycosylated human chorionic gonadotropin. *Journal of Biological Chemistry* **257**: 1446–1452.

Clayton RN & Catt KJ (1981) Gonadotropin-releasing hormone receptors: characterization, physiological regulation and relationship to reproductive function. *Endocrine Reviews* **2**: 186–209.

Dufau ML, Catt KJ & Tsuruhara T (1971a) Gonadotropin stimulation of testosterone production by the rat testis in vitro. *Biochimica et Biophysica Acta* **252**: 574.

Dufau ML, Catt KJ & Tsuruhara T (1971b) Retention of in vitro biological activities by desialylated human luteinizing hormone and chorionic gonadotropin. *Biochemical and Biophysical Research Communications* **44**: 1022–1029.

Dufau ML, Catt KJ & Tsuruhara T (1972) A sensitive gonadotropin response system: radioimmunoassay of testosterone production by the rat testis in vitro. *Endocrinology* **90**: 1032–1040.

Dufau ML, Mendelson CR & Catt KJ (1974) A highly sensitive in vitro bioassay for luteinizing hormone and chorionic gonadotropin: testosterone production by dispersed Leydig cell. *Journal of Clinical Endocrinology and Metabolism* **39**: 610–613.

Dufau ML, Pock R, Neubauer A & Catt KJ (1976a) In vitro bioassay of LH in human serum: the rat interstitial cell testosterone (RICT) assay. *Journal of Clinical Endocrinology and Metabolism* **42**: 958–969.

Dufau ML, Beitins IZ, McArthur JW & Catt KJ (1976b) Effects of luteinizing hormone releasing hormone (LHRH) upon bioactive and immunoreactive serum LH levels in normal subjects. *Journal of Clinical Endocrinology and Metabolism* **43**: 658–667.

Dufau ML, Beitins I, McArthur J & Catt KJ (1977a) Bioassay of serum LH concentration in normal and LHRH stimulated human subjects. In Troen P & Nankin HR (eds) *The Testis in Normal and Infertile Men*, pp 309–325, New York: Raven Press.

Dufau ML, Hodgen GD, Goodman AA & Catt KJ (1977b) Bioassay of circulating luteinizing hormone in the rhesus monkey: comparison with radioimmunoassay during physiological changes. *Endocrinology* **100**: 75–83.

Dufau ML, Nozu K, Dehejia A et al (1982) Biological activity and target cell actions of luteinizing hormone. In Motta M, Zanisi M & Piva F (eds) *Serono Symposium on Pituitary Hormones and Related Peptides*, pp 118–119. New York: Academic Press.

Dufau ML, Veldhuis JD, Fraioli F, Johnson ML & Beitins IZ (1983) Mode of bioactive luteinizing hormone secretion in man. *Journal of Clinical Endocrinology and Metabolism* **57**: 993–1000.

Evans RM, Doelle GC, Lindner J, Bradley V & Rubin D (1984) A luteinizing hormone-releasing hormone agonist decreases biological activity and modified chromatographic behaviour of luteinizing hormone in man. *Journal of Clinical Investigation* **73**: 262–266.

Fabbri A, Gnessi L, Moretti C et al (1986) Idiopathic impotence can be associated with low biological to immunological ratio (B/I) of LH in man. *Psychiatry Research* **16** (4) special supplement (abstract).

Gattuccio F, Bartolo GL, Orlando G & Janni A (1980) Hypogonadism in a male with immunologically active biologically inactive luteinizing hormone. *Acta Europaea Fertilitatis* **11**: 259–268.

Hattori M-A, Sakomato K & Wakabayashi K (1983) The presence of LH components having different ratios of bioactivity to radioimmunoactivity in rat pituitary gonads. *Endocrinologia Japonica* **30**: 289–295.

Kalra SP (1985) Neural circuits involved in the control of LHRH secretion a model for estrous cycle regulation. In Reddy PRK & Dufau ML (eds) Proceedings of the International Symposium on Gonadotrophin Releasing Hormone in Control of Fertility and Malignancy, pp 733–742. *Journal of Steroid Biochemistry* **23**: 5B.

Kalyan NK & Bahl OP (1981) Effect of deglycosylation on the subunit interactions and receptor binding activity of human chorionic gonadotropin. *Biochemical and Biophysical Research Communications* **102**: 1246–1253.

Keel BA & Grotjan HE (1985) Characterization of rat pituitary luteinizing hormone charge microheterogeneity in male and female rat using chromatofocusing: effects of castration. *Endocrinology* **117**: 354–359.

Kessler MJ, Miset, Ghai RD & Bahl, OP (1979) Structure and location of the O-glycosidic carbohydrate units of human chorionic gonadotropin. *Journal of Biological Chemistry* **254:** 7909–7914.

Kohler PO, Ross ET & Odell WD (1968) Metabolic clearance and production rates of human luteinizing hormone in pre and post-menopausal women. *Journal of Clinical Investigation* **47:** 38–44.

Kusuda S & Dufau ML (1986) Purification and characterization of gonadotropin receptors from rat ovary. *Journal of Biological Chemistry* **261:** 16161–16168.

Liu T & Jackson GL (1977) Effect of in vivo treatment with estrogen on luteinizing hormone synthesis and release by rat pituitaries in vitro. *Endocrinology* **100:** 1294–1302.

Loraine JA & Brown JB (1956) Further observations on the estimation of urinary gonadotropins in non-pregnant human subjects. *Journal of Clinical Endocrinology and Metabolism* **16:** 1180–1195.

Lucky AW, Rebar RW, Rosenfield RL, Roche-Bender N & Helke J (1979) Reduction of the potency of luteinizing hormone by estrogen. *New England Journal of Medicine* **300:** 1034–1036.

Lucky AW, Rich BH, Rosenfield RL, Fang VS & Roche-Bender N (1980a) LH bioactivity increases more than immunoreactivity during puberty. *Journal of Pediatrics* **97:** 205–213.

Lucky AW, Rich BH, Rosenfield RL, Fang VS & Roche-Bender N (1980b) Bioactive LH: a test to discriminate the precocious puberty from premature thelarche and adrenarche. *Journal of Pediatrics* **97:** 214–216.

McArthur GW, Ingersoll FM & Worcester, J (1958) Urinary excretion of interstitial-cell stimulating hormone by normal males and females of various ages. *Journal of Clinical Endocrinology and Metabolism* **18:** 460–469.

Manjunath P & Sairam MR (1982) Biochemical, biological, and immunological properties of chemically deglycosylated human choriogonadotropin. *Journal of Biological Chemistry* **257:** 7109–7115.

Marshall JC, Anderson DC, Frazer TR & Harsoulis P (1973) Human luteinizing hormone in man: studies of metabolism and biological action. *Journal of Endocrinology* **56:** 431–439.

Marut EL, Williams RF, Cowan BD et al (1981) Pulsatile pituitary gonadotropin secretion during maturation of the dominant follicle in monkeys. Estrogen positive feedback enhances biological activity of LH. *Endocrinology* **109:** 2270–2272.

Milius RP, Midgley ARJ & Birken S (1983) Preferential masking by the receptor of immunoreactive sites on the α-subunit. *Proceedings of the National Academy of Sciences (USA)* **80:** 7375–7379.

Moyle WR, Bahl OP & Marz L (1975) Role of the carbohydrate of human chorionic gonadotropin in the mechanism of hormone action. *Journal of Biological Chemistry* **250:** 9163–9169.

Nwokoro G, Chen H-C & Chrambach A (1981) Physical, biological and immunological characterization of highly purified urinary human chorionic gonadotropin components separated by gel electrofocusing studies. *Endocrinology* **108:** 291–295.

Parsons TF & Pierce JG (1980) Oligosaccharide moieties of glycoprotein hormones: bovine lutropin resists enzymatic deglycosylation because of terminal O-sulfate N-acetylhexosamine. *Proceedings of the National Academy of Sciences (USA)* **77:** 7089–7093.

Pepperell RJ, de Kretser DM & Burger HG (1975) Studies on the metabolic clearance rate and production rate of human luteinizing hormone and on the initial half-time of its subunits in man. *Journal of Clinical Investigation* **56:** 118–126.

Plourde PV, Dufau M, Plourde N & Santen RJ (1985) Impotence associated with low biological to immunological ratio of luteinizing hormone in a man with pituitary.stone. *Journal of Clinical Endocrinology and Metabolism* **60:** 797–802.

Raiti S, Foley TP, Penny R & Blizzard RM (1975) Measurement of the production rate of human luteinizing hormone using the urinary excretion technique. *Metabolism, Clinical and Experimental* **24:** 937–941.

Reiter EQ, Dufau ML, Root AW & Catt KJ (1978) Bioactive and immunoreactive serum LH in normal prepubertal and pubertal boys. *Pediatric Research* **12:** 330.

Reiter EO, Beitins IZ, Ostrea T & Gutai JP (1982) Bioassayable luteinizing hormone during childhood and adolescence and in patients with delayed pubertal development. *Journal of Clinical Endocrinology and Metabolism* **54:** 155–161.

Reiter EO, Brown RS, Longcope C & Beitins IZ (1984) Male-limited familial precocious puberty in three generations. *New England Journal of Medicine* **311**: 515–519.

Rich BH, Rosenfield RL, Moll GW Jr et al (1982) Bioactive luteinizing hormone pituitary reserves during normal and abnormal male puberty. *Journal of Clinical Endocrinology and Metabolism* **55**: 140–146.

Robertson DM, Van Damme MP & Diczfalusy E (1977) Biological and immunological characterization of human luteinizing hormone: 1. Biological profile in pituitary and plasma samples after electrofocusing. *Molecular and Cellular Endocrinology* **9**: 45–56.

Robertson DM, Fouls LM & Ellis S (1982) Heterogeneity of rat pituitary gonadotropins on electrofocusing differences between axes and after castration. *Endocrinology* **111**: 385–391.

Sairam MR & Fleshner P (1981) Inhibition of hormone-induced cyclic AMP production and steroidogenesis in interstitial cells by deglycosylated lutropin. *Molecular and Cellular Endocrinology* **22**: 41–54.

Sairam MR & Schiller PW (1979) Receptor binding, biological, and immunological properties of chemically deglycosylated pituitary lutropin. *Archives of Biochemistry and Biophysics* **197**: 294–301.

Sairam MR & Bhargavi GN (1985) A role for glycosylation of the α-subunit in transduction of biological signal in glycoprotein hormones. *Science* **229**: 65–67.

Solano AR, Dufau ML & Catt KJ (1979) Bioassay and radioimmunoassay of serum LH in the male rat. *Endocrinology* **105**: 372–381.

Solano AR, Garcia-Vela A, Catt KJ & Dufau ML (1980a) Modulation of serum and pituitary luteinizing hormone bioactivity by androgen in the rat. *Endocrinology* **106**: 1941–1948.

Solano AR, Garcia-Vela A, Catt KJ & Dufau ML (1980b) Regulation of ovarian gonadotropin receptors and LH bioactivity during the estrous cycle. *FEBS Letters* **122**: 184–188.

Swerdloff RS, Handelsman DJ & Bhasin S (1985) Hormonal effects of GnRH agonist in the human male: an approach to male contraception using combined androgen and GnRH agonist treatment. *Journal of Steroid Biochemistry* **23**: 855–861.

Tsuruhara T, Van Hall EV, Dufau ML & Catt KJ (1972a) Ovarian binding of intact and desialylated hCG in vivo and in vitro. *Endocrinology* **91**: 463–469.

Tsuruhara T, Dufau ML, Hickman J & Catt KJ (1972b) Biological properties of hCG after removal of terminal sialic acid and galactose residues. *Endocrinology* **91**: 296–301.

Van Damme M-P, Robertson DM & Diczfalusy E (1974) An improved in vitro bioassay method for measuring luteinizing hormone (LH) activity using mouse Leydig cell preparations. *Acta Endocrinologica* **77**: 655–671.

Van Hall EV, Vaitukaitis JL, Ross GT, Hickman JW & Ashwell G (1971) Immunological and biological activity of HCG following progressive desialylation. *Endocrinology* **89**: 11–15.

Veldhuis JD & Dufau ML (1986) Actions of estradiol on the pulsatile secretion of bioactive luteinizing hormone in man. *Transactions of Association of American Physicians* (in press).

Veldhuis JD, Rogol AD, Johnson ML & Dufau ML (1983) Endogenous opiates modulate the pulsatile secretion of biologically active luteinizing hormone in man. *Journal of Clinical Investigation* **72**: 2031–2040.

Veldhuis JD, Beitins IZ, Johnson ML, Serabian MA & Dufau ML (1984) Biologically active luteinizing hormone is secreted in episodic pulsations that vary in relation to stage of the menstrual cycle. *Journal of Clinical Endocrinology and Metabolism* **58**: 1050–1058.

Veldhuis JD, Rogol AD, Perez Palacios G et al (1985a) Endogenous opiates participate in the regulation of pulsatile luteinizing hormone release in unopposed estrogen milieu. *Journal of Clinical Endocrinology and Metabolism* **61**: 790–792.

Veldhuis JD, Sowers JR, Rogol AD, Klein FA & Dufau ML (1985b) Pathophysiology of a male hypogonadism associated with endogenous hyperestrogenism. *New England Journal of Medicine* **312**: 1371–1375.

Veldhuis JD, Fraioli F, Rogol AD & Dufau ML (1986) Metabolic clearance of biologically active luteinizing hormone in man. *Journal of Clinical Investigation*: **77**: 1122–1128.

Wakabayashi K (1977) Heterogeneity of rat luteinizing hormone revealed by radioimmuno-assay and electrofocusing studies. *Endocrinologia Japonica* **24**: 473–477.

Warner B, Worgul TJ, Diago LD et al (1983) Effect of very high dose D-Leu[6]-GnRH proethylamide on the hypothalamic–pituitary testicular axis as treatment of prostatic cancer. *Journal of Clinical Investigation* **71**: 1842–1853.

Warner BA, Dufau ML & Santen RJ (1985) Effects of aging and illness on the pituitary testicular axis in men: qualitative as well as quantitative changes in luteinizing hormone. *Journal of Clinical Endocrinology and Metabolism* **60:** 163–268.

Yen SSC, Iberena O, Little B & Pearson OH (1968) Disappearance rates of endogenous luteinizing hormone and chorionic gonadotropin in man. *Journal of Clinical Endocrinology and Metabolism* **28:** 1763–1768.

9

Oestrogen replacement therapy: physiological considerations and new applications

HOWARD L. JUDD

According to the Bureau of Census figures for 1980, there were 116 million women in the United States, of whom 32 million were 50 years of age or older. In the industrialized world, this segment of the population increases which each successive decade. Most of these older women have had or shortly will have their last menstrual period, thus becoming postmeno-pausal. There are also younger women who are without ovarian function. With ovarian failure, most women sustain a marked decrease of endogenous oestrogen production, resulting in a constellation of symptoms. Oestrogen replacement therapy can correct many of these, but its use is associated with a number of potentially harmful side-effects. Consequently, it is essential that physicians caring for older women understand the potential benefits and risks of this form of therapy. The following discussion will review these considerations.

CLIMACTERIC SYMPTOMS

Hot flushes

The most common and characteristic symptom of the climacteric is an episodic disturbance consisting of sudden flushing and perspiration, referred to as a 'hot flush' or 'hot flash'. It has been observed in 65–76% of meno-pausal women (Jaszmann et al, 1969; McKinlay and Jefferys, 1974). The severity and frequency of the symptom are variable. They can occur every 20 minutes or as infrequently as once or twice per month (Tataryn et al, 1981). Women with severe flushes have episodes approximately once per hour. Eighty per cent of those having hot flushes will experience the symptoms for longer than 1 year and 25–85% complain of episodes for longer than 5 years (Jaszmann et al, 1969; Thompson et al, 1973).

Measurable changes in physiological function accompany hot flushes supporting the physiological basis of the symptom (Figure 1). Cutaneous vasodilatation, perspiration, decreases in core temperature and increases in pulse rate have been recorded (Molnar, 1979; Tataryn et al, 1981). The cutaneous vasodilatation is generalized and not limited to the upper trunk

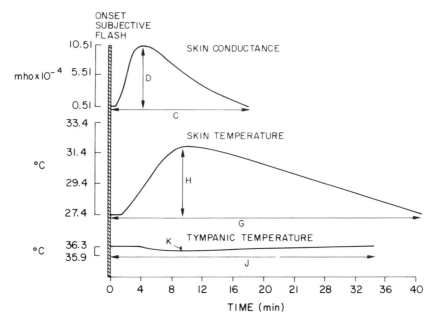

Figure 1. Mean changes in physiological functions associated with 25 menopausal hot flushes. From Tataryn et al (1980), with permission.

and head. Changes of heart rhythm or blood pressure have not been observed (Sturdee et al, 1978; Molnar, 1979).

These alterations in physiological function do not correspond identically to the perception of symptoms. Women first become conscious of symptoms approximately 1 minute after the onset of measurable cutaneous vaso-dilatation and discomfort persists for an average of 4 minutes, whereas physical changes continue for several minutes longer (Ginsberg et al, 1981; Tataryn et al, 1981).

The exact mechanism responsible for hot flushes is not known. Based on physiological and behavioural data, it would appear that the symptom is the result of a defect in central thermoregulatory function. This conclusion is based on several observations.

First, the two major physiological changes associated with hot flushes are the result of different peripheral sympathetic functions. Excitation of sweat glands is by sympathetic cholinergic fibres whereas cutaneous vasocon-striction is under the exclusive control of tonic α-adrenergic fibres. It is difficult to envision some peripheral event, resulting in cholinergic effects on sweat glands and α-adrenergic blockade of cutaneous vessels, but it is well recognized that these are the two basic mechanisms triggered by central thermoregulatory centres to lower core temperature.

Second, during a hot flush, central temperature decreases following cutaneous vasodilatation and perspiration. If hot flushes were the result of some peripheral event, then one would expect the body's regulatory mechanisms to prevent this decrease.

The third indication is the change in behaviour associated with the symptom. Women feel warm and have a conscious desire to cool themselves, by throwing off bedcovers, standing by open windows and doors, fanning themselves, etc. These perceptions occur in the absence of a preceding increase in central temperature.

An analogous dissociation between perception and central temperature is found at the onset of a fever, when the individual feels cold or a 'chill' prior to any change of central temperature. Most investigators working in the field of temperature regulation consider a fever to be the result of an elevation of the set point of central thermoregulatory centres, particularly those in the rostral hypothalamus (Kluger, 1978). A pyrogen elevates the central set point and the febrile organism actively raises the central body temperature, using both physiological (cutaneous vasoconstriction and shivering) and behavioural mechanisms (curling in a ball, putting on more clothes, drinking hot liquids, etc.) (Reynolds et al, 1974).

Based on these observations it is suggested that the climacteric hot flush is triggered by a sudden downward setting of central, hypothalamic thermostats. Subsequently, heat loss mechanisms are activated to bring the core temperature in line with the new set point resulting in the measured fall of core temperature.

Since hot flushes occur after cessation of ovarian function, it has been presumed that the underlying mechanism is endocrinological, and has something to do with either enhanced gonadotrophin secretion or reduced ovarian oestrogen secretion. Studies have now correlated the occurrence of the symptoms with the pulsatile release of luteinizing hormone (LH) from the pituitary (Casper et al, 1979; Tataryn et al, 1979) (Figure 2). Attempts

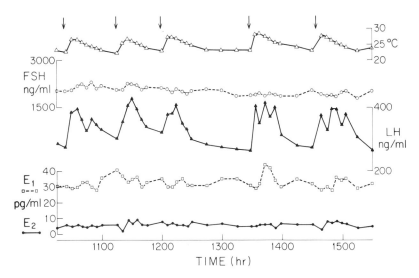

Figure 2. Serial measurements of finger temperature and serum FSH, LH, oestrone (E_1) and oestradiol (E_2) in a woman with severe hot flushes. Arrows mark occurrences of hot flushes. From Meldrum (1980), with permission.

have also been made to correlate symptoms with pulsatile follicle stimulating hormone (FSH) release with some finding and others not finding an association (Casper et al, 1979; Tataryn et al, 1979). This close temporal relationship suggests LH or the factors that initiate pulsatile LH release are involved with the triggering of these thermoregulatory events. LH or increased pituitary activity is not responsible, since hot flushes have been described in patients following surgical hypophysectomy with low gonadotrophin levels and no pulsatile release (Mulley et al, 1977; Meldrum et al, 1981) (Figure 3).

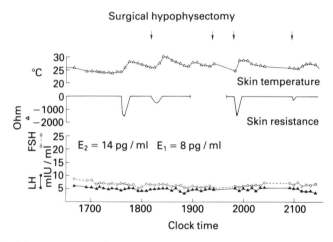

Figure 3. Serial measurements of skin temperature, skin resistance, and serum LH and FSH levels in a woman following partial resection, cryotherapy and radiation of chromophobe adenoma of the pituitary. Arrows mark onset of subjective flushes. From Meldrum et al (1981), with permission.

It is most likely that a suprapituitary mechanism initiates hot flushes and this is somehow influenced by the hypothalamic factors responsible for pulsatile LH release. In monkeys the hypothalamic site governing pulsatile release of LH from the pituitary is the arcuate nucleus through the pulsatile release of gonadotrophin releasing hormone (LH releasing hormone, LHRH) (Plant et al, 1978). Secretion of LHRH is governed by neurotransmitter input, including factors such as noradrenaline (norepinephrine), dopamine, endorphins and prostaglandins (Leblanc et al, 1976; Pang et al, 1977). Thus, LHRH or the neurotransmitters that influence its release may somehow alter the set point of the thermoregulatory centres to trigger hot flushes.

Patients with isolated gonadotrophin deficiency and anosmia (Kallman's syndrome) who have been treated previously with oestrogen replacement have been shown to have objectively measured hot flushes. As the gonadotrophic deficiency in these patients is secondary to absent LHRH release, it is likely LHRH itself is not involved in the hot flush mechanism.

Hypothalamic amenorrhoea is one model of ovarian inactivity that is consistently not accompanied by hot flushes. This syndrome is believed to occur because of alterations of neurotransmitter signals to the LHRH neurons. These data suggest hot flushes are triggered by changes of neuro-transmitter input to the LHRH neurons associated with the menopause. A likely candidate is noradrenaline which is known to be increased in the hyothalamus of castrate animals and has been shown to trigger thermo-regulatory episodes when injected into certain areas of the hypothalamus.

This symptom complex is a greater disturbance than most physicians have recognized. Patients experiencing flushes frequently complain of 'night sweats' and insomnia. Examination of these symptoms has shown a close temporal relationship between the occurrence of hot flushes and waking episodes (Erlik et al, 1981a) (Figure 4). In women with frequent flushes, the average occurrence rate of these symptoms and waking episodes is hourly, resulting in a profound sleep disturbance.

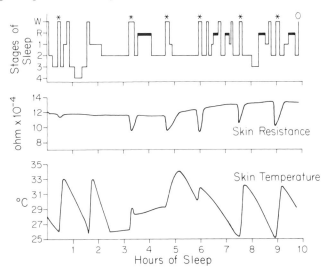

Figure 4. Sleepgram and recordings of skin resistance and temperature in postmenopausal subject with severe flushes. Each * marks the occurrence of an objectively measured hot flush. Open circle indicates arousal of patient by investigator at end of study. From Erlik et al (1981), with permission.

Because of the subjective nature of the complaint, it is not surprising that numerous agents have been used in an attempt to relieve the symptom and many are said to be effective. Adding to the confusion are observations of several investigative teams showing marked effects with placebo (Coope, 1976; Campbell and Whitehead, 1977). Studies showing a placebo action have usually quantitated the occurrence of flushes using subjective criteria. The use of objective measurements of flushes has by and large eliminated this apparent impact of placebo (Erlik et al, 1981b; Laufer et al, 1982).

Oestrogens are the principal medications utilized to relieve hot flushes. There are good randomized, prospective, double-blind, cross-over studies showing beneficial effects (Campbell and Whitehead, 1977) (Figure 5).

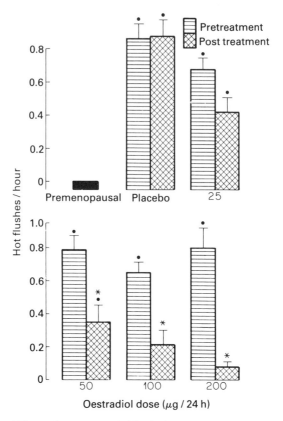

Figure 5. Mean ± SE rate of occurrence of objectively measured hot flushes in five groups of 10 subjects each given placebo and 25, 50, 100, and 200 μg/24 h of oestradiol by transdermal therapeutic systems. From Steingold et al (1985), with permission.

Oestrogens block both the subjective sensation and the physiological changes (Coope, 1976; Campbell and Whitehead, 1977; Tataryn et al, 1981). Daily doses of 0.625 mg of conjugated oestrogens or the equivalent can be effective. Higher doses may be required. Progestins are also effective (Erlik et al, 1981b), with daily doses such as 10–20 mg of medroxyprogesterone acetate being recommended. Clonidine, an α-adrenergic agonist, is partially effective, but at doses (0.2–0.4 mg) that result in frequent side-effects (Laufer et al, 1982). Propranolol, an α-adrenergic antagonist, is not more effective than placebo. Vitamins E and K, mineral supplements, belladonna alkaloids in combination with mild sedatives, tranquillizers, sedatives, and antidepressants have all been used but their efficacies have not been critically evaluated.

Osteoporosis

Osteoporosis is the single most important health hazard associated with the menopause. It has been estimated that 700 000 new fractures due to osteoporosis occur annually in America and cost more than $1 billion in health care yearly for acute care of these fractures (Owens et al, 1980).

Breaking strength of bone is linearly related to its mineral content, and when bone mass falls below a critical threshold level, non-traumatic fractures occur (Figure 6). On the basis of epidemiological data and x-ray appearances of bone, the 'fracture threshold' can be identified at bone mass values that are 1 standard deviation (SD) below the young normal mean in respect to distal forearm fractures and 2.5 SD below the young normal mean for femoral neck fractures (Newton-John and Morgan, 1968). The increased incidence of fractures that are age and sex related can be attributable to the progressive increase in the proportion of the population falling below these thresholds with advancing age.

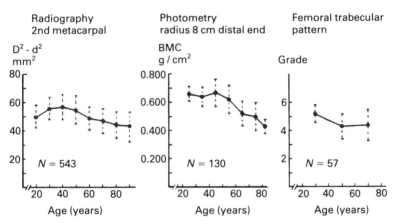

Figure 6. Patterns of bone changes with age in women as measured by radiography at the second metacarpal, by photometry at 8 cm from distal end of the radius, and by trabecular pattern grading at the upper end of the femur. From Dequeber et al (1975), with permission.

Bone mass is determined by two factors, the level of bone mass achieved at skeletal maturity and the rate of bone loss with age. Variance of initial bone density explains in part racial and sexual differences in the occurrence of osteoporotic fractures with white women having the lightest skeletons and black men the heaviest; white men and black women are intermediate (Trotter et al, 1960).

Age-related bone loss is two- to three-fold greater in women than men (Riggs et al, 1982a). This loss is accentuated by the cessation of ovarian function, which is a particular problem in women who have been castrated at an early age or have gonadal dysgenesis. Thus, women are more likely to sustain fractures due to osteoporosis. Cross-sectional studies indicate that one-third of white women in the northern United States sustain a hip fracture by the ninth decade of life (Gallagher et al, 1980a). There is a 10-fold increase of Colles' fractures in women aged 35–65 years, whereas a similar increase is not seen in men (Knowelden et al, 1964) (Figure 7). Over 200 000 women in the USA sustain hip fractures annually (Gordan and

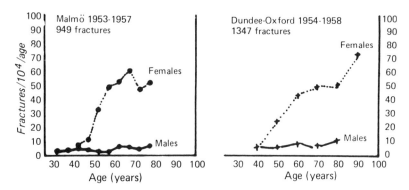

Figure 7. Incidence of Colles' fracture in relation to age in Malmö, Dundee, and Oxford. From Cope (1976), with permission.

Vaughan, 1982). Mortality due to these fractures reaches 12% in the 4–5 months following injury. This represents the number one cause of accidental deaths in women over the age of 75, and falls are the tenth leading cause of death of women in this country (National Safety Council, 1982).

The mechanisms responsible for enhanced bone loss with the menopause have not been completely defined. Initially, it was suggested to be due to decreased bone formation (Albright et al, 1941). Controversy continues on whether osteoporosis results from an absolute increase in bone resorption or an absolute decrease in bone formation. Discrepant results probably can be explained by differences in and limitations of methodologies for assessing bone turnover and also the heterogeneity of the disease. Nevertheless, all studies, regardless of the methodology employed, have shown that bone resorption exceeds formation in osteoporotic patients.

The onset of bone loss is associated with slight rises in plasma calcium, phosphate and alkaline phosphatase concentrations as well as urinary calcium and hydroxyproline (Crilly et al, 1981). The transient increase of serum calcium decreases parathyroid hormone (PTH) secretion. Both the decreased serum PTH and the resultant increase in serum phosphate lower the rate of $1,25(OH)_2$ cholecalciferol production and, thus, reduce calcium absorption from the gut (Gallagher et al, 1979). Low serum PTH also reduces renal tubal reabsorption of calcium. Both decreased calcium absorption from the gut and increased calcium loss through the kidney normalize serum calcium. Thus, serum calcium is maintained but more by bone loss than by absorbed dietary calcium.

PTH plays a central role in the genesis of osteoporosis. It is the principal hormone which stimulates bone resorption. In animal and human studies, osteoporosis does not develop in its absence (Houssain et al, 1970). Measurements of PTH in patients with osteoporotic fractures have shown normal or low levels in the great majority (Gallagher et al, 1980b). This suggests that bone becomes more sensitive to PTH after the menopause.

Reduction of ovarian oestrogen production also plays a key role. This is supported by the measurement of increased bone loss with discontinuation of ovarian function and reductions in parameters of bone resorption with oestrogen replacement (Figure 8). Currently, it is hypothesized that oestrogen decreases the sensitivity of bone to PTH, and the fall of oestrogen at the menopause results in the acceleration of bone loss. The mechanisms by which oestrogen accomplishes this are not clear. In vivo animal studies have shown oestrogens do indeed decrease the effect of PTH on bone (Gallagher and Williamson, 1973), but in vitro data are not as convincing (Atkins et al, 1972). These latter observations are supported by the inability of investigators to document the presence of oestrogen receptors in bone (Chen and Feldman, 1978). Thus, one of the most important questions in the prevention of osteoporosis is what is the mechanism by which oestrogen exerts its action.

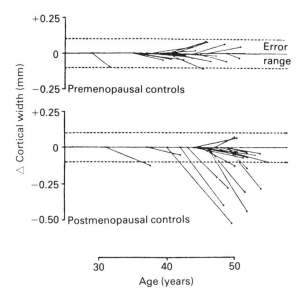

Figure 8. Changes in metacarpal cortical width, as determined by sequential measurements in pre- and postmenopausal women. From Nordin et al (1975), with permission.

A possibility is its effect on the secretion of calcitonin, a potent inhibitor of bone resorption. Calcitonin levels and secretion are lower in women than men, and decrease with age in both sexes (Deftos et al, 1980). After age 50, the response of calcitonin secretion to calcium challenge is negligible. Oestrogen administration enhances calcitonin secretion in both animals and humans (Morimoto et al, 1980). Thus, increased secretion of calcitonin could inhibit calcium loss from bone and possibly prevent the development of osteoporosis.

Several studies indicate low-dose oestrogen therapy can arrest or retard bone loss if begun shortly after the menopause (Figure 9). This effect continues for at least 10 years (Lindsay et al, 1980). The lowest dosage that is effective in most older women is 0.625 mg of conjugated oestrogens or its

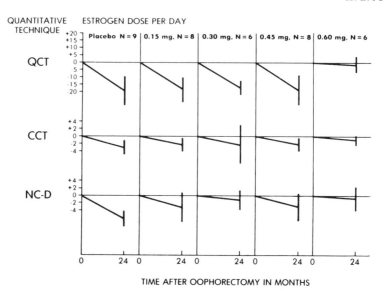

Figure 9. Mean ± SE percentage bone mineral loss at 24 months is shown as a function of different doses of conjugated estrogens. QCT = quantitative computed tomography; CCT = combined cortical thickness; NCD = Norland–Cameron densitometry. From Genant et al (1982), with permission.

equivalent (Genant et al, 1982). Oestrogen therapy also reduces the incidence of fracture. Calcium supplements are said to inhibit bone loss (Recker et al, 1977), but critical studies to address this await publication. Calcium should be given in combination with vitamin D in patients with malabsorption. Doses of elemental calcium of 1000–1500 mg/day are believed to be necessary for this purpose. Administration of vitamin D or its metabolites alone is not successful, possibly because of the bone-resorbing action of these agents. Progestins also appear to have a beneficial effect, but need more thorough evaluation (Lindsay et al, 1978). Small doses of calcitonin combined with calcium administration have resulted in increased total body calcium during the first 24 months of therapy but not thereafter (Jowsey et al, 1978). To date, histological studies of bone have failed to confirm this (Milhaud et al, 1975). Sodium fluoride increases trabecular bone volume, and in high doses may reduce the vertebral fracture rate (Riggs et al, 1982b). Its use has generally been in combination with large doses of vitamin D and calcium which makes the beneficial effects of fluoride difficult to assess. Fluoride also has toxic side-effects at the doses studied. Anabolic steroids have been widely used, and may also be effective, but are associated with severe androgenic symptoms in some patients.

In summary, a growing list of publications indicates that the menopause and the associated reduction of endogenous oestrogens play major roles in the development of osteoporosis in older women. The mechanisms by which oestrogens exert this action have not been defined. Osteoporosis remains responsible for the most serious complication known to result from the loss of ovarian function and represents a major reason to contemplate replacement therapy.

Cardiovascular

In general, the incidence of death from coronary heart disease increases with age in all populations and both sexes. In the United States, cardiovascular disease is the leading cause of death in men and women (World Health Organization, 1980). Cardiovascular disease is less prevalent in women than men before the age of 55, with the chance of a man dying of a heart attack being 5–10 times greater than for a woman before this age (Furman, 1973). The ratio falls off dramatically somewhere between the ages of 55 and 65, and reaches unity in the ninth decade. A closer look at the statistics reveals that the mortality figures among women, when plotted against age, give essentially a curve of steady slope as it passes through the age of the menopause; and it is rather the change in slope of the male curve at this age that results eventually in both curves coinciding.

Two types of studies have been utilized to determine whether cessation of ovarian function is associated with an increased incidence of heart disease. The first type is the examination of the relationship between the menopause and carefully defined cardiovascular disease within the context of an entire population. In Sweden, systematic samples from cohorts of women were examined and classified on the basis of past history of myocardial infarction, angina pectoris and electrocardiographic evidence of ischaemic heart disease (Bengtsson, 1973). The cases found were observed to have undergone an earlier menopause than their cohorts. The Framingham study reported the results of biennial examinations for 24 years on nearly 3000 women (Gordon et al, 1978). These data revealed that, indeed, there was an increased incidence of heart disease in women following the menopause that was not just age-related. The impact of the menopause was substantial, relatively abrupt and augmented afterwards only slowly, if at all. It was unusual to see heart disease in premenopausal women, and when present the disease was usually mild, being just angina pectoris. Other investigators assessed the risk of non-fatal myocardial infarction among groups of American nurses (Rosenberg et al, 1981). Risks were found to be inversely related to age of natural menopause and especially to age of surgical menopause. Women undergoing oophorectomy before the age of 35 had greater than seven times the risk than nurses with intact ovaries.

The second type of study has been case-control studies comparing the degree of coronary heart disease or the incidence of myocardial infarction in women who have undergone early castration with age-matched controls who still had ovarian function (Roberts and Giraldo, 1979). Some of these studies found an increased risk of cardiovascular disease in the castrated subjects. Most reports have been criticized for inadequate numbers of study subjects, imprecise methods for assessing heart disease, or patient selection bias, particularly the controls.

In addition to there being supportive evidence that the menopause is associated with an increased incidence of heart disease, there is a growing list of papers suggesting oestrogen replacement is protective against this type of disease. Again, two types of studies have been performed to support this concept. The first is case-control studies which have been hospital-based or have used the general population as a comparison group (Jick et al, 1978). For the former, relative risk of heart disease in oestrogen users has ranged from 4.2 to 0.6 (Rosenberg et al, 1976; Jick et al, 1978; Adam et al, 1981; Szklo et al, 1984). Results from this type of study are difficult to interpret because oestrogen use may be associated either directly or inversely with diseases or injuries leading to hospitalization. Use of the general population as a comparison group tends to avoid this problem, and the relative risk of heart disease in oestrogen users has always been less than 1 (Pfeffer et al, 1978; Bain et al, 1981; Ross et al, 1981). The second type of study has been prospective follow-up studies in which data on hormone use were obtained before the development of coronary disease (Burch et al, 1974; Gordon et al, 1978; Hammond et al, 1979; Nachtigall et al, 1979; Petitti et al, 1979; Bush et al, 1983; Criqui et al, 1984; Wilson et al, 1984; Paganini-Hill et al, 1985). Six of these nine studies have shown a substantial protective effect of oestrogen against non-fatal myocardial infarction and death due to coronary heart disease. Although none of these studies used a randomized study design, multivariant analysis of known risk factors of coronary disease has failed to show confounding in any of these studies.

One plausible explanation for this protective effect on the development of heart disease is the favourable influence of oestrogens on serum lipid levels. Cross-sectional and prospective studies have demonstrated that oestrogens tend to improve the serum lipid profile by lowering low-density lipoprotein (LDL) and raising the protective high-density lipoprotein (HDL) cholesterol. However, in the Lipid Research Clinics study, adjustment for lipid levels explained only part of the protective effect, suggesting that other mechanisms may also be involved, perhaps alterations in connective tissue or prostaglandins. At least part of the effect seems to be short-acting as the benefits were largely limited to current users, and no effect of duration has been observed.

If a relationship between oestrogen usage and decreased risk of heart disease is correct, it would be consistent with trends in mortality rates. Menopausal oestrogen usage has been widespread in the USA since the early 1960s. Mortality rates from ischaemic heart disease began to decline in white women in this country at the same time, and by 1976 had decreased by over 30%, at a time when rates in white men decreased by almost 20% (US Department of Health, Education and Welfare, 1979). The decrease among men was accompanied by a 26% decline in the proportion of cigarette smokers in the male population, whereas the reduction among women was only 8%.

Since the age-adjusted death rates from heart disease in white women are four times the combined death rates of breast and endometrial cancer, any protective effect of oestrogen replacement on heart disease would far outweigh the carcinogenic effects of this hormone. Clarification of this association is anxiously awaited.

Skin

With ageing, noticeable changes of the skin occur. There is gradual thinning and atrophy, which are more pronounced in areas exposed to light. Wrinkling is seen and attributed to degeneration of elastic and collagenous fibres caused by solar radiation (Punnoven, 1972). There is thinning of the epidermis in old age and the basal layer becomes even. Dehydration and vascular sclerosis are also present to varying degrees. Atrophy of sudoriferous and sebaceous glands with decreased activity is present. According to some investigators these changes begin by age 30, and intensify between 40 and 50 years of age.

Very few studies have been performed to isolate the effect of menopause from ageing on human skin. Several investigators have shown decreased uptake of radiolabelled thymidine (a marker of mitosis) and decreased thickness of the skin following oophorectomy, but appropriate surgical controls were not evaluated (Punnoven, 1972; Rauramo, 1976). More work is clearly needed in this area.

Oestrogen has effects on skin. Using skin from animal and human models, investigators have shown the hormone increases skin thickness, hyaluronic acid and water content, vascularization and tritiated thymidine uptake, and synthesis, maturation and turnover of collagen (Shahrad and Marks, 1976). It also reduces the size and activity of sebaceous glands and the rate of hair growth. It should be noted that some studies have not confirmed these biological actions.

These effects are likely due to direct actions of the hormone on skin elements. Oestrogen receptors have been identified in skin of humans and laboratory animals. In mice, the receptors are localized to specific elements of skin including fibroblasts in the dermis and nuclei of basal cell layers of perineal skin, but not skin from other areas of the body (Stumpf et al, 1974). In humans, high affinity, low capacity, oestrogen-specific binding has been identified (receptor) (Hasselquist et al, 1980). The amount of receptor is highest in facial followed by breast and thigh skins. The number of receptors per cell is considerably lower than other hormone responsive tissues. This may be due to localization of receptors in only a few elements of skin as observed with laboratory animals. Studies are awaited to define this.

A few investigators have examined the effects of oestrogen on skin in vivo (Goldzieher, 1946; Punnoven, 1972; Rauramo, 1976; Shahrad and Marks, 1976). Most of these studies have been troubled by inadequate controls, non-specific changes, or inconsistent results. Thus, a compelling body of data does not exist that shows a beneficial effect of oestrogen on the integument.

Psychological

Several studies have shown an increase in psychological complaints at the time of the menopause (Ballinger, 1975; Bungay et al, 1980). There is an associated increase in consultations for emotional problems and enhanced use of psychotropic drugs (Skegg et al, 1977). Psychological symptoms tend to be maximal just preceding the menopause with the frequency declining during the 1 or 2 years after the cessation of menses. This rise does not appear to be associated with an enhanced occurrence of severe psychiatric illness (Weissman and Klermann, 1977).

There are two physiological alterations related to the menopause which impact on psychological function, and could explain in part the increase of psychological complaints at the climacteric. As mentioned previously, hot flushes occur in a close temporal relationship with waking episodes resulting in a chronic sleep disturbance (Erlik et al, 1981a). Such a disturbance can lead to alterations of psychological function including both cognitive and affective elements. The impact of this on the rate of psychological complaints in perimenopausal women needs to be determined.

Vaginal atrophy can also impact on psychological function. At the time of the menopause, there is an apparent decrease in sexual interest in a majority of women. This decline is not seen in all women with some reporting increased interest, at least temporarily. Vaginal atrophy impacts on sexual interest by its influence on vaginal dryness and dyspareunia. With more prolonged oestrogen deficiency the vaginal epithelium becomes atrophic, there is narrowing and shortening of the vaginal canal, and the thinned epithelium is susceptible to trauma. These all lead to complaints of dyspareunia, resulting in a decline in sexual enjoyment and interest, and impacting on psychological function.

Whether the menopause alters psychological function by mechanisms other than those related to hot flushes and vaginal atrophy is not clear. In the future, investigators will need to control carefully for the confounding effects of these two variables, in order to answer this question.

The influence of oestrogen replacement on psychological symptoms also is not established, and again is influenced by the confounding variables of hot flushes and vaginal atrophy. Oestrogen replacement clearly diminishes the occurrence of hot flushes and improves certain aspects of sleep in comparison to placebo (Campbell and Whitehead, 1977; Erlik et al, 1981a). Beneficial effects include decreases in insomnia, sleep latency and the number and duration of episodes of wakefulness, and increases in length of sleep and the amount of rapid eye movement sleep (Schiff et al, 1979). These actions are different from those observed with most hypnotic agents which reduce both sleep latency and the time of rapid eye movement sleep (Kales et al, 1975). These improvements of sleep presumably explain the measurable improvements of memory, and decreases of anxiety and irritability which occur with oestrogen administration in women with severe flushes (Campbell and Whitehead, 1977).

Oestrogen replacement also diminishes the symptoms of vaginal atrophy leading to improved sexual enjoyment and interest. Whether oestrogen influences other aspects of female sexuality is far less clear. Controlled studies of oestrogen treatment of perimenopausal women have not found an effect on sexuality other than improving vaginal lubrication (Campbell and Whitehead, 1977). Two studies of oophorectomized women have produced conflicting results with one showing no effect on libido whereas the other found oestrogens enhanced the women's sexual interest and enjoyment (Utian, 1972; Dennerstein et al, 1981).

Does oestrogen have mood-elevating effects, other than those exerted by reducing hot flushes or improving vaginal lubrication? Carefully controlled studies will be necessary to answer this question. If oestrogen does, it may exert effects on cerebral function through actions on indoleamine metabolism. Reduced levels of 5-hydroxytryptamine (serotonin) and 5-hydroxy-indoleacetic acid in the brain may lead to depression (Ridges, 1975). Indirect evidence indicates that the rate-limiting step in the synthesis of brain 5-hydroxytryptamine is the concentration of L-tryptophan in the brain (Jequier et al, 1969). Increased availability of tryptophan to the brain could conceivably influence brain function. Most plasma tryptophan is not readily available to the brain because it is bound to albumin (McMenamy and Oncley, 1958). Oestrogen displaces tryptophan from binding sites on albumin which could increase availability of this amino acid to the brain (Aylward, 1976). The validity of this biochemical hypothesis remains uncertain.

COMPLICATIONS OF OESTROGEN REPLACEMENT

Endometrial cancer

Several lines of evidence have examined the possible relationship of oestrogen replacement and the development of endometrial cancer. Although the findings made by each research approach continue to have detractors, the scope of these investigative efforts and the consistent incrimination of oestrogen, leads one to the conclusion that oestrogen stimulation of the endometrium, unopposed by progesterone, leads to endometrial proliferation and hyperplastic and neoplastic transformations of this tissue. The following reviews some of the approaches used to establish this hypothesis.

Endocrinological studies have shown evidence that peripheral conversion of androstenedione to oestrone and subsequently oestradiol is the major source of circulating oestrogens in postmenopausal women (MacDonald et al, 1978; Judd et al, 1982). This conversion is enhanced by several factors, particularly obesity. These observations provide explanations for several hitherto unexplained epidemiological observations, such as the association between obesity and the occurrence of this tumour.

Histological studies have shown the apparent progression of endometrial proliferation from normal to hyperplasia to neoplasia (Gusberg and Kaplan, 1963). The coexistence of hyperplasia and adenocarcinoma of the endometrium has also been described. Opposed to this view are observations showing that endometrial hyperplasia frequently does not accompany adenocarcinoma, and, to date, no one has observed transformation of a specific area of hyperplasia into adenocarcinoma.

Animal studies have not been particularly helpful in studying endometrial cancer since good models of the tumour have been difficult to identify. Older studies in rabbits showed oestrogen administration induced more frequent and earlier carcinomas. Recently, similar and more convincing inductions have been demonstrated using a mouse system (Papadaki et al, 1979).

Biochemical studies have shown that doses of oestrogens used for replacement therapy (0.625 and 1.25 mg conjugated oestrogens) induce growth of endometrial glands and enhance oestrogen receptor content to values equivalent to or greater than those seen during the proliferative phase of the menstrual cycle. This establishes that replacement dosages are clearly able to promote endometrial proliferation (Whitehead et al, 1981). These studies have not addressed the issue of progression to neoplastic growth.

Incidence studies have generally shown increased occurrence of this tumour in several areas of the United States during the 1970s, after many years of relative stability (Weiss et al, 1976; Austin et al, 1979). These increases have been observed particularly in middle-aged women and have been most prominent in white women of high socioeconomic status. Some studies have shown the increase to be confined to localized disease, whereas other investigators have reported no change in the proportion of cases diagnosed in localized or more advanced stages. This enhanced incidence has not been associated with widespread increases in mortality due to this tumour.

The enhanced rate of occurrence has been correlated with a corresponding increase in oestrogen usage. As documented by the Department of Commerce records, the dollar value of oestrogen shipments tripled from 1965 to 1974, only part of which could be accounted for by inflation (US Department of Commerce, 1962–1977). More recent reports indicate a decline in oestrogen usage of 20% from 1975 to 1977 (Jick et al, 1979). A corresponding drop in the incidence of endometrial cancer was also reported.

The enhanced incidence of endometrial cancer could be accounted for by other variables such as changes in case-finding techniques, diagnostic practices and/or fads, and terminology preferences. Of particular concern is that oestrogen usage promotes vaginal bleeding, and one would expect more diagnostic procedures to be used in women taking the medication. Biopsies of oestrogen-stimulated endometrium may result in more false positive diagnoses of endometrial cancer since oestrogen-stimulated endometrial hyperplasia can appear similar microscopically to adenocarcinoma.

Although plausible, the above factors are unlikely to explain all of the recent increase in the occurrence of this tumour. The observations that the increase was in specific groups of women only and in many geographical areas make it unlikely that it is a spurious increase due to case-finding techniques. Changes in terminology preferences is also unlikely, since no alterations in the distribution of diagnostic terminologies have been reported by some authors. Overdiagnosis of oestrogen-stimulated endometrium does appear to inflate current rates. Histological review of cases in the northwest found the rates to be inflated 20% by inclusion of non-malignant hyperplasias (Szekely et al, 1978). However, overdiagnosis accounts for only a minority of the cases observed and is unlikely to be responsible for all of the reported increases in incidence rates.

The studies that have attracted the most attention have been the more than 20 epidemiological reports examining the possible association between oestrogen replacement and endometrial carcinoma (Shapiro et al, 1980). In most, strong associations were found. Overall risk ratios between 2- and 8-fold were reported. Factors contributing to risk included high dosage, and/or prolonged use. The disease found was primarily local, although clearly invasive tumours were observed.

Numerous questions have been raised about these studies, including verification of cases and controls, confirmations of subsequent data, susceptibility bias, retroactive alteration of research hypothesis and detection bias (Horwitz and Feinstein, 1978). Several of these questions have been answered by later studies.

For the studies not showing an association, criticisms have also been raised. These have included small sample size, and very low levels and/or short durations of oestrogen usage. Of particular concern has been the obscuring of possible differences between the cases and controls by the use of controls who themselves had experienced high levels of past oestrogen usage, i.e. all controls had undergone a dilatation and curettage (D&C) which substantiated the absence of disease (Horwitz and Feinstein, 1978).

This issue is of importance to all of the epidemiology studies reported. What is the incidence of endometrial cancer in asymptomatic women? If low, then the necessity of histological examination of the endometrium in asymptomatic controls is not required and use of controls who have undergone a D&C could indeed obscure possible differences in oestrogen usage. If, however, the incidence of silent disease is high, then use of controls whose endometrium has not been evaluated histologically would be unacceptable. Recently, an attempt was made to determine the level of silent disease using autopsy records (Horwitz and Feinstein, 1981). The investigators found that only 44% of all the endometrial cancers observed in the women studied were diagnosed during their lifetime. This report has been questioned because the rate of diagnosis of endometrial cancer during the lifetime of the women studied was very low (2/1000) (Merletti and Cole, 1981). Based on other data, the reviewers of this article suggested that 80–90% of all endometrial tumours are diagnosed during life, and the percentage of undiagnosed cancer is small (10–20%). These latter figures would not support the necessity of restricting controls only to women who had undergone endometrial sampling.

In summary, each line of investigation has repeatedly incriminated constant oestrogen exposure of the endometrium, unopposed by progesterone, as a risk factor for endometrial cancer. Although debates still persist among investigators, a prudent physician should be sufficiently persuaded by the consistent linkage to notify his patient of this probability and undertake steps to prevent it.

A growing body of information now indicates that the addition of progestin therapy to oestrogen replacement lowers the incidence of hyperplastic and neoplastic transformation of the endometrium. Prospective studies from England have shown 15–30% incidences of endometrial hyperplasia in postmenopausal women receiving oestrogen therapy alone with up to one-third having the more sinister atypical pattern, which in its more severe forms is a recognized precursor of corpus cancer (King et al, 1979). These studies and others have shown that the addition of a progestin on a monthly basis reduces the incidence of both carcinoma and hyperplasia (Gambrell, 1978). The incidence of carcinoma in patients receiving oestrogen plus progestin may be less than in subjects receiving no hormonal therapy (Gambrell, 1978). The duration of progestin therapy appears to be critical with the incidence of hyperplasia being 3–4% with 7 days and 0% with 12 days of administration each month (King et al, 1979). Dosage may also be critical. For the 19-norprogestins, DL-norgestrel and norethisterone (norethindrone *USP*), the lowest protective doses are 150 µg and 0.7 µg, respectively (Whitehead et al, 1981). For the C_{21} progestins, such as medroxyprogesterone acetate, the 10 mg dosage is the lowest dosage that is completely protective.

The mechanisms by which progestins oppose the action of oestrogen on the endometrium are elaborate. Withdrawal of oestrogen and progestin support leads to shedding of endometrial tissue. Not only do progestins induce a more complete shedding, but they can also reverse various degrees of hyperplasia to normal (King et al, 1979). However, monthly shedding is not required for protection (King et al, 1979). Progestins also reduce the number of oestrogen receptors in endometrial cells, in both the cytoplasm and nucleus (Whitehead et al, 1981). These agents block oestrogen-induced DNA and RNA synthesis, and alter intracellular enzymes which metabolize oestradiol, the predominant intranuclear oestrogen (Clarke et al, 1982). Oestradiol dehydrogenase and oestrogen sulphotransferase are induced by progestins. The first converts oestradiol to oestrone (a less potent oestrogen) and the second forms sulphated conjugates. This results in rapid elimination of oestrone from endometrial tissue as oestrone sulphate.

It should be recognized that long term usage of progestins may result in its own set of problems. Thus, its use in women without a uterus should not be encouraged. It is known that progestin reduces or eliminates the favourable responses of HDL and LDL cholesterol to oestrogens.

BREAST CANCER

The breast cancer risk factors of early age at menarche and delayed age at menopause have long been known. Early oophorectomy has also been recognized to be strongly protective for this disease. These observations indicate that ovarian activity is an important determinant of risk of this cancer and suggest a critical role for oestrogens. This is strongly supported by findings in the extensive studies of the role of oestrogens in the occurrence of mammary tumours of rodents (International Agency for Research on Cancer, 1979).

Early studies of the possible effects of oestrogen replacement therapy on the risk of breast cancer were largely uncontrolled follow-up studies, which suffered from methodological problems making interpretation difficult. Women treated in two large gynaecological practices appeared to experience a small excess incidence of breast cancer, but in one study there were serious methodological irregularities and both used convenient population-based breast cancer rates for a source of expectation (Burch et al, 1975; Hoover et al, 1976).

A number of case-control studies were performed in this country in the early 1970s (Sartwell et al, 1977). None found an unequivocal association between breast cancer and oestrogen usage, or adequately resolved the methodological difficulties inherent in examining this relationship. These two factors are linked in several important ways (age at menopause, presence of oophorectomy, etc.) whether or not they are linked aetiologically.

More recently, six case-control studies have been reported that overcome some of the methodological difficulties of earlier studies (Hulka et al, 1982). Three of these used healthy population control subjects and found mild increases in breast cancer risks. Another, using a self-referring healthy population as a control, found an increased overall risk only among women with a history of oophorectomy, while another report described an increased risk for women with intact ovaries who received high doses of oestrogen. A fifth, using both hospital and community control subjects, found an overall increased risk for women with a natural menopause. When women who received oestrogen by injection were excluded, the risk estimates were not significant. A final study done as carefully as those just described but employing only hospital controls, showed no association between oestrogen usage and an increased risk of breast cancer.

These inconsistencies cannot be resolved at present. Additionally, the overall risk ratios for oestrogen usage in breast cancer patients are small, and frequently are statistically significant only in certain subsets of patients. Although this potential relationship remains one of the most important issues surrounding hormone replacement, it continues to be unresolved.

Liver

Sex steroids have profound effects on hepatic function. Alterations of hepatic protein and lipid metabolism can lead to various other side-effects. The following is a review of some of these problems.

Hypertension

Hypertension may occur or be exacerbated in women receiving oestrogen replacement therapy (Stern et al, 1976). The elevation of blood pressure is usually reversible when the medication is discontinued. The problem is seen less frequently with oestrogen replacement therapy than with use of oral contraceptives. Although increases of blood pressure have been reported, oestrogen replacement therapy has not been associated with an enhanced risk of cerebral vascular accidents (Pfeffer, 1978).

The mechanism responsible for this increase in blood pressure is believed to be related to the renin–angiotensin–aldosterone system (Laragh et al, 1967). Renin substrate is the rate-limiting step of the renin reaction under physiological conditions (Weir et al, 1917). Oestrogen administration stimulates the hepatic synthesis of this protein (Figure 10). Associated with this are increases of angiotensin I, and aldosterone secretion (Laragh et al, 1967).

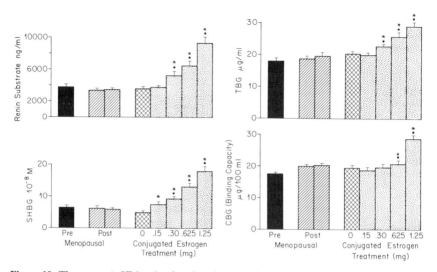

Figure 10. The mean ± SE levels of renin substrate, thyroxine-binding globulin (TBG), sex hormone-binding globulin (SHBG) and cortisol-binding globulin (CBG) in premenopausal women and postmenopausal subjects given placebo or different doses of conjugated oestrogens. From Geola et al (1980), with permission.

Although all women who take a sufficient dosage of oestrogen have increases in renin substrate levels, only a small percentage develop hypertension. There is also no difference in the absolute circulating levels of renin substrate in women with oestrogen-induced hypertension and normotensive women receiving equal doses of the hormone (Eggena et al, 1981). Oestrogen replacement therapy induces synthesis and release of several forms of renin substrate, which are electrophoretically and immunologically distinct from the predominant form of this plasma protein (Eggena et al, 1968). A large molecular weight form (> 150 000) has a greater affinity for the enzyme renin than the predominant form. This large form increases in women with oestrogen-induced hypertension, but not in normotensive subjects on the same dosage of oestrogen (Shionoiri et al, 1983). These data suggest that the composition of renin substrate induced by oestrogen replacement therapy may play an important role in the induction of hypertension in some women on this form of therapy.

Thromboembolic disease

The administration of oral contraceptives increases the risk of overt venous thromboembolic disease and the occurrence of subclinical thrombosis that is extensive enough to be detected by laboratory procedures, such as ^{125}I-labelled fibrinogen uptake (Sagar, et al, 1976) and plasma fibrinogen chromatography (Alkjaersig et al, 1975). In uncontrolled studies thrombophlebitis has been reported with oestrogen replacement therapy, whereas this association has not been present in controlled experiments (Boston Collaborative Drug Surveillance Program, 1974).

Both procoagulant and anticoagulant factors are present in blood to maintain its fluidity while permitting haemostasis with vascular injury. Oestrogen exerts several effects on the clotting mechanism, which may contribute to or be responsible for a generalized hypercoagulable state. The factors influenced include increased vascular endothelial proliferation, decreased venous blood flow, and an increase in the coagulability of blood involving changes in the platelet, coagulation and fibrinolytic systems (Stadel, 1981). Some investigators have reported decreases in platelet counts with oestrogen. Evaluation of clotting factors have shown increases of factors VII, IX, X and X complex (Von Kaulla et al, 1975; Bonnar et al, 1976). These factors are hepatic in origin. Oestrogen replacement therapy can also lower anticoagulant factors such as antithrombin III and anti-Xa (Bonnar et al, 1976). The former is of particular interest. It is also hepatic in origin and inactivates thrombin, activated factor X, and other enzymes involved with the generation of thrombin. The potential importance of a reduction of antithrombin III during oestrogen replacement therapy is suggested by the occurrence of thrombophilia in subjects with a congenital deficiency (Egeberg, 1965). A reduction of 20% or more has been found to be highly predictive of the occurrence of subclinical venous thromboembolic disease that is extensive enough to be detected by ^{125}I-labelled fibrinogen uptake (Stamatakis et al, 1977). Administration of mestranol (up to 0.5 mg/day) has been shown to lower antithrombin III activity by 11% after 2 months, whereas ingestion of conjugated oestrogens (1.25 mg/day) was found to have no effect (Bonnar et al, 1976). This difference presumably reflects differences in dosage since 0.5 mg of mestranol should be equivalent to approximately 5 mg of conjugated oestrogens. This suggests that usual replacement doses of conjugated oestrogen (<1.25 mg/day) should not affect antithrombin III activity, and may also explain the lack of documentation of an increased risk of thromboembolic disease with oestrogen replacement therapy.

The fibrinolytic system is also influenced by oestrogen. This system involves the conversion of plasminogen to plasmin, an enzyme that degrades fibrin and fibrinogen (Stadel, 1981). This conversion is initiated by plasminogen activators released by endothelial cells. Studies in patients with venous or arterial thromboembolic disease have generally found spontaneous fibrolytic activity in blood to be subnormal (Stadel, 1981). The administration of oestrogen increases spontaneous fibrinolytic activity and the fibrinolytic response to venous occlusion. Fibrin degradation products also increase in the circulation with oestrogen replacement therapy (Stadel, 1981). These effects are accompanied by a reduction in circulating plasminogen and the plasminogen activator content of endothelium. Increased fibrinolytic activity with oestrogen administration probably represents increased release of plasminogen activators from endothelium in response to increased intravascular coagulation.

All studies have not shown effects of oestrogen replacement therapy on the above clotting parameters. The differences in findings may result from the fact that different oestrogen preparations were evaluated. The relative potencies of these preparations are being defined at present. Until this is accomplished, it will be difficult to determine if discrepancies between studies are due to methodological problems, variable effects of the different types of oestrogen preparations on clotting parameters, or different potencies of the preparations.

Lipids

Oestrogen replacement therapy also influences hepatic lipid metabolism. An increased incidence of gall bladder disease has been reported with oral contraceptive usage and oestrogen replacement therapy (Boston Collaborative Drug Surveillance Program, 1974; Honore, 1980). Because bile saturation of cholesterol is between 75% and 90%, small increases of cholesterol in bile can initiate precipitation leading to stone formation. Increased amounts of cholesterol in bile is a common finding in gall bladder disease. Oestrogen replacement therapy increases the cholesterol fraction of bile (Sagar et al, 1976). Proposed mechanisms for this include increased turnover of body cholesterol and increased hepatic synthesis. Cholesterol synthesis is regulated by the enzyme hydroxymethylglutamyl-CoA reductase, which is inhibited by chenodeoxycholate. A decrease of chenodeoxycholate and an increase of cholate occur in bile of women on oestrogen replacement therapy (Heuman et al, 1979), which may explain the increase of cholesterol in bile.

As mentioned previously, circulating lipids are also influenced by oestrogen replacement therapy. Decreases of LDL, reductions or no changes of cholesterol and very low density lipoproteins, and increases of HDL and triglycerides (Wahl et al, 1983) being associated with oestrogen usage.

In patients with familial defects of lipoprotein metabolism, oestrogen replacement therapy has been associated with massive elevations of plasma triglycerides, which have led to pancreatitis and other complications (Glueck et al, 1972). The effects of oestrogen on circulating lipids are also believed to be related to changes in hepatic synthesis, although altered clearance of these substances may be involved.

Route of administration

Oral administration of oestrogens is associated with enhanced hepatic effects as compared with other systemic sites of action (Geola et al, 1980; Mandel et al, 1982) (Figure 10). To date, the mechanism responsible for these enhanced actions has been ascribed to a so-called 'first pass' effect of orally administered oestrogens on hepatocytes (Geola et al, 1980). According to this concept, ingested hormones are absorbed by the intestines, delivered directly to the liver through the portal vein, exert actions on hepatic functions and undergo partial metabolism to less active forms before entry into the general circulation.

If this concept is correct, then administration of oestrogens by non-oral routes should reduce if not eliminate these enhanced hepatic effects. However, studies to compare the effects of oestrogens administered by oral and non-oral routes have not revealed consistent responses. Oestradiol (E_2)

(Thom et al, 1978), but not conjugated equine oestrogens (CE) (Mandel et al, 1983) or ethinyloestradiol (EE) (Goebelsmann et al, 1985), administered by mouth has been shown to elicit similar reductions of gonadotrophin levels but greater actions on hepatic protein and lipid metabolism than those induced by the non-oral application of the hormone. The failure to alter the relative potencies of CE and EE on hepatic compared with non-hepatic functions with the use of a non-oral route of administration indicates that the 'first pass' mechanism is not the sole explanation for the exaggerated responses of the liver to oestrogen administration.

Using an in vivo rat model, recent studies indicate the exit from the circulation of all major types of oestrogens used for replacement therapy is much greater into the liver than into two other important organs of oestrogen action, the brain and uterus (Steingold et al, 1986) (Figure 11).

The data may help explain the apparent dichotomy of effects of CE and EE as opposed to E_2 on hepatic as compared to non-hepatic markers of oestrogen action when the preparations are given orally versus systemically. The major oestrogen in CE is oestrone sulphate (E_1-S). Based on these in vivo studies, very little circulating E_1-S is available to the brain or uterus. E_1-S also does not interact with the oestrogen receptor (Brooks et al, 1978). It is possible the small amount of E_1-S that crosses the blood–brain barrier is converted to unconjugated oestrogens locally and these could have function. More likely the major mechanism by which E_1-S suppresses LHRH release is through conversion to unconjugated oestrogens, principally E_1

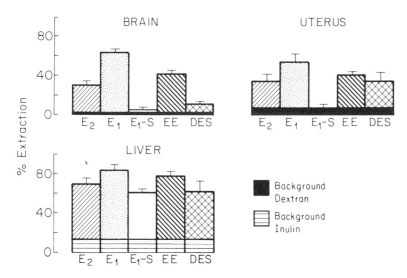

Figure 11. The mean ($\pm$ SE) tissue extractions (percentage) by the brain, uterus and liver of [^{3}H]oestrone (E_1), oestradiol (E_2), oestrone sulphate (E_1-S), ethinyloestradiol (EE), and stilboestrol (diethylstilbestrol *USP*, DES) from postmenopausal serum relative to that of [^{14}C]butanol. The background values of dextran for the brain and uterus and inulin for the liver correspond to non-specific isotope remaining 15 s after injection in the brain and uterus and 18 s after injection in liver capillaries, respectively. From Steingold et al (1986), with permission.

and E_2, in the liver (Pardridge and Landaw, 1984). The large extraction of E_1-S by the liver allows accessibility of the hepatocyte for this conversion. Based on this concept, CE must enter the liver to be converted to its active forms. The route of administration then should have little impact on changing the relative potency of this preparation on hepatic and non-hepatic markers of oestrogen action.

For EE, the preparation is orally active because it is rapidly and almost completely absorbed from the stomach and undergoes limited hepatic metabolism before entry into the general circulation (Helton and Goldzieher, 1977). This limited hepatic metabolism should reduce if not eliminate the impact of the so-called 'first pass' mechanism of orally administered EE. Thus, the major explanation for enhanced hepatic action of EE is the increased influx of the hormone into the liver compared to non-hepatic sites of action.

For E_2, the oral preparation undergoes substantial hepatic metabolism to less active forms, principally oestrogen conjugates (Spona and Schneider, 1977). The amount of E_2 leaving the liver following oral administration is substantially less than that which enters it through the portal vein. The systemic administration of E_2 avoids this initial hepatic metabolism and this reduces the exaggerated hepatic responses in comparison to non-hepatic actions (Fahraeus and Wallentin, 1983). Use of transcutaneous administration of E_2 appears to come closest to reproducing ovarian function.

SUMMARY

The total impact of the menopause on the health of women and the ultimate benefit/risk ratio of oestrogen replacement therapy are yet to be defined completely. Until these are accomplished, broad general guidelines for the use of oestrogen replacement therapy in all patients cannot be given. Treatment should be individualized to the patient's specific needs. Use of appropriate dosages of oestrogen in combination with progestin administration should reduce risk and enhance benefits for those subjects requiring its use. The development of new non-oral methods of administration should also help.

Acknowledgements

I would like to thank Drs E. Barrett-Connor, L. L. Judd, M. C. Pike, and B. L. Riggs for review of and suggestions about specific sections of this manuscript.
Supported in part by USPHS Grants CA 23093 and RR 865.

REFERENCES

Adam S, Williams V & Vessey MP (1981) Cardiovascular disease and hormone replacement treatment: a pilot case–control study. *British Medical Journal* **282:** 1277–1278.
Albright F, Smith PH & Richardson AM (1941) Postmenopausal osteoporosis. *Journal of the American Medical Association* **116:** 2465–2474.

Alkjaersig N, Fletcher A & Burstein R (1975) Association between oral contraceptive use and thromboembolism: a new approach to its investigation based on plasma fibrinogen chromatography. *American Journal of Obstetrics and Gynecology* **122:** 199–211.

Atkins D, Zanelli JM, Peacock M & Nordin BEC (1972) The effect of oestrogens on the response of bone to parathyroid hormone in vitro. *Journal of Endocrinology* **54:** 107–117.

Austin DF, King M & Roe K (1979) Cancer incidence trends in white women in the San Francisco Bay area. *National Cancer Institute Monographs* **53:** 95–101.

Aylward M (1976) Estrogens, plasma tryptophan levels in perimenopausal patients. In Campbell S (ed.) *The Management of the Menopause and the Postmenopausal Years*, pp 135–140. Lancaster: MTP Press.

Bain C, Willett W, Hennekens CH et al (1981) Use of postmenopausal hormones and risk of myocardial infarction. *Circulation* **64:** 42–46.

Ballinger CB (1975) Psychiatric morbidity and the menopause: screening of a general population sample. *British Medical Journal* **3:** 344–346.

Bengtsson C (1973) Ischemic heart disease in women. *Acta Medica Scandinavica, Supplementum* **549:** 75–81.

Bonnar J, Haddon M, Hunter DH, Richards DH & Thornton C (1976) Coagulation system changes in postmenopausal women receiving oestrogen preparations. *Postgraduate Medical Journal* **52**(supplement 6): 30–34.

Boston Collaborative Drug Surveillance Program (1974) Surgically confirmed gallbladder disease, venous thromboembolism, and breast tumors in relation to postmenopausal estrogen therapy. *New England Journal of Medicine* **290:** 15–19.

Brooks SC, Rozhin J, Pack BA et al (1978) Role of sulphate conjugation in estrogen metabolism and activity. *Journal of Toxicology and Environmental Health* **4:** 283–290.

Bungay GT, Vessey MP & McPherson CK (1980) Study of symptoms in the middle life with special reference to the menopause. *British Medical Journal* **281:** 181–183.

Burch JC, Byrd BF & Vaughn WK (1974) The effects of long-term estrogen on hysterectomized women. *American Journal of Obstetrics and Gynecology* **118:** 778–782.

Burch JC, Byrd BF & Vaughn WK (1975) The effects of long-term estrogen administrated to women following hysterectomy: estrogens in the post-menopause. *Frontiers of Hormone Research* **3:** 208–214.

Bush T, Cowan LD, Barrett-Connor E et al (1983) Estrogen use and all-cause mortality: preliminary results from the Lipid Research Clinics Program follow-up study. *Journal of the American Medical Association* **249:** 903–906.

Campbell S & Whitehead M (1977) Estrogen therapy and the postmenopausal syndrome. *Clinics in Obstetrics and Gynaecology* **4:** 31–47.

Casper RF, Yen SSC & Wilkes MM (1979) Menopausal flushes: a neuroendocrine link with pulsatile luteinizing hormone secretion. *Science* **205:** 823–825.

Chen TL & Feldman D (1978) Distinction between alpha-fetoprotein and intracellular estrogen receptors: evidence against the presence of estradiol receptors in bone. *Endocrinology* **102:** 236–242.

Clarke CL, Adams JB & Wren BG (1982) Induction of estrogen sulfotransferase in the human endometrium by progesterone in organ culture. *Journal of Clinical Endocrinology and Metabolism* **55:** 70–75.

Coope J (1976) Double-blind cross-over study of estrogen replacement therapy. In Campbell S (ed.) *The Management of the Menopause and Postmenopausal Years*, pp 159–168. Lancaster: MTP Press.

Cope E (1976) Physical changes associated with postmenopausal years. In Campbell S (ed.) *Management of the Menopause and Postmenopausal Years*, p 4. Lancaster: MTP Press.

Crilly RG, Francis RM & Nordin BEC (1981) Ageing, steroid hormones and bone. *Clinics in Endocrinology and Metabolism* **10:** 115–139.

Criqui M, Suarez L, Barrett-Connor E, Wingard D & Garland C (1984) Postmenopausal estrogen use and mortality: a prospective study. *American Journal of Epidemiology* **120:** 466. (abstract).

Deftos LJ, Weisman MH, Williams GW et al (1980) Influence of age and sex on plasma calcitonin in human beings. *New England Journal of Medicine* **302:** 1351–1353.

Dennerstein L, Burrows GD, Wood C & Hyman G (1981) Hormones and sexuality: the effects of estrogen and progestogen. *Obstetrics and Gynecology* **56:** 316–322.

Dequeber J et al (1975) Aging of bone: its relation to osteoporosis and osteoarthritis in postmenopausal women. *Frontiers of Hormone Research* **3**: 116.

Egeberg O (1965) Inherited antithrombin deficiency causing thrombophilia. *Thrombosis et Diathesis Haemorrhagica* **15**: 516–530.

Eggena P, Hidaka H, Barrett JD & Sambhi MP (1968) Multiple forms of human plasma renin substrate. *Journal of Clinical Investigation* **62**: 367–372.

Eggena P, Barrett JD, Shioniori H et al (1981) The influence of estrogens on plasma renin substrate. In Sambhi MP (ed.) *Heterogeneity of Renin and Renin Substance*, pp 256–260. New York: Elsevier.

Erlik Y, Tataryn IV, Meldrum DR et al (1981a) Association of waking episodes with menopausal hot flushes. *Journal of the American Medical Association* **245**: 1741–1744.

Erlik Y, Meldrum DR, Lagasse LD & Judd HL (1981b) Effect of megestrol acetate on flushing and bone metabolism in postmenopausal women. *Maturitas* **3**: 167–172.

Fahraeus L & Wallentin L (1983) High density lipoprotein subfractions during oral and cutaneous administration of 17 β-estradiol to menopausal women. *Journal of Clinical Endocrinology and Metabolism* **56**: 797–803.

Furman RH (1973) Coronary heart disease and the menopause: menopause and aging. In Ryan KJ & Gibson DC (eds) *Menopause and Aging: Summary Report and Selected Papers from a Research Conference on Menopause and Aging.* DHEW Publication No. (NIH) 73-319, pp 39–55. Washington DC: US Government Printing Office.

Gallagher JC & Williamson R (1973) Effect of ethinyl estradiol on calcium and phosphorus metabolism in postmenopausal women with primary hyperparathyroidism. *Clinical Science and Molecular Medicine* **45**: 785–802.

Gallagher JC, Riggs BL, Eisman J et al (1979) Intestinal calcium absorption and serum vitamin D metabolites in normal subjects and osteoporotic patients: effective age and dietary calcium. *Journal of Clinical Investigation* **64**: 729–736.

Gallagher JC, Melton LJ, Riggs BL & Bergstralh E (1980a) Epidemiology of fractures of the proximal femur. *Clinical Orthopaedics* **150**: 163–171.

Gallagher JC, Riggs BL, Jerpbak CM & Arnaud CD (1980b) The effect of age on serum immunoreactive parathyroid hormone in normal and osteoporotic women. *Journal of Laboratory and Clinical Medicine* **95**: 373–385.

Gambrell RD Jr (1978) The prevention of endometrial cancer in postmenopausal women with progestogens. *Maturitas* **1**: 107–112.

Genant HK, Cann C, Ettinger B & Gordan GS (1982) Quantitative computed tomography of vertebral spongiosa: a sensitive method for detecting early bone loss after oophorectomy. *Annals of Internal Medicine* **97**: 699–705.

Geola FL, Frumar AM, Tataryn IV et al (1980) Biological effects of various doses of conjugated equine estrogens in postmenopausal women. *Journal of Clinical Endocrinology and Metabolism* **51**: 620–625.

Ginsberg J, Swinhoe J & O'Reilly B (1981) Cardiovascular responses during menopausal hot flush. *British Journal of Obstetrics and Gynaecology* **88**: 925–930.

Glueck CJ, Scheel D, Fishback J & Steiner P (1972) Estrogen-induced pancreatitis in patients with previously covert familial type V hyperlipoproteinemia. *Metabolism* **21**: 657–666.

Goebelsmann U, Mashchak CA & Mishell DR Jr (1985) Comparison of hepatic impact of oral and vaginal administration of ethinyl estradiol. *American Journal of Obstetrics and Gynecology* **151**: 868–874.

Goldzieher J (1946) The direct effect of steroids on the senile human skin. *Journal of Gerontology* **1**: 104–112.

Gordan GS & Vaughan C (1982) Sex steroids in the clinical management of osteoporosis. *Current Problems in Obstetrics and Gynecology* **V**: 6–45.

Gordon T, Kannel WB, Hjortland MC & McNamara PM (1978) Menopause and coronary heart disease: the Framingham study. *Annals of Internal Medicine* **89**: 157–161.

Gusberg SB & Kaplan AL (1963) Precursors of corpus cancer. IV. Adenomatous hyperplasia as Stage 0 carcinoma of the endometrium. *Journal of Obstetrics and Gynecology* **87**: 662–678.

Hammond CB, Jelovsek FR, Lee KL, Creasman WT & Parker RT (1979) Effects of long-term estrogen replacement therapy. I. Metabolic effects. *American Journal of Obstetrics and Gynecology* **133**: 525–536.

Hasselquist MG, Goldberg N, Schroeter A & Spelsberg TC (1980) Isolation and characterization of the estrogen receptor in human skin. *Journal of Clinical Endocrinology and*

Metabolism **50:** 76–82.

Helton ED & Goldzieher JW (1977) The pharmacokinetics of ethinyl esti **15:** 255–282.

Heuman R, Larsson-Cohn U, Hammar M & Tiselius HG (1979) Effects ethinyl estradiol treatment on gallbladder bile. *Maturitas* **2:** 69–72.

Honore LH (1980) Increased incidence of symptomatic cholesterol chc menopausal women receiving estrogen replacement therapy: a rei *Journal of Reproductive Medicine* **25:** 187–190.

Hoover R, Gray LA, Cole P & MacMahon B (1976) Menopausal estrogens ai *New England Journal of Medicine* **295:** 401–405.

Horwitz RI & Feinstein AR (1978) Alternative analytic methods for case-co .uies of estrogens and endometrial cancer. *New England Journal of Medicine* **229:** 1089–1094.

Horwitz RI & Feinstein AR (1981) Necropsy diagnosis of endometrial cancer and detection-bias in case/control studies. *Lancet* **ii:** 66–68.

Houssain M, Smith DA & Nordin BEC (1970) Parathyroid activity and postmenopausal osteoporosis. *Lancet* **i:** 809–811.

Hulka BS, Chambless LE, Deubner DC & Wilkinson WE (1982) Breast cancer and estrogen replacement therapy. *American Journal of Obstetrics and Gynecology* **143:** 638–644.

International Agency for Research on Cancer (1979) Sex Hormones (II). *IARC Monographs on the Evaluation of Carcinogenic Risk of Chemicals to Humans* **21.**

Jaszmann L, Van Lith ND & Zaat JCA (1969) The perimenopausal symptoms. *Medical Gynaecology, Andrology, and Sociology* **4:** 268–276.

Jequier E, Robinson DS, Levenberg W & Sjverdsma A (1969) Tryptophan-5-hydroxylase activity and brain tryptophan metabolism. *Biochemical Pharmacology* **18:** 1071–1081.

Jick H, Dinan B & Rothman KJ (1978) Noncontraceptive estrogens and nonfatal myocardial infarction. *Journal of the American Medical Association* **240:** 2548–2552.

Jick H, Watkins RN, Hunter JR et al (1979) Replacement estrogens and endometrial cancer. *New England Journal of Medicine* **300:** 218–222.

Jowsey J, Riggs BL, Kelly PJ & Hoffman DL (1978) Calcium and salmon calcitonin in treatment of osteoporosis. *Journal of Clinical Endocrinology and Metabolism* **47:** 633–639.

Judd HL, Shamonki IM, Frumar AM & Lagasse LD (1982) Origin of serum estradiol in postmenopausal women. *Obstetrics and Gynecology* **59:** 680–686.

Kales A, Kales JD, Bixler EO & Scharf MB (1975) Effectiveness of hypnotic drugs with prolonged use: flurozepan and pentobarbital. *Clinical Pharmacology and Therapeutics* **18:** 356–363.

King RJB, Whitehead MI, Campbell S & Minardi J (1979) Effect of estrogen and progestin treatments on endometria from postmenopausal women. *Cancer Research* **39:** 1094–1101.

Kluger MJ (1978) The evolution and adaptive value of fever. *Annals of Science* **66:** 38–43.

Knowelden J, Buhr AJ & Dunbar O (1964) Incidence of fractures in persons over 35 years of age. *British Journal of Preventive and Social Medicine* **18:** 130–141.

Laragh JH, Sealey JE, Ledingham JG & Newton MA (1967) Oral contraceptives: renin, aldosterone and high blood pressure. *Journal of the American Medical Association* **201:** 918–922.

Laufer LR, Erlik Y, Meldrum DR & Judd HL (1982) Effect of clonidine on hot flashes in postmenopausal women. *Obstetrics and Gynecology* **60:** 583–586.

Leblanc H, Lachelin GCL, Abu-Fadil S & Yen SSC (1976) Effects of dopamine agonists on LH release in women. *Journal of Clinical Endocrinology and Metabolism* **44:** 728–732.

Lindsay R, Hart DM, Purdie D et al (1978) Comparative effects of oestrogen and a progestogen on bone loss in postmenopausal women. *Clinical Science and Molecular Medicine* **54:** 193–195.

Lindsay R, Hart DM, Forrest C & Baird C (1980) Prevention of spinal osteoporosis in oophorectomized women. *Lancet* **ii:** 1151–1154.

MacDonald PC, Edman CD, Hemsell DL, Porter JC & Siiteri PK (1978) Effect of obesity on conversion of plasma androstenedione to estrone in postmenopausal women with and without endometrial cancer. *American Journal of Obstetrics and Gynecology* **130:** 448–455.

Mandel FP, Geola FL, Lu JKH et al (1982) Biological effects of various doses of ethinyl estradiol in postmenopausal women. *Obstetrics and Gynecology* **59:** 673–679.

Mandel FP, Geola FL, Meldrum DR et al (1983) Biological effects of various doses of vaginally ministered conjugated equine estrogens in postmenopausal women. *Journal of Clinical Endocrinology and Metabolism* **57:** 133–139.

McKinlay S & Jefferys M (1974) The menopausal syndrome. *British Journal of Preventive and Social Medicine* **28:** 108–115.

McMenamy RH & Oncley JL (1958) Specific binding of L-tryptophan to serum albumin. *Journal of Biological Chemistry* **233:** 1436–1447.

Meldrum DR (1980) Gonadotropins, estrogens, and adrenal steroids during the menopausal hot flash. *Journal of Clinical Endocrinology and Metabolism* **50:** 687.

Meldrum DR, Erlik Y, Lu JHK & Judd HL (1981) Objectively recorded hot flashes in patients with pituitary insufficiency. *Journal of Clinical Endocrinology and Metabolism* **52:** 684–687.

Merletti F & Cole P (1981) Detection bias and endometrial cancer. *Lancet* **ii:** 579–580.

Milhaud G, Talbot JN & Coutris G (1975) Calcitonin treatment of postmenopausal osteoporosis: evaluation of efficacy by principal components analysis. *Biomedicine* **22:** 223–232.

Molnar GW (1979) Investigation of hot flashes by ambulatory monitoring. *American Journal of Physiology* **237:** R306–310.

Morimoto S, Tsuji M, Okada Y, Onishi T & Kumahara Y (1980) The effect of oestrogens on human calcitonin secretion after calcium infusion in elderly female subjects. *Clinical Endocrinology* **13:** 135–143.

Mulley G, Mitchell JRA & Tattersall RB (1977) Hot flushes after hypophysectomy. *British Medical Journal* **ii:** 1062.

Nachtigall LE, Machtigall RH, Machtigall RD & Beckman EM (1979) Estrogen replacement therapy II: a prospective study in the relationship to carcinoma and cardiovascular and metabolic problems. *Obstetrics and Gynecology* **54:** 74–79.

National Safety Council (1982) *Accident Facts.* Chicago, Illinois.

Newton-John HF & Morgan DB (1968) Osteoporosis disease or senescence? *Lancet* **i:** 232–233.

Nordin BEC et al (1975) Post-menopausal osteopenia and osteoporosis. *Frontiers of Hormone Research* **3:** 131.

Owens RA, Melton LJ III, Gallagher JC & Riggs BL (1980) National cost of acute case of hip fractures associated with osteoporosis. *Clinical Orthopaedics* **150:** 172–176.

Paganini-Hill A, Ross RK & Henderson BE (1985) Protection from acute myocardial infarction among users of estrogen replacement therapy. *American Journal of Epidemiology* **122:** 512 (abstract).

Pang CN, Zimmerman E & Sawyer CH (1977) Morphine inhibition of the preovulatory surges of plasma luteinizing hormone and follicle stimulating hormone in the rat. *Endocrinology* **101:** 1726–1732.

Papadaki L, Balby OW, Chowaviec J et al (1979) Hormone replacement therapy in the menopause: a suitable animal model. *Journal of Endocrinology* **83:** 67–77.

Pardridge WM & Landaw EM (1984) Tracer kinetic model of blood–brain barrier transport of plasma protein-bound ligands. Empiric testing of the free hormone hypothesis. *Journal of Clinical Investigation* **74:** 745–752.

Petitti DB, Wingerd J, Pellegrin F & Ramcharan S (1979) Risk of vascular disease in women: smoking, oral contraceptives, noncontraceptive estrogens, and other factors. *Journal of the American Medical Association* **242:** 1150–1154.

Pfeffer RI (1978) Estrogen use, hypertension and stroke in postmenopausal women. *Journal of Chronic Diseases* **31:** 389–399.

Pfeffer TI, Whipple GH, Kurosaki TT & Chapman JM (1978) Coronary risk and estrogen use in postmenopausal women. *American Journal of Epidemiology* **107:** 479–487.

Plant TM, Krey LC, Moossy J et al (1978) The arcuate nucleus and the control of gonadotropin and prolactin secretion in the female rhesus monkey. *Endocrinology* **102:** 52–62.

Punnoven R (1972) Effect of castration and peroral estrogen therapy on the skin. *Acta Obstetrica et Gynecologica Scandinavica Supplement* **21**(5): 1–44.

Rauramo L (1976) Effect of castration and peroral estradiol valerate and estriol succinate therapy on the epidermis. In Campbell S (ed.) *The Management of the Menopause and Postmenopausal Years*, pp 253–262. Lancaster: MTP Press.

Recker RR, Saville PD & Heaney RP (1977) Effect of estrogens and calcium carbonate on bone loss in postmenopausal women. *Annals of Internal Medicine* **87:** 649–655.

Reynolds WW, Casterlin ME & Covert JB (1974) Behavioral fever in teleost fishes. *Nature* **259:** 41–42.

Ridges AP (1975) Biochemistry of depression: a review. *Journal of International Medical Research Supplement* **3**(2): 42–54.

Riggs BL, Wahner HW, Seeman E et al (1982a) Changes in bone mineral density of the proximal femur and spine with aging: differences between the postmenopausal and senile osteoporosis syndrome. *Journal of Clinical Investigation* **70**: 716–723.

Riggs BL, Seeman E, Hodgson SF, Taves DR & O'Fallon WM (1982b) Effect of fluoride/calcium regimen on vertebral fracture occurrence in postmenopausal osteoporosis. *New England Journal of Medicine* **306**: 446–450.

Roberts WC & Giraldo AA (1979) Bilateral oophorectomy in menstruating women and accelerated coronary atherosclerosis: an unproved connection. *American Journal of Medicine* **67**: 363–365.

Rosenberg L, Armstrong B & Jick H (1976) Myocardial infarction and estrogen therapy in post-menopausal women. *New England Journal of Medicine* **194**: 1256–1259.

Rosenberg L, Hennekens CH, Rosner B et al (1981) Early menopause and the risk of myocardial infarction. *American Journal of Obstetrics and Gynecology* **139**: 47–51.

Ross RK, Paganini-Hill A, Mack TM, Arthur M & Henderson BE (1981) Menopausal oestrogen therapy and protection from death from ischaemic heart disease. *Lancet* **i**: 858–860.

Sagar S, Stamatakis JD, Thomas DP & Kakkar VV (1976) Oral contraceptives, antithrombin III activity, and postoperative deep-vein thrombosis. *Lancet* **i**: 509–511.

Sartwell PE, Arthes FG & Tonascia JA (1977) Exogenous hormones, reproductive history and breast cancer. *Journal of the National Cancer Institute* **59**: 1589–1592.

Schiff I, Regestein Q, Tulchinsky D & Ryan KJ (1979) Effects of estrogens on sleep and psychological state of hypogonadal women. *Journal of the American Medical Association* **242**: 2405–2407.

Schwenk M, López Del Pino V & Bolt HM (1979) The kinetics of hepatocellular transport and metabolism of estrogens (comparison between estrone sulphate, estrone and ethinyl estradiol). *Journal of Steroid Biochemistry* **10**: 37–42.

Shahrad P & Marks R (1976) The effects of estrogens on the skin. In Campbell S (ed.) *The Management of the Menopause and Postmenopausal Years*, pp 243–251. Lancaster: MTP Press.

Shapiro S, Kaufman DW, Slone D et al (1980) Recent and past use of conjugated estrogens in relation to adenocarcinoma of the endometrium. *New England Journal of Medicine* **303**: 485–489.

Shionoiri H, Eggena P, Barrett JD et al (1983) An increase in high molecular weight renin substrate associated with estrogenic hypertension. *Biochemical Medicine* **29**: 14–22.

Skegg DC, Doll R & Perry J (1977) Use of medicine in general practice. *British Medical Journal* **i**: 1561–1563.

Spona J & Schneider WHF (1977) Bioavailability of natural estrogens in young females with secondary amenorrhea. *Acta Obstetricia et Gynecologica Scandinavica Supplement* **65**: 33–40.

Stadel BV (1981) Oral contraceptives and cardiovascular disease. *New England Journal of Medicine* **305**: 612–618.

Steingold KA et al (1985) Treatment of hot flashes with transdermal estradiol administration. *Journal of Clinical Endocrinology and Metabolism* **61**: 630.

Steingold KA, Cefalu W, Pardridge W, Judd HL & Chaudhuri G (1986) Enhanced hepatic extraction of estrogens used for replacement therapy. *Journal of Clinical Endocrinology and Metabolism* **62**: 761–766.

Stern MP, Brown BW, Haskell WL et al (1976) Cardiovascular risk and use of estrogens or estrogen–progestagen combinations. *Journal of the American Medical Association* **235**: 811–815.

Stumpf WE, Sar M & Joshi SG (1974) Estrogens target cells in the skin. *Experientia* **30**: 196–198.

Sturdee DW, Wilson KA, Pipili E & Crocker AD (1978) Physiological aspects of menopausal hot flush. *British Medical Journal* **ii**: 79–80.

Szekely DR, Weiss NS & Schweid AI (1978) Incidence of endometrial carcinoma in King County, Washington: a standardized histologic review. Brief Communication. *Journal of the National Cancer Institute* **60**: 985–989.

Szklo M, Tonascia J, Gordis L & Bloom I (1984) Estrogen use and myocardial infarction risk: a case-control study. *Preventive Medicine* **13**: 510–516.

Tataryn IV, Lomax P, Meldrum DR et al (1981) Objective techniques for the assessment of postmenopausal hot flashes. *Obstetrics and Gynecology* **57**: 340–344.

Tataryn IV, Meldrum DR, Lu KH, Frumar AM & Judd HL (1979) LH, FSH, and skin temperature during the menopausal hot flash. *Journal of Clinical Endocrinology and Metabolism* **49**: 152–154.

Tataryn IV et al (1980) Postmenopausal hot flushes: a disorder of thermoregulation. *Maturitas* **2**: 104.

Thom M, Dubiel M, Kakkar VV & Studd JWW (1978) The effect of different regimens of estrogen on the clotting and fibrinolytic system of the post-menopausal woman. *Frontiers of Hormone Research* **5**: 192–199.

Thompson B, Hart SA, Durno D (1973) Menopausal age and symptomatology in general practice. *Journal of Biological Sciences* **5**: 71–82.

Trotter M, Broman GE & Peterson RR (1960) Densities of bones of white and negro skeletons. *Journal of Bone and Joint Surgery* **42A**: 50–58.

U.S. Department of Commerce, Bureau of the Census, Industry Division (1962–1977) *Current Industrial Reports: Pharmaceutical Preparators Except Biologicals*. Series MA-28G (62)-1 through MA-28G (77)-1, Washington DC: US Government Printing Office.

U.S. Department of Health, Education and Welfare (1979) *Healthy People–The Surgeon General's Report on Health, Promotion and Disease Prevention* (DHEW [PHS] Publication No. 79-55071). Washington DC: US Government Printing Office.

Utian WH (1972) The true clinical features of postmenopausal and oophorectomy, and their response to estrogen therapy. *South African Medical Journal* **46**: 732–737.

Von Kaulla E, Droegmueller W & Van Kaulla KN (1975) Conjugated oestrogens and hyper-coagulability. *American Journal of Obstetrics and Gynecology* **122**: 688–692.

Wahl P, Walden C, Knopp R et al (1983) Effect of estrogen/progestin potency on lipid/lipoprotein cholesterol. *New England Journal of Medicine* **308**: 862–867.

Weir RJ, Briggs E, Mack A et al (1917) Blood pressure in women after one year of oral contraception. *Lancet* **i**: 467–470.

Weiss NS, Szekely DR & Austin DF (1976) Increasing incidence of endometrial cancer in the United States. *New England Journal of Medicine* **294**: 1259–1262.

Weissman MM & Klermann GL (1977) Sex differences and the epidemiology of depression. *Archives of General Psychiatry* **34**: 98–111.

Whitehead MI, Townsend PT, Pryse-Davies J, Ryder TA & King RJB (1981) Effects of estrogens and progestins on the biochemistry and morphology of the postmenopausal endometrium. *New England Journal of Medicine* **305**: 1599–1605.

Wilson PWF, Garrison RJ & Castelli WP (1984) Postmenopausal estrogen use and cardio-vascular morbidity: the Framingham study. *CVD Epidemiology News* **35**: 35. abstract.

World Health Organization (1980) *Sixth Report on the World Health Situation*. Part I. Global analysis. Geneva: World Health Organization.

10

The antiprogesterone steroid RU 486: a short pharmacological and clinical review, with emphasis on the interruption of pregnancy

R. E. GARFIELD
E. E. BAULIEU

It has long been recognized that oestrogen and progesterone are involved in the normal physiological control of many different types of target tissues. These hormones regulate a variety of cell functions including growth and differentiation by stimulating or inhibiting the synthesis of structural and functional proteins. It has also been realized that many pathological conditions, such as some abnormal growths, are associated with changes in the action or synthesis of the steroid hormones.

Certainly a significant contribution to our understanding of how hormones act in target tissues was the identification and quantification of receptor binding sites for the hormones during the early 1960s. We now acknowledge that oestrogen and progesterone bind to specific receptor molecules within target cells. The interaction of steroid molecules with their receptors leads to selective action in the nucleus to regulate protein synthesis through an effect at the genomic level.

During the fertile period in adult women, oestrogen and progesterone levels fluctuate in a cyclic manner. The changes in the levels of the steroid hormones during the cycle regulate the synthesis of gonadotrophins from the pituitary, which in turn control ovulation. The steroid hormones have tremendous effects on the structure and function of both the endometrium and the myometrial layers of the uterus to prepare the tissues for the fertilized ovum. Oestrogens stimulate growth of the glandular epithelium of the endometrium and the uterine muscle mass. Progesterone, on the other hand, is essential for the formation of the secretory endometrium which is required for nidation and nourishment of the trophoblast. In addition, progesterone inhibits uterine muscle and thereby insures that the muscle does not contract during development of the fetus (Csapo, 1981). Because the steroid hormones are intricately involved in various steps preceding and following fertilization, changes in their levels and/or action will influence either the progression of the cycle or postfertilization phenomena (Pincus, 1965).

Recently an antiprogesterone compound (RU 486 or mifepristone,

Roussel Uclaf) has been synthesized. This antihormone binds to the progesterone receptor and prevents progesterone action by a competitive mechanism (Baulieu, 1985). One application of this new compound has been in the area of fertility control because progesterone action is essential for the implantation of the embryo in the uterine wall and to maintain uterine quiescence throughout pregnancy (Baulieu and Segal, 1985). Certainly the antihormone will prove efficacious for many other purposes, and it is a very powerful tool to help define the molecular events involved in steroid-regulated reactions. In this chapter we will briefly review the antiprogestin RU 486, with an emphasis on its effect on the termination of pregnancy.

THE ANTIPROGESTIN RU 486—CLINICAL APPLICATIONS

RU 486 is the first antiprogesterone compound to be used clinically. The data on RU 486 have been obtained through physiopharmacological, endocrinological and biochemical studies. The development of the antihormone represents a classic example of a concerted research effort between chemistry, biology and medicine. RU 486's action is particularly significant on the uterus (Baulieu, 1985). Many studies indicate that the compound can be used clinically for: (1) voluntary interruption of pregnancy at early and late stages, (2) induction of menstruation during the fourth and fifth weeks of amenorrhoea, (3) post-coital contraception (see Table 1).

Other possibilities include its use as a once-a-month menses inducer and adjuvant treatment in some cases of cancers.

More than 1000 pregnancy terminations have been successfully obtained with RU 486. A dose of ≈ 400–600 mg of RU 486, given once in the evening, is more efficient than 50–200 mg/day for 3–7 days as indicated by initial trials

Table 1. Clinical uses of RU 486.

1. Interruption of pregnancy	
Early stage (5–10 weeks)	Herrmann et al (1982)
	Kovacs et al (1984)
	Vervest and Haspels (1985)
Late stage (30 weeks) (dead or abnormal fetuses)	Cabrol et al (1985)
2. Induction of menstruation	Herrmann et al (1982)
	Healy et al (1983)
	Schaison et al (1985)
	Baulieu and Ulmann (1986)
3. Postcoital contraception	Haspels (1985)
	Schaison et al (1985)
	Baulieu and Ulmann (1986)
4. Other possible uses	
Once-a-month pill	Baulieu (1985)
Adjuvant treatment for some endocrine-influenced cancers	Bardon et al (1985)
Advanced breast cancer	Baulieu and Ulmann (1986)
Ectopic pregnancy extraction	Paris et al (1984)
Cushing's syndrome	Nieman et al (1985)

(Herrmann et al, 1982; Kovacs et al, 1984; Vervest and Haspels, 1985). Such low dosages had been defined in view of the fear of an antiglucocortico-steroid effect, which, however, is only detectable with dosages greater than those leading to an antiprogesterone effect at the uterine level. In any case, the adrenal–pituitary feedback compensating system (Gaillard et al, 1984) has always worked perfectly, and no peripheral sign of adrenal insufficiency has ever been noticed. The results are particularly satisfying when the compound is administered within the days following the assumed date of menstruation (fifth week of amenorrhoea). Several cases of normal preg-nancies have been reported after using RU 486, including one as early as starting during the following month (Hermann et al, 1982).

RU 486 may also be used for postcoital contraception of occasionally exposed patients, who often are very young women. Just as RU 486 may disrupt the cycle in the luteal phase, by directly provoking bleeding at the endometrial level, and indirectly affecting luteolysis by depression of gonadotrophins (Herrmann et al, 1982; Schaison et al, 1985), it may also be used in this particular case. Trials, which are still limited, have shown the feasibility of this approach. The monthly use of RU 486, at each cycle, as a menses inducer for women who lead a regular sexual life, is still under study: potential advantages are obvious, but it is preferable to avoid an effect on the follicular development in the following cycle. A study as to how much and for how long RU 486 is to be prescribed should permit the definition of conditions for maintaining a regular menstrual cycle.

RU 486 also makes it possible to provoke the therapeutic abortion of dead or abnormal fetuses, even at a late date (Cabrol et al, 1985), and it is better tolerated than oxytocic drugs currently used. Owing to its remarkable property of softening and dilating the cervix and inducing uterine con-tractility, it is even being considered to induce labour at term (see Csapo, 1979). All precautions would obviously have to be taken to prevent any possible action on the newborn. Trials have also been carried out for ectopic pregnancies (Paris et al, 1984), and seem to indicate an effect which makes the embryo extraction easier under coelioscopy. At no time has toxicity been reported, and a woman who had previously undergone an operation on a sole tube, and who had received RU 486 for facilitating the treatment of an ectopic pregnancy, later carried a normal pregnancy to term (Paris et al, 1984).

MECHANISM OF ACTION OF RU 486

The RU 486 steroid (17-β-hydroxy-11β-(4-dimethyl-aminophenyl)-17α-(1-propynyl)-oestra-4,9-dien-3-one) (Figure 1) prevents progesterone action by taking its place at the receptor level in target cells. Indeed, steroids act in target cells through an intranuclear receptor (Figure 2) (Gasc et al, 1984) and an antihormone binds to the same site as the corresponding hormone, yet without provoking the biological response. Thus the anti-hormone structure resembles that of the hormone in order to substitute for it, and it is different so as not to 'activate' the receptor (Baulieu and Mester,

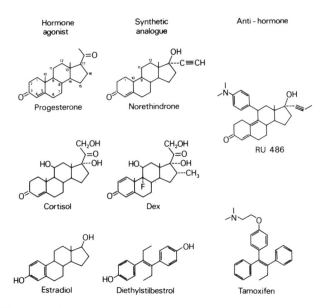

Figure 1. Hormones (natural), synthetic agonistic derivatives and corresponding anti-hormones. Note the analogy of antihormones with a phenolic ring in the region corresponding to C-11β of steroids that is probably responsible for the antihormonal effect.

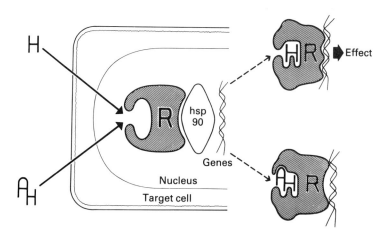

Figure 2. Mechanism of action of steroid hormones and their antihormones. The nuclear receptor is made up of one subunit 'R', binding the hormone, and two subunits 'hsp 90', heat-shock protein of MW ≈ 90 000 (Catelli et al, 1985). This stoichiometry is that found for the progesterone receptor in chick oviduct (Renoir et al, 1984), but all non-transformed receptors show an oligo–heteromeric structure including hormone binding subunit and hsp 90. The hormone H which binds to the receptor provokes its 'transformation' with release of hsp 90, and the 'activated' subunit R modifies the transcription of specific genes. An antihormone AH binding to the receptor may also provoke a transformation with dissociation of R from hsp 90, but R is not activated and does not mediate a biological response. If AH is abundant and/or has high affinity for the receptor, it binds preferentially to R and thus precludes H activity.

1985). This is the case for antioestrogens (Figure 1) with a triphenylethylenic structure, and for steroids with a phenylic nucleus in C-11β position, as synthesized by G. Teutsch and Roussel Uclaf's researchers (Teutsch, 1985). RU 486 is a derivative of norethindrone, the historical progestagen of oral contraception (Pincus, 1965). Its affinity for the progesterone receptor is high, it is orally active, and toxicology studies do not show any effects other than the endocrine consequences which may be expected from the anti-hormone (Baulieu and Segal, 1985; Deraedt et al, 1985; Philibert et al, 1985).

The mechanism by which RU 486 stimulates menses has been considered in several studies. Treatment of women during the luteal phase of the cycle results in endometrial bleeding, irreversible luteolysis with rapid decline in plasma levels of progesterone and oestradiol and also decreases in LH and FSH (Herrmann et al, 1982). These results suggest that RU 486 effects are mediated at the endometrial level causing increased synthesis and release of prostaglandins (Healy, 1985; Secchi et al, 1985; Kelly et al, 1986) and haemorrhage. At the hypothalamus/pituitary level it produces a decrease in LH and subsequent luteolysis with a decrease in synthesis of progesterone. Treatment of patients during the follicular phase of the normal cycle does not cause uterine bleeding but RU 486 may interfere with follicle maturation and ovulation. These effects form the bases for application of RU 486 for postcoital contraception (possibly a once-a-month fertility agent) and menses induction, if given late in the cycle a few days before the expected date of menstruation.

The mechanism by which RU 486 interrupts early pregnancy is probably similar to the way it induces menses. The blockade of progesterone activity by RU 486 on the decidualized endometrium causes bleeding, increased prostaglandin release (Herrmann et al, 1985; Healy et al, 1983), separation of the conceptus from the uterine wall, a drop in human chorionic gonado-trophin (hCG) production and secondary luteolysis (Figure 3). These changes are accompanied by increased myometrial contractility and soften-ing of the cervix. Measurements of hormonal levels in pregnant women treated with RU 486 do not show any significant changes until after the interruption of pregnancy has begun (Figure 4). This indicates that RU 486 action is not mediated by changes in hormonal levels.

Prostaglandins have been used to terminate pregnancy for some time (Bygdeman et al, 1983). Therefore the fact of adding, on the fourth day of the RU 486 treatment, a small dosage of synthetic prostaglandin equal to one-sixth of that used alone when inducing abortions, made it possible to clearly improve the results (Swahn et al, 1985). Since this does not cause pain or digestive problems as observed when prescribing an abortive dosage of prostaglandin alone, associations of RU 486 and prostaglandins are being tested in several centres to find the most efficient formula.

The fact that RU 486 is effective in producing delivery of the conceptus in all species studied, even in late pregnancy, may exemplify the necessity for the action of progesterone for the maintenance of pregnancy. Indeed, there was never any consensus on the need for progesterone in human pregnancy. Therefore the demonstration that RU 486 induces labour and delivery in

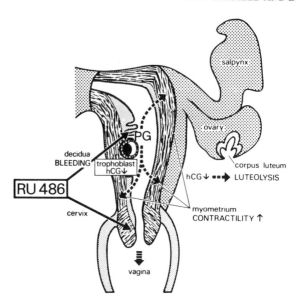

Figure 3. Mechanism of action of RU 486 in early pregnancy. The antiprogesterone provokes the increase of prostaglandin (PG) production and in turn PG stimulates uterine contractility. Alteration of decidualized endometrium leads to separation of the blastocyst, decrease in hCG and consequently luteolysis. The mechanism of the dilatation and softening of the cervix is not well understood (direct or via PG release).

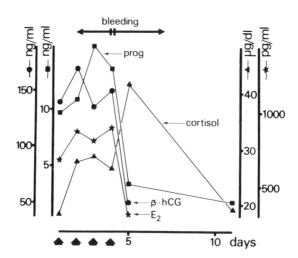

Figure 4. Seven-week pregnancy terminated by the administration of four doses of 200 mg of RU 486. The horizontal line indicates the length of the bleeding, and the double vertical line signals the abortion itself. Plasma concentrations are shown for progesterone ■, E_2 (oestradiol) ★, cortisol ▲, β-hCG ●.

humans helps to demonstrate that progesterone action is required. Below we consider in greater detail the possible mechanisms of this action, because they are fundamental to our understanding of the systems which maintain pregnancy and those that terminate it normally at term.

Induction of labour during late gestation

It is probable that the mechanism by which RU 486 interrupts late pregnancy is somewhat different from that of early gestation. The former may involve an effect more on muscular activity whereas the latter action of RU 486 is thought to be directed mainly on the endometrium (see above). The uterus, with its muscle the myometrium, grows tremendously during pregnancy (at term the human uterus is about 15 times the non-pregnant weight and 500–1000 times the internal volume) to support the growing fetus. The myometrium, which contains the same progesterone receptors as the endo-metrium, is relatively inactive throughout most of pregnancy so that a tranquil environment is maintained within the uterine cavity for the developing fetus. Normally at term the muscle becomes increasingly active and reactive to stimulants, eventually contracting rhythmically and force-fully. This pattern of contractility aids in retracting the cervix and expelling the fetus. Any compound which initiates delivery late in pregnancy probably has a major effect on the contractility of the myometrium.

The changes in hormonal levels that precede normal labour and that are thought to be responsible for the conversion of the myometrium from inactive to active have been the subject of much discussion. Changes in the synthesis of the steroid hormones, as reflected in tissue and plasma levels, occur before normal or premature labour in most animal species (Csapo, 1981). In many elegant studies of uterine contractile patterns and hormonal levels, Csapo showed that, when progesterone levels decline either at term or preterm, the myometrium becomes increasingly active. These observations led Csapo to propose the progesterone block theory. The theory stated that the maintenance of pregnancy was determined by the ability of progesterone to suppress myometrial contractility, and when the hormone declined myometrial activity gradually intensified to produce labour contractions. The theory was later expanded to the 'seesaw theory' to include the effects of stimulants (oestrogens, prostaglandins, oxytocin, and stretching) on myometrial activity during the onset of parturition. The seesaw theory predicted that the maintenance of pregnancy involved a balance in the myometrium of opposing forces, between stimulants and suppressors, whereas the onset and progression of labour depended upon a regulatory imbalance (decrease in progesterone) in favour of the stimulants (increase in oestrogen and prostaglandins).

However, prior to the development and application of RU 486 Csapo's theories did not seem to apply to humans. Progesterone does not seem to decline significantly prior to human labour, although oestrogen rises. Also, progesterone administration does not seem to inhibit premature labour except possibly in very high doses. What is clearly apparent is that, if progesterone levels decline in humans during early pregnancy, labour followed by abortion ensues. This has been adequately documented following lutectomy before the luteal–placental shift in the synthesis of the steroid hormones (Csapo and Pulkkinen, 1978). The studies with RU 486 show that this agent is an efficient abortifacient at any time during human pregnancy (see above), and this evidence strongly supports the role of progesterone in the maintenance of pregnancy, because the antiprogesterone agent binds to the steroid receptor and prevents its action and effectively produces the same effect as progesterone withdrawal. Furthermore, the studies with RU 486 imply that normally, at term, there must be some mechanism for down-regulation of progesterone action to initiate labour.

Many studies show that the initiation of labour occurs during a change of a state dominated by progesterone to a state dominated by oestrogens. It is probable, therefore, that the capacity of the muscle to contract is mediated through the control of protein synthesis. Oestrogens provoke the synthesis of proteins necessary for stimulation (receptors for oxytocin and possibly other stimulants, Alexandrova and Soloff, 1980) and conduction (gap junctions, see below) within the muscle cells. The oestrogen effects are opposed by progesterone. Oestrogens also increase the production of stimulatory prostaglandins (PGE_2 and $PGF_{2\alpha}$); this effect may be inhibited by progesterone and/or progesterone could be responsible for maintaining levels of inhibitory prostaglandins (possibly PGI_2, Thorburn and Challis, 1979). The levels of stimulatory prostaglandins are probably controlled through the same steroid receptor mechanisms that regulate the synthesis of gap junctions, oxytocin receptors and probably other proteins important for contractility.

Gap junctions—specific genomic products regulated by progesterone

Uterine contractions require the coordination or synchronization of all the smooth muscle cells of the uterus (Csapo, 1981). Propagation of electrical activity along the cell surface occurs by a local circuit mechanism when an active region directly activates the surrounding resting membrane to change the membrane potential or generate action potentials. The propagation of current between cells is thought to occur by the same mechanism and involves the flow of ions (ionic current) between cell interiors. Gap junctions are believed to be the sites of continuity between cells and the loci of electrical coupling between cells (Meda et al, 1984; Peracchia, 1980). A gap junction is a structure composed of identical portions of the plasma membranes from two closely apposed cells. The gap junction is characterized by close regions of plasma membranes of two cells, at a distance of $\approx 2\,nm$ (Figure 5). Intramembranous particles (proteins or connexons) penetrate through each membrane at the junction to form channels between the cell interiors.

The onset and progression of labour is associated with the appearance of large numbers of gap junctions between myometrial cells in rats (Garfield et al, 1977, 1978), other species (see Garfield, 1984), including humans (Garfield and Hayashi, 1981). The junctions develop immediately prior to term, are present in large sizes and increased number during labour and

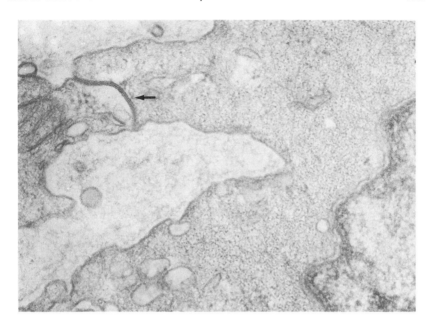

Figure 5. Electron micrograph of portion of two myometrial cells from rat uterus. Note the gap junction (arrow). × 84 000. (R. E. Garfield, J. M. Gasc and E. E. Baulieu, 1986, unpublished observation.)

delivery, then decline rapidly postpartum. During delivery, the gap junctions occupy about 0.3% of the surface of each smooth muscle cell (Figure 6); this value represents about 500 gap junctions per cell. The increased area of the junctions may be necessary for the initiation and maintainance of labour since all conditions which induce the premature appearance of the gap junctions provoke early labour and delivery, and treatments which prevent junction development inhibit parturition. The formation of the junctions appears to be the structural basis for synchronized contractile activity of labour (Garfield, 1984), providing a pathway for current flow stimulated by prostaglandins and/or oxytocin.

The development of gap junctions is accompanied by an increase in the ability of spontaneous and evoked electrical activity to propagate between myometrial cells (Sims et al, 1982). Furthermore, the presence of the junctions is accompanied by a 10-fold increase in the ability of 2-deoxyglucose to diffuse between the muscle cells (Cole et al, 1985). These studies show that the muscle is coupled electrically and metabolically when gap junctions are present during parturition. The data show that the presence of gap junctions converts the myometrium to a functional syncytium during labour.

The presence of gap junctions is regulated by the steroid hormones, and this may explain how they control the contractile activity of the myometrium during labour. The results of several studies show that the steroid hormones regulate the synthesis and assembly of gap junctions by receptor-operated mechanisms. Figure 7 shows the changes in the steroid hormones and PGF

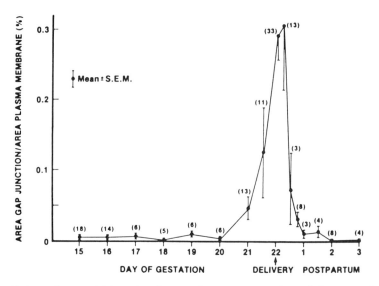

Figure 6. Area of myometrial gap junction membrane as a percentage of plasma membrane area before, during and following parturition in rats. The numbers in brackets indicate the number of tissues studied at each point. From Garfield (1984), with permission.

that precede and accompany the increase in gap junctions in the rat uterus. Evidence that oestrogens stimulate and progesterone inhibits gap junction synthesis is considerable:

1. Oestradiol and other oestrogen agonists which bind to its receptor increase gap junctions in vivo and in vitro in myometrium from pregnant and non-pregnant animals.
2. Tamoxifen, cycloheximide and actinomycin D prevent oestrogen effects.
3. Progesterone inhibits gap junctions in all models studied (Garfield 1984).

Recently we have concentrated on the mechanism of induction of delivery in pregnant rats treated with RU 486. Treatment of animals with a single injection of RU 486 (10 mg/kg) on day 7 or day 16 of gestation is followed by delivery of the fetuses before any changes in steroid levels. The delivery of the fetuses in animals treated with RU 486 at 16 days gestation (24–48 hours afterwards) was accompanied by the appearance of large numbers of gap junctions (650–800/cell) between the myometrial cells. By contrast, there was no increase in gap junctions in non-pregnant immature or mature cycling rats and little increase in pregnant animals treated at day 7 of gestation (Table 2). We have also demonstrated that an analogue of progesterone (R 5020) with a high affinity for the progesterone receptor, prevents labour, delivery and the development of gap junctions induced in rats after RU 486 treatment in late pregnancy. Moreover, the use of prostaglandin synthesis inhibitors with RU 486 suggests that prostaglandins are

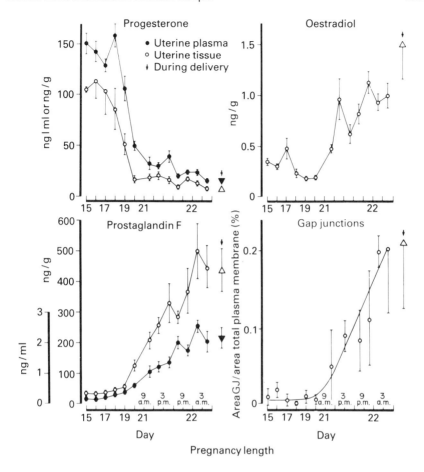

Figure 7. Changes (mean ± SEM) in levels of progesterone, oestradiol, and PGF in uterine vein plasma (●) and uterine tissues (○) and myometrial gap junctional area during the latter days of pregnancy and delivery (▲) in rats. Note that the axis of the time scale is expanded from day 21 onward to delivery. The number of samples at each point is three or four. (From Puri and Garfield, 1982; with permission).

not involved in the increase in gap junctions, even though the prostaglandins play an important role in increasing myometrial contractility. These results support the hypothesis that gap junctions are necessary for labour and show that progesterone may normally repress the receptor-regulated expression of gap junctions between myometrial cells to maintain pregnancy. Furthermore these studies show that there are differences between early and late gestation. Since gap junctions are also present between myometrial cells of the human uterus during labour and delivery (Garfield and Hayashi, 1981), we suggest that this may be one of the important mechanisms of action of RU 486 in women.

Table 2. Number and area of gap junctions (GJs) in non-pregnant and pregnant rat myometrium.

Treatment	n	No. GJs	Length of plasma membrane surveyed (μm)	Area GJs (% membrane) Mean ± SEM	Approximate No. GJs/cell
Nonpregnant					
Immature					
Control	4	0	5187	—	—
RU 486 × 3 d					
30 mg/kg	4	0	5850	—	—
3 mg/kg	4	1	5533	0.010 ± 0.010	17
0.3 mg/kg	4	0	5187	—	—
Mature cycling					
Control	6	1	7320	0.008 ± 0.008	13
RU 486 × 3 d					
10 mg/kg	6	0	7688	—	—
Pregnant (10 mg/kg as one injection)					
Day 7					
Control (12 h)	4	0	6058	—	—
RU 486 (12 h)	6	0	8741	—	—
Day 8					
Control (24 h)	5	0	7398	—	—
RU 486 (24 h)	6	31	8424	0.105 ± 0.038	175
Day 9					
Control (48 h)	2	0	3212	—	—
RU 486 (48 h)	6	4	8948	0.006 ± 0.004	10
Day 16					
Control (6 h)	2	0	2570	—	—
RU 486 (6 h)	2	2	2572	0.013 ± 0.013	22
Control (12 h)	4	1	5009	0.002 ± 0.002	3
RU 486 (12 h)	5	15	5642	0.090 ± 0.051	150
Day 17					
Control (24 h)	6	3	7778	0.005 ± 0.005	8
RU 486 (24 h)	8	75	8486	0.393 ± 0.018*	655
Control (30 h)	2	1	2566	0.009 ± 0.009	15
RU 486 (30 h)	5	60	5546	0.488 ± 0.129*	813
Day 18					
Control (48 h)	5	4	6391	0.015 ± 0.013	25
RU 486 (48 h)	6	19	6774	0.158 ± 0.060*	263

n = number of tissues examined, No. of GJs refers to total number of gap junctions found in 22 photographs of all tissues. Length of membrane is the length of plasma membrane of smooth muscle cells in all photos. Area of GJs is the percentage area = length of gap junction membrane divided by length of plasma membrane for each group of tissues. * indicate significant differences ($P<0.05$). The approximate number of GJs was estimated from the value of the surface area of a smooth muscle cell ($\approx 5000\,\mu m^2$), the area of plasma membrane occupied by gap junctions (fourth column), and the average area of a gap junction ($\approx 0.03\,\mu m^2$).

SUMMARY

In this review we have briefly outlined the clinical applications and mechanism of action of the progesterone antagonist RU 486. RU 486 has been successfully used in a variety of conditions to regulate the reproductive cycle and to control fertility in women. We suggest that the mechanism by which

RU 486 acts during the cycle and early pregnancy is probably by affecting mainly the endometrium. During late pregnancy, the compound has significant effects on the myometrium including the induction of gap junctions between myometrium cells, which is required for muscle contractility during labour. The use of RU 486 has helped to demonstrate that progesterone is required for maintenance of the late stages of pregnancy in women.

REFERENCES

Alexandrova M & Soloff MS (1980) Oxytocin receptors and parturition. I. Control of oxytocin receptor concentration in the rat myometrium at term. *Endocrinology* **106**: 730–748.
Bardon S, Vignon F, Chalbos D & Rochefort H (1985) RU 486 a progestin and glucocorticoid antagonist inhibits the growth of breast cancer cells via the progesterone receptor. *Journal of Endocrinology and Metabolism* **60**: 692–697.
Baulieu EE (1985) RU 486: an antiprogestin with contragestive activity in women. In Baulieu EE & Segal SJ (eds) *The Antiprogestin Steroid RU 486 and Human Fertility Control*, pp 1–25. New York: Plenum Press.
Baulieu EE & Mester J (1985) Steroid hormone receptors. In DeGroot LJ (ed.) *Endocrinology* Orlando: Grune & Stratton.
Baulieu EE & Segal SJ (1985) *The Antiprogesterone Steroid RU 486 and Human Fertility Control.* New York: Plenum Press. 353 pp.
Baulieu EE & Ulmann A (1985) Anti-hormones stéroides: l'activité antiprogestérone du RU 486 et ses applications contragestive et autres. *Bulletin de l'Académie Nationale de Médecine* **169**: 1191–1199.
Baulieu EE & Ulmann A (1986) Antiprogesterone activity of RU 486 and its contragestive and other applications. *Human Reproduction* **1**: 107–110.
Bygdeman M, Christensen N, Green K, Zheng S & Lundstrom V (1983) Termination of early pregnancy: future developments. *Acta Obstetrica et Gynecologica Scandinavica Supplement* **113**: 125–129.
Cabrol D, Bouvier d'Yvoire M, Mermet E et al (1985) Induction of labor with mifepristone after intrauterine fetal death. *Lancet* **ii**: 1019.
Catelli MG, Binart N, Jung-Testas I et al (1985) The common 90-kd protein component of non-transformed '8S' steroid receptors is a heat-shock protein. *EMBO Journal* **4**: 3131–3135.
Cole WC, Garfield RE & Kirkaldy JS (1985) Gap junctions and direct intercellular communication between rat uterine smooth muscle cells. *American Journal of Physiology* **249**: C20–C31.
Csapo AI (1979) Antiprogesterone in fertility control. In Zatuchni GI, Sciarra JJ & Spiedel JJ (eds) *Pregnancy Termination: Procedures, Safety and New Developments*, pp 16–34. Hagerstown: Harper Row.
Csapo AI (1981) Force of labor. In Iffy L & Kaminetzky HA (eds) *Principles and Practice of Obstetrics and Perinatology*, pp 761–799. New York: John Wiley.
Csapo AI & Pulkkinen M (1978) Indispensability of the human corpus luteum in the maintenance of early pregnancy: luteectomy evidence. *Obstetrical and Gynecological Survey* **33**: 69–81.
Deraedt R, Bonnat C, Busigny M et al (1985) Pharmacokinetics of RU 486 In Baulieu EE & Segal JJ (eds) *The Antiprogestin Steroid RU 486 and Human Fertility Control*, pp 103–126. New York: Plenum Press.
Gaillard RC, Riondel A, Muller AF, Herrmann W & Baulieu EE (1984) RU 486: a steroid with antiglucocorticosteroid activity that only disinhibits the human pituitary–adrenal system at a specific time of day. *Proceedings of the National Academy of Sciences (USA)* **81**: 3879–3882.
Garfield RE (1984) Control of myometrial junction in preterm versus term labor. *Clinical Obstetrics and Gynecology* **27**: 572–591.

Garfield RE & Hayashi RH (1981) Appearance of gap junctions in the myometrium of women during labor. *American Journal of Obstetrics and Gynecology* **140:** 254–260.

Garfield RE, Sims S & Daniel EE (1977) Gap junctions: their presence and necessity in myometrium during parturition. *Science* **198:** 958–960.

Garfield RE, Sims S, Kannan MS & Daniel EE (1978) Possible role of gap junctions in activation of myometrium during parturition. *American Journal of Physiology* **235:** C168–179.

Gasc JM, Renoir JM, Radanyi C et al (1984) Progesterone receptor in the chick oviduct: an immunohistochemical study with antibodies to distinct receptor components. *Journal of Cell Biology* **99:** 1193–2101.

Haspels AA (1985) Interruption of early pregnancy by the antiprogestational compound RU 486. In Baulieu EE & Segal SJ (eds) *The Antiprogestin Steroid RU 486 and Human Fertility Control*, pp 199–209. New York: Plenum Press.

Healy DL, Baulieu EE & Hodhen GD (1983) Induction of menstruation by an anti-progesterone steroid (RU 486) in primate: site of action, dose–response relationships and hormonal effects. *Fertility and Sterility* **40:** 253–257.

Healy DL (1985) Clinical status of antiprogesterone steroids. *Clinical Reproduction and Fertility* **3:** 277–296.

Herrmann W, Wyss R, Riondel A et al (1982) Effect d'un steroide antiprogesterone chez la femme: interruption du cycle menstruel et de la grossesse au debut *Comptes Rendus des Séances de l'Académie des Sciences* **294:** 933–938.

Herrmann WL, Schindler AM, Wyss R & Bischof P (1985) Effects of the antiprogesterone RU 486 in early pregnancy and during the menstrual cycle. In Baulieu EE & Segal SJ (eds) *The Antiprogestin Steroid RU 486 and Human Fertility Control*, pp 179–198. New York: Plenum Press.

Kelly RW, Healy DL, Cameron MJ & Baird DT (1986) The stimulation of prostaglandin production by two antiprogesterone steroids in human endometrial cells. *Journal of Clinical Endocrinology and Metabolism* **62:** 1116–1123.

Kovacs L, Sar M, Resch BA et al (1984) Termination of very early pregnancy by RU 486, and antiprogestational compound. *Contraception* **29:** 399–410.

Meda P, Perrelet A & Orci L (1984) Gap junctions and cell to cell coupling in endocrine glands. *Modern Cell Biology* **3:** 131–196.

Nieman LK, Chrousos GP, Kellner C et al (1985) Successful treatment of Cushing's syndrome with the glucocorticoid antagonist RU 486. *Journal of Clinical Endocrinology and Metabolism* **61:** 536.

Paris FX, Henry-Suchet J, Tesquier L et al (1984) Le traitement médical des grossesses extra-utérines par le RU 486. *La Presse Médicale* **13:** 1219.

Peracchia C (1980) Structural correlates of gap junction permeation. *International Review of Cytology* **66:** 81–146.

Philibert D, Moguilewsky M, Mary I et al (1985) Pharmacological profile of RU 486 in animals. In Baulieu EE & Segal SJ (eds) *The Antiprogestin Steroid RU 486 and Human Fertility Control*, pp 49–78. New York: Plenum Press.

Pincus G (1965) *The Control of Fertility*. London: Academic Press. 360 pp.

Puri CP & Garfield RE (1982) Changes in hormone levels and gap junctions in the rat uterus during pregnancy and parturition. *Biology of Reproduction* **27:** 967–975.

Renoir JM, Buchou T, Mester J, Radanyi C & Baulieu EE (1984) Oligomeric structure of the molybdate-stabilized, non-transformed '8S' progesterone receptor from chick oviduct cytosol. *Biochemistry* **23:** 6016–6023.

Schaison G, George M, Lestrat N, Reinberg A & Baulieu EE (1985) Effects of the anti-progesterone steroid RU 486 during midluteal phase in normal women. *Journal of Clinical Endocrinology and Metabolism* **61:** 484–489.

Secchi J, Lecaque D, Tournemine C & Philibert D (1985) Histopharmacology of RU 486. In Baulieu EE & Segal J (eds) *The Antiprogestin Steroid RU 486 and Human Fertility Control*, pp 79–97. New York: Plenum Press.

Sims S, Daniel EE & Garfield RE (1982) Improved electrical coupling in uterine smooth muscle in associated with increased members of gap junctions at parturition. *Journal of General Physiology* **80:** 353–375.

Swahn ML, Cekan S, Wang G, Lundstrom V & Bygdeman M (1985) Pharmacokinetic and clinical studies of RU 486 for fertility regulation. In Baulieu EE & Segal J (eds) *The*

Antiprogestin Steroid RU 486 and Human Fertility Control, pp 249–258. New York: Plenum Press.

Teutsch G (1985) Analogues of RU 486 for the mapping of the progestin receptor: synthetic and structural aspects. In Baulieu EE & Segal J (eds) *The Antiprogestin Steroid RU 486 and Human Fertility Control*, pp 27–47. New York: Plenum Press.

Thorburn GD & Challis JRG (1979) Endocrine control of parturition. *Physiological Reviews* **59:** 863–918.

Vervest HAM & Haspels AA (1985) Preliminary results with the antiprogestational compound RU 486 (mifepristone) for interruption of early pregnancy. *Fertility and Sterility* **44:** 627–632.

11

Intragonadal control mechanisms

J. K. FINDLAY
G. P. RISBRIDGER

The necessity of the pituitary hormones follicle stimulating hormone (FSH) and luteinizing hormone (LH), and in some cases prolactin, for normal gonadal function is beyond dispute (Greep, 1961). Neither the gametogenic nor the endocrinological functions of the testes and ovaries are normal in the absence of this pituitary gonadotrophic influence. Indeed, the correct sequence and ratio of FSH and LH secretion, controlled mainly by the feedback influence of the gonads, are needed to achieve successful gameto-genesis and fertility.

Notwithstanding this requirement for gonadotrophins, there are events of gametogenesis and endocrine function to be outlined below which do not necessarily have a direct relationship to the known hormonal milieu being determined by pituitary secretion rates and the afferent blood supply to the gonad. This leads to the conclusion that there are local chemical messages being generated by the gonad which act within and between the gonads. At this point it should be clearly emphasized that these local factors act in conjunction with the pituitary hormones and in some cases are the proxi-mate regulators for the gonadotrophins.

Local regulators can be divided into two classes (Sporn and Todaro, 1980). Those which are secreted by one cell and move through the interstitial spaces to act on neighbouring target cells are called paracrine regulators. Those which act on the same cells that are secreting them are called auto-crine regulators. Both paracrine and autocrine regulators can have stimu-latory and inhibitory influences, in some cases both, depending on the presence of other regulators acting on the cell (Roberts et al, 1985). The regulators can be steroids, prostaglandins, polypeptides or glycoproteins, although in many cases their true identity is still unknown.

The purpose of this review is to outline those processes of gonadal function which appear to be under the influence of local regulators. This is not an exhaustive review of the literature but a selection of reports which exemplify the points we wish to make, together with material from pre-viously published reviews on the broader principles of regulation of gonadal function.

INTRAGONADAL CONTROL MECHANISMS IN THE OVARY

Control of folliculogenesis and determination of ovulation rate

Initiation and maintenance of the growth of preantral follicles

The postnatal ovary of mammals contains a large pool of non-proliferating primary follicles, each consisting of an oocyte arrested in meiotic prophase surrounded by a single or several layers of squamous granulosa cells. The initiation of growth of these follicles is characterized by an increase in size of the oocyte (still arrested in meiotic prophase) and proliferation and differentiation of the surrounding granulosa cells; subsequently, the thecal cells organize external to the basement membrane of the granulosa cells (Peters and McNatty, 1980; Richards, 1980).

Once initiation of growth of primary follicles begins late in fetal or early in postnatal life, it is continuous throughout life. Every day, a certain number of primary follicles begin to grow. For example, follicle growth is initiated and maintained through most of the preantral stages on all days of the ovarian cycle and pregnancy, during seasonal and postpartum anovulation and after hypophysectomy.

The processes by which primary follicles are chosen from the pool, the hormonal and/or intraovarian factors regulating this choice and the subsequent mechanisms controlling initiation and maintenance of preantral growth are not known. The rete ovarii has been implicated in selecting primary follicles for growth. It has been observed that the first germ cells to enter meiosis and then form follicles with the oocyte arrested in prophase were the first to contact the mesonephric-derived rete cells in the ovarian medulla (Byskov, 1975). Both meiosis-inducing (MIS) and meiosis-preventing substances (MPS) which act on the oocyte, were attributed to the rete system and there is good evidence that granulosa cells may be derived from the same mesonephric cells as the rete (Byskov, 1981). The growth of primary follicles begins in the centre of the ovary in proximity to the rete. It is implied therefore that the trigger for growth may arise from the association of the oocyte and granulosa cells with the rete and that subsequent responsibility for meiotic arrest of the oocyte lies with the somatic (? granulosa) cells of the follicle, until the LH surge and ovulation when meiosis recommences (see below).

Initiation of growth and subsequent differentiation of the somatic cells of follicles requires the presence of an oocyte (Franchi et al, 1962), supporting the hypothesis that the oocyte is an active partner in the initiation process and may control the early stages of somatic cell division and differentiation. The fact that the oocyte enlarges in size (Lintern-Moore et al, 1974; Cahill and Mauleon, 1980) and has evidence of being metabolically active at this time (Moore et al, 1974) attests to its lack of dormancy in the early stages of follicular growth. Dunbar and Wolgemuth (1984) have described an oocyte antigen which is localized on the granulosa layer of preantral rabbit follicles that may influence the early differentiation of these cells.

Although initiation of follicular growth is continuous throughout life, the number of follicles beginning to grow each day does vary (Peters and McNatty, 1980; Richards, 1980). It is related to the age of the animal and to the number of follicles in the non-growing pool. The larger the pool, the greater the number of follicles which begin to grow in mice (Peters and McNatty, 1980). In different genetic strains of the some species, for example sheep, there is an inverse relationship between the number of primary and growing follicles (Driancourt et al, 1985). However, the number of primary follicles initiating growth is relatively constant during adult reproductive life of an animal while the total number of primordial follicles continues to decline (Peters and McNatty, 1980; Driancourt et al, 1985).

Peters et al (1973b) have shown that follicular fluid aspirated from antral cow follicles and injected into neonatal mice between days 3 and 5 of age caused a reduction in the number of follicles starting to grow. They concluded that antral follicles can influence the rate of growth initiation. This could be a direct intraovarian effect on primary follicles or it could result from an effect of the follicular fluid on small growing follicles (see below) which in turn may influence the rate of initiation. It is unlikely to be an effect exerted via the pituitary secretion of gonadotrophin, FSH in particular, as suggested by Jones (1978). Initiation of growth of primordial follicles can occur independently of gonadotrophins (Peters et al, 1973a) (although they may facilitate the process), and mouse ovaries show no in vivo response to exogenous gonadotrophin at that age (Greenwald, 1978).

Other evidence of intragonadal regulation of initiation of folliculogenesis comes from studies involving surgical manipulation of the ovaries. Unilateral ovariectomy in sheep (Dufour et al, 1979), pigs, rats, cats and rabbits (see Jones, 1978), but apparently not in mice (Peters and Braathen, 1973), results in an increase in the proportion of growing preantral follicles in the remaining ovary. Since this procedure is not associated with a sustained increase in gonadotrophins (Jones, 1978), it is suggested that there is communication within and between ovaries with respect to the rate of initiation of growth of primordial follicles. If women with one ovary also have an increased rate of follicle growth initiation compared to those with two ovaries, and they have had the one ovary for most of their adult life, one might expect them to deplete their pool of follicles more quickly and therefore become menopausal at an earlier age than women with two ovaries. There is some evidence for this suggestion (Rozewicki et al, 1979).

In summary, it would appear that the initiation of growth of primordial follicles, maintenance of the oocyte in meiotic arrest and organization of the basement membrane and theca layer are controlled within the ovary and do not require the obligatory influence of the pituitary gland. There is evidence to suggest that the initiation process involves an interaction between the rete ovarii, the somatic granulosa cells and the oocyte, but the nature of the agents responsible is not yet known.

Development of the granulosa cells in a growing preantral follicle is characterized by mitotic division, such that by the time of antrum formation there are at least four or five layers of granulosa cells surrounding the oocyte. Because treatment of immature or hypophysectomized laboratory rodents with oestrogens enhanced mitotic division of granulosa cells in preantral follicles, oestrogen has been implicated in the control of preantral folliculogenesis (see Richards, 1980). Preantral follicles apparently have an inherent capacity to synthesize oestrogen with little or no pituitary support (Ingram and Mandl, 1958), and the oestrogen is believed to act locally, presumably within the follicle, to support development to the antral stage.

Relatively little is known about the cellular origin and control of steroidogenesis, particularly oestrogen production, in preantral follicles. Granulosa cells of antral follicles from all species have aromatase activity which requires stimulation by FSH. There may be receptors for FSH on granulosa cells during the latter stages of normal preantral growth as there are in the oestrogen-treated hypophysectomized rat (Richards, 1980). An alternative site of oestrogen production is the theca cells, but not all species express detectable aromatase activity in the theca of antral follicles and similar studies have not been reported on preantral follicles.

It is possible that oestrogen is not the proximal regulator of mitosis of granulosa and theca cells in preantral follicles, and that this role is served either by a 'non-steroidal' mitogenic agent(s) or by removal of a mitotic inhibitor, both under regulation by oestrogen. Of interest in this regard is the recent identification of growth factors in antral follicles (Hammond, 1981), including fibroblast growth factor, which have a mitogenic action on granulosa cells in vitro (Gospordarowicz et al, 1985).

Control of growth and differentiation of antral follicles

Although the formation, growth and differentiation of antral follicles require gonadotrophic support and stimulation (Greep, 1961; Richards, 1980), there are several aspects of antral folliculogenesis which cannot be explained simply by changes in the amounts and ratios of FSH and LH which reach the ovary, implying communication between follicles and local control within follicles.

Recruitment and selection of the dominant follicle(s) are the processes by which the ovaries adjust the cohorts of follicles available for ovulation to contain the number consistent with the ovulation rate of the species (Goodman and Hodgen, 1983), known as the law of follicular consistency (Lipschutz, 1928). In species such as primates, sheep and cows which generally ovulate only one to three eggs, the adjustment is likely to involve the ovulatory follicle in a single cohort becoming dominant and suppressing development of other antral follicles of the cohort (Goodman and Hodgen, 1983; Driancourt et al, 1985). In polyovular species such as pigs and rodents, recruitment and selection of ovulatory follicles may be from more than one cohort and continue over the whole follicular phase or longer until the required number is reached or recruitment is terminated by the onset of the ovulatory surge of LH (Greenwald, 1978; Foxcroft and Hunter, 1985). This implies a less important role for dominance and a more important role for recruitment in these species. In both situations, recruitment and selection are taking place during changing profiles of both gonadotrophins. One can envisage intra- and interovarian regulation operating to determine the final number of ovulations from within a framework (or cohort) of follicles originally set by pituitary stimulation of the ovary. Dominance could be exerted at two levels, not mutually exclusive, (a) by reducing the availability of gonadotrophic support to other antral follicles by increasing the feedback inhibition of pituitary FSH in particular, with steroids and inhibin (Baird, 1983) and (b) by intra- and interovarian regulation which modifies the number of large antral follicles allowed to develop (Hammond, 1981).

Communications between follicles. It is possible to modify the follicular response to exogenous (pregnant mare serum gonadotrophin) and endogenous gonadotrophin in intact (diZerega and Wilks, 1984; Cahill et al, 1985b) and hypophysectomized animals (diZerega et al, 1984; Cahill et al, 1985a) by coadministration of ovarian follicular fluid of sheep, pigs and humans or ovarian venous plasma draining the human ovary containing the dominant follicle. The active principle(s) in follicular fluid or plasma responsible for these effects have not been fully characterized, but they could act by inhibiting steroidogenesis in the follicle, particularly oestrogen production (diZerega et al, 1984), FSH binding to granulosa cells (Reichert et al, 1981) and mitosis of granulosa cells (Cahill et al, 1985a,b). An hypothesis of modification of the follicular response to gonadotrophin stimulation by local intraovarian regulators, particularly from the dominant follicle, could explain such phenomena as the variation in ovarian response to exogenous and endogenous gonadotrophins, the frequency of multiple ovulators in a population, ovarian compensatory hypertrophy and interrelationships between follicle size classes during growth.

There is an increased frequency of dizygotic twinning in older women, particularly around 35–40 years of age (Parkes, 1976), which is before the time when FSH secretion is expected to increase (World Health Organization, 1981). This suggests a local influence within the ovary, perhaps associated with the depletion of the follicular pool. The increased frequency of multiple ovulations in other animals which are attributed to breed, nutrition and season (see Jones, 1978; Scaramuzzi and Radford, 1983) could also result from inter- and intragonadal modulating mechanisms, since it has not always been possible to relate increased ovulation rate to concentrations of gonadotrophins in peripheral blood. Only modest changes in FSH are required to promote recruitment and selection of follicles in women. Brown (1978) concluded that within an individual, the difference in dose of gonadotrophin between no effect and stimulation may be as little as 20% and that the threshold dose necessary to maintain follicular development changes between individuals and with the size of the follicle within an individual.

Unilateral ovariectomy in a number of mammals including women leads to compensatory ovarian hypertrophy and a doubling of the ovulations on the remaining ovary so that litter size is held more or less constant (Lipschutz, 1928; Jones, 1978). Because removal of one ovary is followed by no change in LH and a transient rise in FSH with concentrations returning to presurgical levels within hours or several days (Jones, 1978), it is unlikely that the increased ovulation rate is due to persistently higher FSH levels. Several days after unilateral ovariectomy in sheep, Dufour et al (1979) observed an increase in recruitment of small preantral follicles, an increased number of antral follicles in the remaining ovary and no significant change in the rate of atresia to account for the observed ovulation rates. In the pig, removal of antral follicles on one side leads to compensation on the same side (Brinkley and Young, 1969), whereas the same treatment in anoestrous ewes leads to compensation on the contralateral ovary (Dufour et al, 1971). Assuming no persistent increase in FSH after this type of treatment (Cahill et al, 1985b), it can be argued that there is regulation within and between ovaries leading to compensatory hypertrophy. Jones (1978) has put forward the hypothesis that the compensation occurs as a result of increased access of gonadotrophin to the remaining ovary because vascular access and permeability increase and there is a lower utilization rate of FSH. An equally plausible hypothesis is that unilateral ovariectomy results in a change in the modulating influence of intraovarian regulators in the remaining ovary. Cahill et al (1979) observed that, as follicle size increased, the number of follicles per size class in each ovary became similar. This was interpreted to mean that as follicles grow, communication between ovaries and follicles increases until dominance is assumed.

In summary, there is evidence that control of follicular growth after antrum formation involves communication between follicles such that local ovarian factors can modify the response of the follicle to stimulation by pituitary hormones. It is conceivable that these processes involve communication within and between ovaries, and provide mechanisms for recruitment, selection and dominance of follicles.

Communication within follicles. There are well-documented examples of both paracrine and autocrine regulation within the follicle. Undoubtedly, some of the regulators are the proximal agents of gonadotrophin action on the follicle and represent a further stage of differentiation of the cells producing them.

Paracrine interaction between the theca and granulosa is best characterized by the steroids, which can either act as substrates for further metabolism or have a direct action on the target cells. Falck (1959) provided the first experimental evidence supporting an interaction between theca and granulosa cells to produce oestrogens. This two-cell hypothesis has been verified subsequently in that granulosa cells rely on the theca for androgen substrate to produce oestrogens because granulosa cells lack the 17,20-lyase activity required to convert C_{21}- to C_{19}-steroids (Leung and Armstrong, 1980; Richards, 1980). The direct paracrine actions of steroids on follicular cells include inhibition of enzyme activities such as the competitive effects of reduced androgens on aromatase activity (Hillier et al, 1980), and actions as a result of binding of the steroid to receptors. Examples include the stimulatory action of androgens on FSH-induced progesterone production and aromatase activity by granulosa cells (Richards, 1980). Oestrogens can negatively influence androgen production by thecal cells (Leung and Armstrong, 1980), although the source of oestrogen could be either the granulosa or theca cells.

There is also evidence of a paracrine interaction between the granulosa cells, including the cumulus cells, and the oocyte, to prevent the resumption of meiosis and maturation of the oocyte until after the preovulatory surge of gonadotrophins (Byskov 1979; Tsafriri et al, 1982). Removal of oocytes from their follicles, particularly the association of the oocyte with the granulosa cells, results in spontaneous maturation of the oocyte in vitro, even in hormone-free media. This led to the concept that the follicle cells of mammals 'supply to the ovum a substance or substances which directly inhibit nuclear maturation' (Pincus and Enzmann, 1935). That activity, termed oocyte maturation inhibitor (OMI; Tsafriri et al, 1982), is synthesized by the granulosa cells and is present in the follicular fluid, particularly in small follicles. OMI is thought to be a peptide of molecular weight less than 2000, which acts on the cumulus cells to impose meiotic arrest on the oocyte by a mechanism still not understood. LH induces the resumption of meiosis by either eliminating the cumulus signal, blocking transfer of the inhibitory signal from cumulus cells to oocyte or terminating OMI production. Alternatively, LH may generate a positive signal.

Byskov (1979) proposed that meiosis in mammalian gonads is regulated by a balance between MIS and MPS. Meiosis is arrested by the presence of MPS in the follicle and resumption of the meiosis is facilitated by increasing amounts of MIS in the preovulatory follicle (Westergaard et al, 1984), particularly in those healthy human follicles in which the oocyte can be fertilized and undergo cleavage in vitro (Westergaard et al, 1985). MPS activity could not be demonstrated by Westergaard et al (1984) in any samples from large follicles, suggesting it was either absent or it was present in amounts below the level of detection of the assay system. The relationship, if any, between OMI (molecular weight <2000) and MPS (molecular weight >5000) is uncertain. MIS has a molecular weight <5000 and has the characteristics of a lipid, but is unlikely to be progesterone (Westergaard et al, 1984).

Maturation of the oocyte just prior to ovulation involves much more than just resumption of meiosis to the second metaphase and exclusion of the first polar body (Crosby and Moor, 1984). It also involves the oocyte acquiring a sensitivity to the LH stimulus and, subsequently includes changes in a wide variety of cellular activities, including transcription, synthesis and post-translational modifications of proteins, energy metabolism, and membrane transport in cooperation with the surrounding follicle cells. Interruption of these processes will inhibit fertilization and subsequent development.

Recent evidence supports a paracrine influence of granulosa cells on the vascular endothelium of the theca leading to angiogenesis during follicular growth (see Findlay, 1986). There are several reports of angiogenic activity in ovarian follicles but the factor(s) responsible has not been isolated and characterized.

There are several examples of autocrine effects of granulosa cells based on in vivo and in vitro studies. Oestradiol causes mitotic division of granulosa cells and facilitates the induction of LH receptors by FSH, an effect thought to be mediated by an interaction of oestradiol with its receptor in granulosa cells (Richards, 1980). There is also evidence of autocrine effects of growth factors in the ovarian follicle (Hammond, 1981). Granulosa cells secrete the growth factor, insulin-like growth factor I (IGF-I), have receptors for IGF-I and respond to IGF-I by an augmentation of FSH-induced progesterone production, aromatase activity and proteoglycan synthesis (Adashi et al, 1985). Granulosa cells also secrete in vitro, and probably in vivo, an inhibitor of aromatase activity (diZerega et al, 1984) and a mitotic inhibitor (Cahill et al, 1985a,b) of granulosa cells.

These few examples of paracrine and autocrine interactions within ovarian follicles serve to emphasize the complex nature of the control processes which are operating at the local ovarian level in the face of relatively constant gonadotrophin stimulation. There is an ever-increasing list of factors, activities and substances being identified in the ovarian follicle (see Sharpe, 1984), some of which have no known function; many have no chemical identity.

Corpus luteum formation and regulation

There are several examples of local regulators controlling the formation and function of the corpus luteum.

Neovascularization of the new corpus luteum is one example (see Findlay, 1986). At about the time of follicular rupture, capillaries and arterioles of the theca begin to sprout and when the folds of theca interdigitate with the luteinizing membrana granulosa these sprouts penetrate the granulosa layers to form a dense vascular network. The process is quite rapid and the vascular supply is established within several days of ovulation. There is in vivo and in vitro evidence for the presence of angiogenic activity in the follicular fluid after an ovulatory dose of human chorionic gonadotrophin (hCG) and in the luteal tissue (Gospodarowicz et al, 1985; Findlay, 1986). The available evidence suggests that this activity arises as a result of luteinization of the granulosa cells and that it acts locally to control neovascularization.

The second example concerns the relationships between the two major cell types of the corpus luteum, the theca-derived small luteal cell and the granulosa-derived large luteal cell (Rodgers et al, 1985; Schwall et al, 1986). The small luteal cell is characterized by being the more abundant type with an ability to respond to LH by increasing progesterone production, by the absence of receptors for prostaglandin and, according to one body of opinion (see Schwall et al, 1986), an ability to transform into large luteal cells as the corpus luteum ages. The large luteal cell, on the other hand, is less abundant, does not respond to LH but can produce progesterone, has receptors for prostaglandins and an ability to synthesize and secrete proteins, such as relaxin and oxytocin, the latter peptide in response to prostaglandin. There is the possibility that the control of progesterone production by the corpus luteum may rest partly with an interaction between these two cell types, particularly at the time of luteolysis (Rodgers et al, 1985). The luteolysin in primates remains elusive despite extensive studies on prostaglandins and steroids. Perhaps attention should be focused on other non-steroidal products of large luteal cells that might modulate progesterone production of the small cells by a paracrine action.

The final example of local regulatory mechanisms in the corpus luteum concerns an interaction between luteal cells and macrophages. Coculture of peritoneal macrophages with mouse luteal cells (Kirsch et al, 1981) or human granulosa cells harvested after an ovulatory dose of hCG (Halme et al, 1985) enhanced progesterone production by the luteal cells. Macrophages found within the corpus luteum (Kirsch et al, 1981) and blood monocytes have a similar action (Halme et al, 1985), which apparently requires contact between the macrophages and luteal cells to be effective (Kirsch et al, 1983). This appears to be the first evidence that a cell of the immune system communicates directly with a steroid-secreting cell of the ovary.

INTRAGONADAL CONTROL MECHANISMS IN THE TESTIS

The requirement for local factors regulating and coordinating the numerous functions of different cell types within the testis is self-evident when one considers the following points. Firstly, the maintenance of spermatogenesis is controlled by the Sertoli cells under the influence of testosterone produced by the Leydig cells. Thus it is logical that the Sertoli and Leydig cells should interact and influence each others' function; and indeed there is growing evidence to support this concept. Similarly, there are complex cell–cell interactions in the seminiferous epithelium. Cyclical activity of Sertoli cells has been correlated with differing stages of spermatogenesis, but these changes in activity occur during the constant (but episodic) secretion of pituitary gonadotrophins. Thus it is logical that the germ cells and Sertoli cells must interact to locally regulate each other's functions.

Tubule–Leydig cell interactions

Historically the first demonstration of local communication between the seminiferous tubules and Leydig cells was described by Aoki and Fawcett in 1978. These workers had implanted capsules of antiandrogens in the testes and recorded focal areas of damage to the seminiferous epithelium; adjacent to these areas the interstitial tissue was hypertrophied. In unaffected areas of the same testes, the appearance of the interstitial tissue was normal. These data were interpreted as a demonstration of a local mechanism of controlling Leydig cell function. This study was complemented by a series of articles on the effects of experimental disruption of spermatogenesis induced by vitamin A deficiency, x-irradiation, cryptorchidism, efferent duct ligation or heat treatment (see Sharpe, 1984). Each treatment resulted in morphological changes to the Leydig cells which became hypertrophied, the organelles associated with steroidogenesis were more prominent, and in vitro the capacity to secrete testosterone was enhanced compared to normal.

More recent studies by Bergh (1982) have examined the normal seminiferous tubules and shown that Leydig cells lying close to tubules vary in phase with the spermatogenic cycle, being largest when adjacent to tubules at stage VII–VIII. He thus proposed that there was cyclic, stage-dependent paracrine regulation of Leydig cells by seminiferous tubules. It is not known whether the factor responsible for cyclic changes in Leydig cell size in the normal testis is the same as that which causes Leydig cell hypertrophy caused by damage to the seminiferous tubule.

Most of the studies from which this information has been accumulated have been performed in the laboratory rat. As in most mammals, the seminiferous epithelium exhibits a regular pattern consisting of character-istic germ cell associations (stage of spermatogenesis), which occupy the complete circumference of a tubular cross-section, and which are arranged in serial continuity in the longitudinal course of the tubule (wave of spermatogenesis). In contrast however, the regular pattern of the epi-thelium in the human is not immediately obvious as, for example, more than one spermatogenic stage is present in a tubular cross-section or atypical or heterogeneous stages are observed. Thus observations of the type described in the rat using a conventional stage concept have not been completed. Recently however Schulze and Rehder (1984) have reported that the arrangement of germ cells in the human seminiferous epithelium is not irregular or chaotic, but exhibits a complex organizational pattern that is based on the geometry of spirals, thus the seminiferous epithelium in all mammals, including humans, may be subjected to a uniform principle of morphogenesis and autoregulation. Further examination is required to determine if similar data can be derived concerning the stage-dependent regulation of Leydig cell function by the seminiferous epithelium using human testicular tissues. Nevertheless there is evidence in the human male that disorders of spermatogenesis are associated with altered Leydig cell function. For example, men with Sertoli-cell-only syndrome exhibit impaired Leydig cell function (de Kretser et al, 1975).

The quest for factors which may be the agents of communication between the seminiferous tubules and Leydig cells has been disappointing to date. On the one hand a diffusible product from the tubule could act to inhibit and thus regulate androgen synthesis in the normal animal. Alternatively, damage to the tubules could interfere with the production of this agent and Leydig cells would become hypertrophic as they are released from this inhibitory influence. The first candidate suggested for this role was oestra-diol. However, in the adult testis the Leydig cell, not the Sertoli cell, is the principal site of oestradiol production (Valladares and Payne, 1979). Thus it is unlikely that oestradiol would have a local regulatory role in the testis.

Speculation that luteinizing hormone releasing hormone (LHRH) was involved in the local control of Leydig cell function arose from the obser-vations that LHRH and its agonists had inhibitory effects on testicular function in man and the rat (see review by Sharpe, 1984). The role of LHRH as an intragonadal hormone in the rat was proposed on the basis that LHRH was produced in the testis, that there were specific LHRH receptors and that biological actions of the hormone were detected (e.g. effects on testicular blood flow and capillary permeability) (see Sharpe, 1984). However, it has been established that the measurement of LHRH in extracts of rat testicular tissue by radioimmunoassay or in vitro bioassay techniques is complicated by the presence of testicular proteases, multiple LHRH-immunoactive species, factors which non-specifically stimulate the release of anterior pituitary hormones in vitro, and by low levels of LHRH in these extracts (Hedger et al, 1985). Thus, extensive extraction/fractionation procedures which have not been previously employed are required to minimize inter-ference by non-specific factors in immuno- or bioassays. Secondly, the testes of the human do not appear to possess specific high affinity LHRH receptors (Clayton and Huhtaniemi, 1982) and there is no effect of LHRH agonists on reproductive function in the mouse (Wang et al, 1983). These observations suggest that studies on the direct effects of LHRH and its agonists on reproductive function in the rat may not necessarily be relevant to other species including man. Nevertheless it has been established that the adult rat testis contains approximately 1 pg LHRH; as it is unlikely that this is due simply to contamination of the extracts by hypothalamic LHRH from the circulation, the source and physiological role of LHRH in the extracts remain to be resolved.

More recently there have been numerous reports of factors emanating from tubules which can affect Leydig cell steroidogenesis in vitro (Parvinen et al, 1984; Janecki et al, 1985; Syed et al, 1985; Verhoeven and Cailleau 1985). These studies have been performed in the rat and a factor in rat testicular interstitial fluid (IF) has been identified (Sharpe and Cooper, 1984) which is non-gonadotrophic and capable of stimulating steroido-genesis by Percoll-purified Leydig cells in vitro. The levels of this stimu-latory factor in IF have been shown to alter according to changes in the intratesticular environment, which may be a consequence of decreased intratesticular testosterone levels, altered FSH levels or Sertoli cell mal-functions (Sharpe and Bartlett, 1985; Sharpe et al, 1986).

The identity of factors in testicular IF which stimulate steroidogenesis is unknown. Recently Valenca and Negro-Vilar (1986) have measured the pro-opiomelanocortin (POMC)-derived peptide, adenocorticotrophic hormone and β-endorphin, in testicular IF and have suggested that they may be important local regulators of testicular function. These findings support earlier studies that these peptides were present in the testis (Margioris et al, 1983; Fabbri et al, 1985) and that the POMC gene was expressed in testicular tissue indicating that it was synthesized locally (Chen et al, 1984). The apparent molecular weight of the factor in testicular IF which stimulates steroidogenesis has been shown to be ≈ 58 000 and thus it is unlikely that the activity in IF is due to POMC-derived peptides.

Finally it is possible that a local regulatory factor may emanate from the macrophage population present in the interstitium. It has been shown that media from testicular macrophage cultures stimulate Leydig cell steroido-genesis and the potency of the media is increased after culturing the macro-phages with FSH (Yee and Hutson, 1985). Thus Leydig cell steroidogenesis could be regulated by FSH-stimulated products from testicular macro-phages.

Whilst the most common effect of substances in Leydig cells has been to stimulate steroidogenesis, arginine vasopressin (AVP)-like peptides inhibit gonadotrophin-induced androgen production (Adashi and Hseuh, 1981). AVP-like peptides and AVP receptors have been described in both Sprague-Dawley and Battleboro rats (Kasson et al, 1985; Kasson and Hseuh, 1986) and it has been proposed that AVP could be an intratesticular modulator of steroidogenesis.

Sertoli–germ cell interactions

Clearly Leydig cell function is influenced by factors emanating from the seminiferous tubules, in addition to LH. Likewise, the functioning of the Sertoli cells is principally regulated by FSH and androgens, but other factors may play a role in the local control of spermatogenesis. The requirement for specific local mechanisms of control is necessary in order to achieve the remarkably high degree of synchronous proliferation and differentiation of germ cells in the epithelium of all species studied so far. The Sertoli cells are believed to play a key role in regulating the process of spermatogenesis as they partially or completely surround every germ cell (Fawcett, 1975). The requirements of germ cells change as they develop at each stage of the spermatogenic cycle, therefore it is apparent that the function of the Sertoli cells will vary in cyclical fashion.

Morphological evidence for cyclical activity of Sertoli cells in the rat has been demonstrated (see Parvinen, 1982) but in the monkey and human testis no clear relationship between Sertoli cell ultrastructure and particular stages of the spermatogenic cycle has emerged (Dym, 1973; Kerr and de Kretser, 1981). These tissues were fixed by perfusion rather than immersion and contemporary morphometric techniques were not employed. The application of these techniques combined with superior methods of fixation of tissue may yield similar information in species other than the laboratory rat.

The stage-dependent cyclical variation of the functional activities of the Sertoli cells has been vigorously investigated. These studies progressed rapidly due to the development of a transillumination-assisted microdissection technique in the rat which was poineered by Parvinen (1982). This technique allowed the collection of seminiferous tubule fragments of defined stages of the cycle for organ culture, or biochemical analysis of hormone or protein content. Application of this technique is possible in all mammalian species which have a wave-like arrangement of the seminiferous epithelium except of course the human male, which as discussed previously has a different spatial arrangement. Using this technique, the pattern of production of a number of substances has been shown to be cyclical. For example, receptors for FSH and the activities of adenyl cyclase and aromatase show stage-dependent variations and substances such as androgen binding protein (ABP), transferrin, somatomedins and plasminogen activator exhibit a stage-dependent variation in production (see Ritzen, 1983). Therefore both morphological and biochemical data show evidence for the cyclical activity of the Sertoli cell, despite the facts that firstly, adjacent Sertoli cells may be performing different functions, and secondly, that all cells are exposed to the same level of pituitary gonadotrophins.

One method of achieving stage-dependent changes in the action of FSH, for example, on the seminiferous tubules would be to engage local mechanisms of altering the ability of the cells to detect and respond to FSH. Maximum binding of FSH and enhanced response to FSH stimulation occur in stages I–V, whereas stages VII–VIII are almost insensitive to FSH (see Parvinen, 1982). The precise reasons for this local variation in response to FSH are not certain. Nevertheless it is noteworthy that the distribution of two spermatid-specific enzymes, Mn^{2+}-dependent adenyl cyclase and protein carboxyl methylase closely follows that of FSH-stimulated cyclic adenosine monophosphate secretion (see Parvinen, 1982). It was suggested that these enzymes may be required for the activation of cytoskeletal components of the Sertoli cells resulting in the deep location of the tight bundles of maturing spermatids close to Sertoli cell nuclei. Maximum formation of spermatid bundles intimately associated with Sertoli cells coincides exactly with maximum response to FSH in stages II–V. Thus it is tempting to conclude that the differential sensitivity of Sertoli cells to FSH may be a local mechanism associated with spermatid maturation and release.

The preferential requirement for androgens in stages VII and VIII of the cycle of the seminiferous epithelium has been clearly demonstrated by observing the effects of hypophysectomy or the administration of LH antiserum (Dym et al, 1977; Russell and Clermont, 1977). This requirement for androgen at stage VII and VIII coincides with the times at which intratubular levels of testosterone are highest (Parvinen and Ruokonen, 1982), when peritubular Leydig cells in the interstitium are largest (Bergh, 1982) and the rate of secretion of ABP (Ritzen et al, 1982), which is believed to transport testosterone within the tubule, is maximal. It is tempting therefore to speculate that at stages VII and VIII when there is the greatest need for testosterone by the germ cells, the Leydig cells can produce higher levels of testosterone transported by ABP for utilization in the seminiferous epithelium—thus demonstrating local interaction between tubules and Leydig cells and Sertoli and germ cells.

Clearly there are FSH- and androgen-sensitive stages of the seminiferous cycle of the rat which are the result of the operation of local mechanisms within the tubule. There are numerous other examples of the interaction of Sertoli and germ cells. Consider first the process of mitotic proliferation of spermatogonia in the basal compartment of the tubule. What causes the reactivation of mitosis at puberty? What controls the ratio of active to resting spermatogonia? What causes type A spermatogonia to 'drop out' of the sequence of differentiation and division in order to conserve their numbers? Little is known about these processes although they must be controlled within the testis. Indeed Feig et al (1980) have reported the presence of a mitogenic polypeptide in mouse Sertoli cells, thus supporting the hypothesis that a local mitogenic factor(s) could stimulate germ cell proliferation and be of fundamental importance in regulating mammalian spermatogenesis. Conversely, an inhibitor of spermatogonial mitosis has been detected in crude extracts of rat seminiferous tubules (Clermont and Mauger, 1974).

At the next stage of spermatogenesis, the primary spermatocytes enter the adluminal compartment of the testis and undergo meiotic division. The control of meiosis is not understood. MIS and MPS have been detected in the mouse (Byskov, 1978) and human (Grindsted and Byskov, 1981) and are thought to interact with one another to regulate meiosis in the adult male. Parvinen (1982) reported that, whereas MPS was secreted at a relatively constant level at all stages of the cycle in the rat, MIS was maximally secreted in stages VII and VIII and therefore speculated that MPS was preventing cells from entering meiosis at stages other than VII and VIII, but that during these stages MIS could stimulate the cell to enter meiosis. The entry of cells into meiosis also occurs with the movement of the primary spermatocytes through the tight junctions of the Sertoli cells. The transfer of the germ cells is thought to involve the secretion of plasminogen activator and this idea was supported by the detection of maximal levels of plasminogen activator at stages VII and VIII (Lacroix et al, 1981). Furthermore, at these stages step 19 spermatids eliminate their cytoplasm as residual bodies and spermatozoa are released from the seminiferous epithelium; and it has been proposed that phagocytosis of the residual bodies represents a stimulus to increase Sertoli cell production of plasminogen activator (Lacroix et al, 1981).

Another fine example of the symbiotic functional relationship between Sertoli and germ cells is the regulation of the survival of rat pachytene spermatocytes by lactate supplied from the Sertoli cells. Using techniques of tissue culture, Jutte et al (1981) showed that lactate was essential for the metabolic activities of isolated rat spermatocytes and spermatids which could not themselves survive in glucose alone; whereas the Sertoli cells have an enormous capacity to convert glucose to lactate (Jutte et al, 1982), which was stimulated by FSH (Jutte et al, 1983). Thus the activity and survival of pachytene spermatocytes is regulated by Sertoli cells via conversion of glucose to lactate. In addition to FSH, insulin and IGF-I can stimulate the production of lactate by immature rat Sertoli cells cultured in vitro (Borland et al, 1984; Mita et al, 1985). The exact role of insulin and IGF-I in promoting the synthesis of lactate remains to be determined.

The cyclic activity of proteins such as ABP and plasminogen activator has long been documented (see Parvinen, 1982). However numerous other proteins are secreted by the Sertoli cells. Wright et al (1983) used the technique of dissecting stage-specific tubular segments and determined that, in the rat, at least 15 different proteins were secreted in a cyclical fashion, including transferrin and ceruloplasmin. Testicular transferrin appears to be secreted by both rat (Skinner and Griswold, 1980) and human (Holmes et al, 1984) Sertoli cells in culture. The exact role of transferrin in the regulation of spermatogenesis is uncertain, but it may provide iron for haem proteins or non-haem metalloproteins for the developing germ cells. Ceruloplasmin is a major copper transport protein in serum and can act as a ferroxidase. Since germ cells develop in a unique microenvironment created by the formation of the blood–testis barrier, ceruloplasmin produced by Sertoli cells could be involved in the maintenance of germ cell viability by providing copper or acting as a ferroxidase (Skinner and Griswold, 1983).

The demonstration that Sertoli cell proteins are secreted in a cyclical fashion reinforces the view that the functional activity of Sertoli cells must be coordinated over space and time. Other Sertoli cell proteins have been identified, for example spectrin and clusterin, but their patterns of secretion during the cycle of the seminiferous epithelium have not been analysed.

The synthesis of some glycoproteins proceeds at a constant rate during the cycle of the seminiferous epithelium (Lalli et al, 1984). However it appears that changes in the synthesis of specific glycoproteins of rat Sertoli cells cultured in vitro may be influenced by the association with germ cells (Galdieri et al, 1984). Glycoproteins are thought to be involved in recognition and adhesion between adjacent cells and this view is supported by the observation that the attachment of pachytene spermatocytes and round spermatids to Sertoli cells in vitro is enhanced in the presence of concanavalin A (Grootegoed et al, 1982). Perhaps future investigations will delineate the role of glycoproteins in the interaction between Sertoli and germ cells and the stage-dependent production of newly identified proteins will be characterized. Nevertheless it is obvious that the Sertoli cells recognize differences in the maturation of the developing germ cells that they surround. The cyclical activity of the Sertoli cells may be inherent or dictated by germ cell products which stimulate Sertoli cell activity. Alternatively the cytoplasmic bridges between spermatocytes and the gap junctions between Sertoli cells could permit the transfer of messages between the cells of the seminiferous epithelium.

Sertoli–peritubular cell interactions

The previous paragraphs have emphasized the local interaction between the Sertoli and germ cells, but there is a growing body of evidence to demonstrate the cooperation between Sertoli cells and peritubular cells. The seminiferous epithelium rests upon the basal lamina and one or more layers of myoid cells bounded peripherally by lymphatic endothelial cells separate the seminiferous tubules from the interstitial tissue. The peritubular myoid cells meet edge-to-edge, the majority forming tight junctions and represent a component of the blood–testis barrier. However, the role of these cells in promoting the integrity and function of Sertoli cells is novel.

Tung and Fritz (1980) first reported that cocultures of immature rat Sertoli cells and peritubular myoid cells resulted in the formation of a basal lamina and the architecture of the Sertoli cells resembled that in the seminiferous tubules, whereas Sertoli or peritubular cells in monocultures form relatively uniform layers. Later studies revealed that the morphology and function of Sertoli cells was greatly influenced by the substratum upon which they were placed (Tung and Fritz, 1984; Hadley et al, 1985). Although Sertoli and peritubular cells independently produce components of the extracellular matrix (ECM), together in culture the levels of ECM components are quantitatively altered (Skinner and Fritz, 1985a; Skinner et al, 1985). This suggests that the two cell types act cooperatively in culture in the formation and deposition of ECM which permits both cell types to maintain their structural and functional integrity. The presence of peritubular cells or ECM also enhances the production of Sertoli cell ABP and transferrin secretion (Hutson and Stocco, 1981; Hadley et al, 1985; Skinner and Fritz, 1985b).

The peritubular cells are thought to produce a modulating protein(s) (P-Mod-S) which stimulates Sertoli cell ABP and transferrin secretion; the formation of P-Mod-S itself may be controlled by androgens (Skinner and Fritz, 1985c). At this time it is not known if the nature of the ECM components produced by these two cell types varies during the stages of spermatogenesis to modify their structural or functional activities.

SUMMARY

On the weight of the evidence presented above, it is concluded that regulation at a local, intragonadal level is an integral part of the overall regulation of gonadal function in both sexes. The interaction between cells within a gonad extends beyond the same cell type to include germ cell–somatic cell inter-actions as well. We believe this local interaction between cell types facilitates the differing requirements of the various developmental stages of germ cells within the gonad, which would not be possible by simply varying the afferent pituitary hormone supply. We re-emphasize that the local factors responsible for these interactions are acting in conjunction with the pituitary hormones, and, in some cases, may be their proximate regulators.

A more controversial phenomenon is the possibility of an interaction between the gonads which does not involve the hypothalamic–pituitary axis. The little evidence which is available to support this hypothesis comes mainly from studies on ovarian function, particularly recruitment and selection of follicles. More research on this phenomenon is warranted.

Not surprisingly there are many parallels between the testes and ovaries with respect to the nature and action of local regulators. For example, the intragonadal action of steroids, the local modulation of the response of target cells to FSH, the influence of macrophages on steroidogenesis and the presence of mitotic and meiotic regulators are common to both sexes. It would not be surprising if the chemical nature of these factors in the ovary and testes are similar.

If the ever-increasing list of factors and activities being discovered in the gonads is any guide, the phenomena outlined in this review are just the beginning of an extensive list of cell–cell interactions occurring within and between the gonads. No doubt the gonads will share with other organs the same interactions between cells which are required for normal cellular function. The uniqueness of the gonads lies in their protection and pro-duction of germ cells. The challenge of the future for reproductive biologists will be to discover and describe the interactions within and between germ cells which are obligatory for normal reproductive function, and to apply that information to devising ways of overcoming infertility and regulating fertility.

Acknowledgements

We are grateful to Jenny Judd for secretarial assistance. The authors are supported financially by a Programme Grant from the National Health and Medical Research Council of Australia.

Part of this review was prepared while J. K. Findlay was on leave as a consultant to the Special Programme of Research, Development and Research Training in Human Reproduction, World Health Organization, Geneva, Switzerland.

REFERENCES

Adashi EY & Hseuh AJ (1981) Direct inhibition of testicular androgen biosynthesis revealing antigonadal activity of neurohypophyseal hormones. *Nature* **293:** 650–652.

Adashi EY, Resnick CE, D'Ercole AJ, Svoboda ME & van Wyk JJ (1985) Insulin-like growth factors as intraovarian regulators of granulosa cell growth and function. *Endocrine Reviews* **6:** 400–420.

Aoki A & Fawcett DW (1978) Is there a local feedback from the seminiferous tubules affecting activity of the Leydig cell? *Biology of Reproduction* **19:** 144–158.

Baird DT (1983) Factors regulating the growth of the preovulatory follicle in the sheep and human. *Journal of Reproduction and Fertility* **69:** 343–352.

Bergh A (1982) Local differences in Leydig cell morphology in the adult rat testis: evidence for a local control of Leydig cells by adjacent seminiferous tubules. *International Journal of Andrology* **5:** 325–330.

Borland K, Mita M, Oppenheimer CL et al (1984) The actions of insulin-like growth factors I and II on cultured Sertoli cells. *Endocrinology* **114:** 240–246.

Brinkley HJ & Young EP (1969) Effects of unilateral ovariectomy or unilateral destruction of ovarian components on the follicles and corpora lutea of the non pregnant pig. *Endocrinology* **84:** 1250–1256.

Brown JB (1978) Pituitary control of ovarian function-concepts derived from gonadotrophin therapy. *Australian and New Zealand Journal of Obstetrics and Gynaecology* **18:** 47–54.

Byskov AG (1975) The role of the rete ovarii in meiosis and follicle formation in the cat, mink and ferret. *Journal of Reproduction and Fertility* **45:** 201–209.

Byskov AG (1978) Regulation of initiation of meiosis in fetal gonads. *International Journal of Andrology* (supplement 2, part 1) 29–38.

Byskov AG (1979) Regulation of meiosis in mammals. *Annales de Biologiè Animale, Biochemie, Biophysique* **19:** 1251–1261.

Byskov AG (1981) Gonadal sex and germ cell differentiation. In Austin CR & Edwards RG (eds) *Mechanisms of Sex Differentiation in Animals and Man*, pp 145–164. London: Academic Press.

Cahill LP & Mauleon P (1980) Influence of season, cycle and breed on follicular growth rates in sheep. *Journal of Reproduction and Fertility* **58:** 321–328.

Cahill LP, Mariana JC & Mauleon P (1979) Total follicular populations in ewes of high and low ovulation rates. *Journal of Reproduction and Fertility* **55:** 27–36.

Cahill LP, Clarke IJ, Cummins JT et al (1985a) An inhibitory action at the ovarian level of ovine follicular fluid on PMSG-induced folliculogenesis in hypophysectomized ewes. In Toft D & Ryan RH (eds) *Proceedings of the Fifth Ovarian Workshop*, pp 35–38. New York: Plenum Press.

Cahill LP, Driancourt MA, Chamley WA & Findlay JK (1985b) Role of intrafollicular regulators and FSH in growth and development of large antral follicles in sheep. *Journal of Reproduction and Fertility* **75:** 599–607.

Chen CLC, Mather J, Morris PL & Bardin CW (1984) Expression of proopiomelanocortin-like gene in the testis and epididymis. *Proceedings of the National Academy Sciences (USA)* **81:** 5672.

Clayton RN & Huhtaniemi IT (1982) Absence of gonadotropin-releasing hormone receptors in human gonadal tissue. *Nature* **299:** 56–59.

Clermont Y & Mauger A (1974) Existence of a spermatogonial chalone in the rat testis. *Cell and Tissue Kinetics* **7:** 165–172.

Crosby IM & Moor RM (1984) Oocyte maturation. In Trounson A & Wood C (eds) *In Vitro Fertilization and Embryo Transfer*, pp 19–31. Edinburgh: Churchill Livingstone.

de Kretser DM, Burger HG, Hudson B & Keogh GJ (1975) The hCG stimulation test in men with testicular disorders. *Clinical Endocrinology* **4:** 591–596.

diZerega GS & Wilks JW (1984) Inhibition of the primate ovarian cycle by a porcine follicular fluid protein(s). *Fertility and Sterility* **41:** 635–638.

diZerega GS, Campeau JD, Ujita EL et al (1984) Follicular regulatory proteins: paracrine regulators of follicular steroidogenesis. In Sairam MR & Atkinson LE (eds) *Gonadal Proteins and Peptides and Their Biological Significance*, pp 215–228. Singapore: World Scientific Publications.

Driancourt MA, Cahill LP & Bindon BM (1985) Ovarian follicular populations and pre-ovulatory enlargement in Booroola and control Merino ewes. *Journal of Reproduction and Fertility* **73:** 93–107.

Dufour J, Ginther OJ & Casida LE (1971) Compensatory hypertrophy after unilateral ovari-ectomy and destruction of follicles in the anestrous ewe. *Proceedings of the Society for Experimental Biology and Medicine* **138:** 1068–1072.

Dufour J, Cahill LP & Mauleon P (1979) Short- and long-term effects of hypophysectomy and unilateral ovariectomy on ovarian follicular populations in sheep. *Journal of Reproduction and Fertility* **57:** 301–309.

Dunbar BS & Wolgemuth DJ (1984) Structure and function of the mammalian zona pellucida, a unique extracellular matrix. *Modern Cell Biology* **3:** 77–111.

Dym M (1973) The fine structure of the monkey (*Macaca*) Sertoli cell and its role in maintaining the blood tests barrier. *Anatomical Record* **175:** 639–656.

Dym M, Raj HGM & Chernes HG (1977) Response of the testis to selective withdrawal of LH or FSH using antigonadotropic sera in the testis in normal and infertile men. In Mancini RE & Martin L (eds) *The Testis in Normal and Infertile Men*, pp 97–124. New York: Academic Press.

Fabbri A, Tsai-Morris CH, Luna S, Fraioli F & Dufau ML (1985) Opiate receptors are present in rat testis: identification and localization in Sertoli cells. *Endocrinology* **117:** 2544–2546.

Falck B (1959) Site of production of oestrogen in rat ovary as studied by microtransplants. *Acta Physiologica Scandinavica* **47**(supplement 163): 1–101.

Fawcett DW (1975) Ultrastructure and function of the Sertoli cell. In Hamilton DW & Greep RO (eds) *Handbook of Physiology: Male Reproductive System*, vol. 5, pp 21–55. Bethesda: American Physiological Society.

Feig LA, Bellve AR, Erickson NH & Klagsbrun M (1980) Sertoli cells contain a mitogenic polypeptide. *Proceedings of the National Academy of Sciences (USA)* **77:** 4774–4778.

Foxcroft GR & Hunter MG (1985) Basic physiology of follicular maturation in the pig. *Journal of Reproduction and Fertility Supplement* **33:** 1–19.

Findlay JK (1986) Angiogenesis in reproductive tissues. *Journal of Endocrinology* (in press).

Franchi LL, Mandl AM & Zuckerman S (1962) The development of the ovary and process of oogenesis. In Zuckerman S (ed.) *The Ovary*, vol. 1, p 27. London: Academic Press.

Galdieri M, Monaco L & Stefanini M (1984) Secretion of androgen binding protein by Sertoli cells is influenced by contact with germ cells. *Journal of Andrology* **5:** 409–415.

Goodman AL & Hodgen GD (1983) The ovarian triad of the primate menstrual cycle. *Recent Progress in Hormone Research* **39:** 1–73.

Gospodarowicz D, Cheng J, Liu G et al (1985) Corpus luteum angiogenic factor is related to fibroblast growth factor. *Endocrinology* **117:** 2383–2391.

Greenwald GS (1978) Follicular activity in the mammalian ovary. In Jones RE (ed.) *The Vertebrate Ovary*, pp 639–689. New York: Plenum Press.

Greep RO (1961) Physiology of the anterior hypophysis in relation to reproduction. In Young WWC (ed.) *Sex and Internal Secretions*, vol. 1, 3rd edn, pp 240–301. Baltimore: Williams & Wilkins.

Grindsted J & Byskov AG (1981) Meiosis inducing and meiosis preventing substances in human male reproductive organs. *Fertility and Sterility* **35:** 199–204.

Grootegoed JA, Jutte NHPM, Rommerts FFG, van der Molen HJ & Ohno S (1982) Concana-valin A-induced attachment of spermatogenic cells to Sertoli cells in vitro. *Experimental Cell Research* **139:** 472–475.

Hadley MA, Byers SW, Suarez-Quian CA, Kleinman HK & Dym M (1985) Extracellular matrix regulates Sertoli cell differentiation, testicular cord formation, and germ cell development in vitro. *Journal of Cell Biology* **101:** 1–12.

Halme J, Hammond MG, Syrop CH & Talbert LM (1985) Peritoneal macrophages modulate human granulosa–luteal cell progesterone production. *Journal of Clinical Endocrinology and Metabolism* **61:** 912–916.

Hammond JM (1981) Peptide regulators in the ovarian follicle. *Australian Journal of Biological Sciences* **34:** 491–504.

Hedger MP, Robertson DM, Browne CA & de Kretser DM (1985) The isolation and measurement of luteinizing hormone-releasing hormone (LHRH) from rat testis. *Molecular and Cellular Endocrinology* **42:** 163–174.

Hillier SG, van den Boogaard AMJ, Reichart LE Jr & van Hall EV (1980) Alterations in granulosa cell aromatase activity accompanying preovulatory follicular development in the rat ovary with evidence that 5α-induced C_{19} steroids inhibit the aromatase reaction in vitro. *Journal of Endocrinology* **84:** 409–419.

Holmes SD, Lipshultz LI & Smith RG (1984) Regulation of transferrin secretion by human Sertoli cells cultured in the presence or absence of human peritubular cells. *Journal of Clinical Endocrinology and Metabolism* **59:** 1058–1062.

Hutson JC & Stocco DM (1981) Peritubular cell influence on the efficiency of androgen binding protein secretion by Sertoli cells in culture. *Endocrinology* **108:** 1362–1368.

Ingram DL & Mandl AM (1958) The secretion of oestrogen after hypophysectomy. *Journal of Endocrinology* **17:** 13–16.

Janecki A, Jakubowiak A & Lukaszyk A (1985) Stimulatory effect of Sertoli cell secretory products in testosterone secretion by purified Leydig cells in primary culture. *Molecular and Cellular Endocrinology* **42:** 235–243.

Jones RE (1978) Control of follicular selection. In Jones RE (ed.) *The Vertebrate Ovary*, pp 763–788. New York: Plenum Press.

Jutte NHPM, Grootegoed JA, Rommerts FFG & van der Molen HJ (1981) Exogenous lactate is essential for metabolic activity in isolated rat spermatocytes and spermatids. *Journal of Reproduction and Fertility* **62:** 399–405.

Jutte NHPM, Jansen R, Grootegoed JA et al (1982) Regulation of survival of rat pachytene spermatocytes by lactate supply from Sertoli cells. *Journal of Reproduction and Fertility* **65:** 431–438.

Jutte NHPM, Jansen R, Grootegoed JA, Rommerts FFG & van der Molen HJ (1983) FSH stimulation of the production of pyruvate and lactate by rat Sertoli cells may be involved in hormonal regulation of spermatogenesis. *Journal of Reproduction and Fertility* **68:** 219–226.

Kasson B & Hseuh AJW (1986) Arginine vasopressin as an intragonadal hormone in Battleboro rats: presence of a testicular vasopressin like peptide and functional vasopressin receptors. *Endocrinology* **118:** 23–31.

Kasson BG, Meidan R & Hseuh AJW (1985) Identification and characterization of arginine vasopressin-like substances in the rat testis. *Journal of Biological Chemistry* **260:** 5302–5306.

Kerr JB & de Kretser DM (1981) The cytology of the human testis. In Burger HG & de Kretser DM (eds) *The Testis*, pp 141–169. New York: Raven Press.

Kirsch TM, Friedman AC, Vogel RI & Flickinger GL (1981) Macrophages in corpora lutea of mice: characterization and effects on steroid secretion. *Biology of Reproduction* **25:** 629–638.

Kirsch TM, Vogel RL & Flickinger GL (1983) Macrophages: a source of luteotropic cybernins. *Endocrinology* **113:** 1910–1912.

Lacroix M, Parvinen M & Fritz IB (1981) Localisation of testicular plasminogen activator in discrete portions (stage VII & VIII) of the seminiferous tubule. *Biology of Reproduction* **25:** 143–146.

Lalli MF, Tang X-M & Clermont Y (1984) Glycoprotein synthesis in Sertoli cells during the cycle of the seminiferous epithelium of adult rats: a radioautographic study. *Biology of Reproduction* **30:** 493–505.

Leung PCK & Armstrong DT (1980) Interactions of steroids and gonadotrophins in the control of steroidogenesis in the ovarian follicle. *Annual Reviews of Physiology* **42:** 71–82.

Lintern-Moore S, Peters H, Moore GPM & Faber M (1974) Follicular development in the human infant ovary. *Journal of Reproduction and Fertility* **39:** 53–64.

Lipschutz A (1928) New developments in ovarian dynamics and the law of follicular consistency. *Journal of Experimental Biology* **5:** 283–291.

Margioris AN, Liotla AS, Vaudry H, Barden CW & Kreiger DT (1983) Characterization of immunoreactive proopiomelanocortin-related peptides in rat testis. *Endocrinology* **113:** 663.

Mita M, Borland K, Price JM & Hall PF (1985) The influence of insulin and insulin-like growth factor-I on hexose transport by Sertoli cells. *Endocrinology* **116**: 987–992.

Moore GPM, Lintern-Moore S, Peters H & Faber M (1974) RNA synthesis in the mouse oocyte. *Journal of Cell Biology* **60**: 416–422.

Parkes AS (1976) *Patterns of Sexuality and Reproduction*. London: Oxford University Press. 148 pp.

Parvinen M (1982) Regulation of the seminiferous epithelium. *Endocrine Reviews* **3**: 404–417.

Parvinen M & Ruokonen A (1982) Endogenous steroids in the rat seminiferous tubule. Comparison of the stages of the epithelial cycle isolated by transillumination-assisted microdissection. *Journal of Andrology* **3**: 211–220.

Parvinen M, Nikula H & Huhtaniemi I (1984) Influence of rat seminiferous tubules on Leydig cell testosterone production in vitro. *Molecular and Cellular Endocrinology* **37**: 331–336.

Peters H & Braathen B (1973) The effect of unilateral ovariectomy in the neonatal mouse on follicular development. *Journal of Endocrinology* **56**: 85–89.

Peters H & McNatty KP (1980) The ovary: a correlation of structure and function in mammals. London: Paul Elek.

Peters H, Byskov AG, Lintern-Moore S, Faber M & Andersen M (1973a) The effect of gonadotrophin on follicle growth initiation in the neonatal mouse ovary. *Journal of Reproduction and Fertility* **35**: 139–141.

Peters H, Byskov AG, Lintern-Moore S & Faber M (1973b) Follicle growth initiation in the immature mouse ovary: extraovarian or intraovarian control? *Journal of Reproduction and Fertility* **35**: 619–620.

Pincus G & Enzmann EV (1935) The comparative behaviour of mammalian eggs in vivo and in vitro. 1. The activation of ovarian eggs. *Journal of Experimental Medicine* **62**: 665–675.

Reichert LE Jr, Sanzo MA, Fletcher PW, Dias JA & Lee CY (1981) Properties of follicle stimulating hormone binding inhibitors found in physiological fluids. *Advances in Experimental Medicine and Biology* **147**: 135–144.

Richards JS (1980) Maturation of ovarian follicles: actions and interactions of pituitary and ovarian hormones on follicular cell differentiation. *Physiological Reviews* **60**: 51–89.

Ritzen EM (1983) Chemical messengers between Sertoli cells and neighbouring cells. *Journal of Steroid Biochemistry* **19**: 499–504.

Ritzen EM, Boitani C, Parvinen M, French FS & Feldman M (1982) Stage dependant secretion of ABP by rat seminiferous tubules. *Molecular and Cellular Endocrinology* **25**: 25–33.

Roberts AB, Anzano MA, Wakefield LM et al (1985) Type B transforming growth factor: a bifunctional regulator of cell growth. *Proceedings of the National Academy of Sciences (USA)* **82**: 119–123.

Rodgers RJ, O'Shea JD & Findlay JK (1985) Do small and large luteal cells of the sheep interact in the production of progesterone? *Journal of Reproduction and Fertility* **75**: 85–94.

Rozewicki K, Rzepka I, Rozewicki S & Strzelecki E (1979) Menopause after unilateral ovariectomy. *Ginekologia Polska* (supplement): 130–132.

Russell LD & Clermont Y (1977) Degeneration of germ cells in normal, hypophysectomized and hormone treated hypophysectomized rats. *Anatomical Record* **187**: 347–366.

Scaramuzzi RJ & Radford HM (1983) Factors regulating ovulation rate in the ewe. *Journal of Reproduction and Fertility* **69**: 51–89.

Schwall RH, Sawyer HR & Niswender GD (1986) Differential regulation by LH and prostaglandins of steroidogenesis in small and large luteal cells of the ewe. *Journal of Reproduction and Fertility* **76**: 821–829.

Schulze W & Rehder V (1984) Organization and morphogenesis of the human seminiferous epithelium. *Cell and Tissue Research* **237**: 395–407.

Sharpe RM (1984) Intragonadal hormones. *Bibliography of Reproduction* **44**: C1–C16.

Sharpe RM & Bartlett JMS (1985) The intratesticular distribution of testosterone and the relationship to the levels of a peptide that stimulates testosterone production. *Journal of Reproduction and Fertility* **73**: 223–236.

Sharpe RM & Cooper I (1984) Intratesticular secretion of a factor(s) with major stimulatory effects on Leydig cell testosterone secretion in vitro. *Molecular and Cellular Endocrinology* **37**: 159–168.

Sharpe RM, Kerr JB, Fraser HM & Bartlett JMS (1986) Intratesticular factors and testosterone secretion: effect of treatments which alter the level of testosterone within the testis.

Journal of Andrology **7**: 180–189.

Skinner MK & Fritz IB (1985a) Structural characterization of proteoglycans produced by testicular peritubular cells and Sertoli cells. *Journal of Biological Chemistry* **260**: 11874–11883.

Skinner MK & Fritz IB (1985b) Androgen stimulation of Sertoli cell function is enhanced by peritubular cells. *Molecular and Cellular Endocrinology* **40**: 115–122.

Skinner MK & Fritz IB (1985c) Testicular peritubular cells secrete a protein under androgen control that modulates Sertoli cell functions. *Cell Biology* **82**: 114–118.

Skinner MK & Griswold MD (1980) Sertoli cells synthesize and secrete transferrin-like protein. *Journal of Biological Chemistry* **255**: 9523–9525.

Skinner MK & Griswald MD (1983) Sertoli cells synthesize and secrete a ceruloplasmin-like protein. *Biology of Reproduction* **28**: 1225–1229.

Skinner MK, Tung PS & Fritz IB (1985) Cooperativity between Sertoli cells and testicular peritubular cells in the production and deposition of extracellular matrix components. *Journal of Cellular Biology* **100**: 1941–1947.

Sporn MB & Todaro GJ (1980) Autocrine secretion and malignant transformation of cells. *New England Journal of Medicine* **303**: 878–880.

Syed V, Kahn SA & Ritzen GM (1985) Stage specific inhibition of interstitial cell testosterone secretion by rat seminiferous tubules in vitro. *Molecular and Cellular Endocrinology* **40**: 257–264.

Tsafriri A, Dekel N & Bar-Ami S (1982) The role of oocyte maturation inhibitor in follicular regulation of the oocyte maturation. *Journal of Reproduction and Fertility* **64**: 541–551.

Tung PS & Fritz IB (1980) Interaction of Sertoli cells with myoid cells in vitro. *Biology of Reproduction* **23**: 207–217.

Tung PS & Fritz IB (1984) Extracellular matrix promotes rat Sertoli cell mitotypic expression in vitro. *Biology of Reproduction* **30**: 213–229.

Valenca MM & Negro-Vilar A (1986) Proopiomelanocortin-derived peptides in testicular interstitial: characterization and changes in secretion after human chorionic gonadotropin or luteinizing hormone-releasing hormone analog treatment. *Endocrinology* **118**: 32–37.

Valladares LT & Payne AH (1979) Induction of testicular aromatization by luteinizing hormone in mature rats. *Endocrinology* **105**: 431–436.

Verhoeven G & Cailleau J (1985) A factor in spent media from Sertoli cell-enriched cultures that stimulates steroidogenesis in Leydig cells. *Molecular and Cellular Endocrinology* **40**: 57–68.

Wang NG, Sundaram K, Pavlou S et al (1983) Mice are insensitive to the antitesticular effects of luteinizing hormone releasing hormone agonists. *Endocrinology* **112**: 331–335.

Westergaard L, Byskov AG, Yding Anderson C, Grinsted J & McNatty KP (1984) Is resumption of meiosis in the human preovulatory oocyte triggered by a meiosis inducing substance (MIS) in the follicular fluid? *Fertility and Sterility* **41**: 377–384.

Westergaard L, Byskov AG, Van Look PFA et al (1985) Meiosis-inducing substances in human preovulatory follicular fluid related to time of follicle aspiration and to the potential of the oocyte to fertilize and cleave in vitro. *Fertility and Sterility* **44**: 663–667.

World Health Organization (1981) Research on the menopause. *Technical Report Series* No. 679, p 12, Geneva: World Health Organization.

Wright WW, Parvinen M, Musto NA et al (1983) Identification of stage-specific proteins synthesized by rat seminiferous tubules. *Biology of Reproduction* **29**: 257–270.

Yee JB & Hutson JC (1985) Effects of testicular macrophage-conditioned medium on Leydig cells in culture. *Endocrinology* **116**: 2682–2684.

Index

Note: Page numbers of article titles are in **bold** type

Anadur, 119–121
Andriol, *see* Testosterone undecanoate
Androgen binding protein (ABP), 75, 234, 238
Androgens, oral, 116
Antiandrogens, 116–117
Arginine vasopressin (AVP)-like peptides, 283–284
Azoospermia, *see* Spermatogenesis

Bioactive:immunoactive ratios, 157–161, 164–167, 169–172
Blood clotting, and ORT, 196–198
Bone strength, *see* Osteoporosis
Bovine follicular fluid, 89, 91
  and inhibin, 99
Breast cancer, 51, 60–62, 194–195
Bromocriptine, 145
Buserelin, 122–125, 147–148

Calcitonin, 185
Cardiovascular disease, and ORT, 187–188
Clomiphene citrate, 133, 136–139
Clonidine, 182
Contraception—
  and inhibin, 105–106
  with LHRH analogues, 52–55
Corpus luteum, 230–231
Cryptorchidism, 84
Cyproterone acetate, 116–117
Cystic ovaries, 38

Danazol, 119
Deca-Durabolin, 119
Depot medroxyprogesterone acetate, *see* DMPA
DHNT, 119
Dihydronortestosterone, *see* DHNT
Dihydrotestosterone, 74, 75
DMPA, 117–118
Dysmenorrhoea, 58

Endometrial cancer, 191–194

Endometriosis, 55–56
Extracellular matrix, 237

Fibromyomata, 56–57
Flushes, hot, 177–182
Follicle-stimulating hormone (FSH), 31, 35, 39, 40, 45–47, 72, 76–84, 135, 141, 143, 147–148
  and follicular control, 223–229
  and inhibin, **89–112**
  and Sertoli cells, 234–236
Follicles, 224–230
  antral, 226–227
  communication between 227–228
  communication within, 228–230
  preantral, 224–226
Follicular fluid inhibins, 99–101
  bovine, 99
  human, 100
  immunology of, 100–101
  porcine, 99–100
  seminal plasma, 101–102
Follicular phase, of cycle, and IVF, 136–144
Folliculogenesis, 224–230

Gap junction, 214–218
Gestagens, combined with testosterone, 117–118
Glycoproteins, 237
Gonadotrophins, and pulsatility, 1–2
Granulosa cell cultures, and inhibin, 92–93
Growth hormone (GH), 28–29

Heart disease, 51
  and ORT, 187–188
Hirsutism, 58
Human chorionic gonadotrophin (hCG), 77–84, 133–134, 136, 145–146, 153–157
Human follicular fluid, 91
  inhibin, 100
Human menopausal gonadotrophin (hMG), 58–59, 79, 81–83, 136–138, 148
Hypertension, and ORT, 195–196
Hypogonadotrophic hypogonadism, 76–84

244

Hypothalamic–pituitary–testicular axis, **71–87**
  physiology of, 71–75
Hypothalamus, and pituitary gonadotrophin secretion, 72–73

Infertility, female, 35–37
Inhibin, **89–112**
  α-, 102
  β-, 102
  bioassays for, 90–91
  female physiology and, 92–93, 95–97
  in fertility regulation, 105–106
  and FSH, **89–112**
  and IVF, 139–143
  male physiology and, 91–95
  peptides related to, 102–105
  purification of, 97–102
  roles for, 105–106
  subunit A, 100
  subunit B, 100, 103–104
  subunit dimers, 103–105
Insulin-like growth factor-I, 229–230
Ischaemic heart disease, 51
Intragonadal control mechanisms, **223–243**
  ovary, 224–231
  testes, 231–238
In vitro fertilization (IVF), 58–59, **133–152**
  abandoned treatments, 146–148
  follicular phase and, 136–144
  inhibin and, 139–143
  and LH, 143
  luteal phase and, 145–146
  oestradiol, 136–139
  oocytes, 143–145
  progesterone and, 144–145
  prolactin and, 145
IVF, *see In vitro* fertilization

Kallman's syndrome, 82, 180
Ketoconazole, 63

Labour induction, with RU-486, 213–214
Leydig cells, 231–234
  and LHRH, 232–234
LH, 1–14, 72–75, **153–176**
  bioactivity, 157–172
  bioassay for, 153–154
  and follicular control, 223–231
  and infertility, female, 35–37
  and inhibin, 89–91, 95, 97, 140–142
  and IVF, 143
  LHRH, bioactivity, 157–163, 167–172
  in normal women, 35–37
  and oestradiol, 136–137
  structure–function, 154–157
LHRH, 1–14
  in abnormal reproduction function, 37–40
  agonists, and B:I ratio, 159–160

and hot flushes, 180–181
and hypothalamic–pituitary–testicular axis, 72–73
and infertility, female, 35–37
and inhibin, 90, 91, 93, 95, 97, 103, 104
and Leydig cells, 232–234
and LH, bioactivity, 157–163, 167–172
puberty and, 23–25
pulsatility, 1–12
LHRH analogues—
  agonists, in male, 55
  agonists, with testosterone, 121–125
  antagonists, in female, 54
  antagonists, in male, 55
  antagonists, with testosterone, 125
  breast cancer, 61–62
  clinical uses of, **43–70**
    agonists, action, 45–49
    in combination therapy, 49
    in contraception, 52–55
    dosing, 45–48
    implants, 47–48
    side-effects, 49–51
    therapeutic applications, 55–64
  in endometriosis, 55–56
  in fibrinomyomata, 56–57
  in IVF, 58–59
  in menstrual disorders, 58
  in PCO, 58–59
  in PMS, 59–60
  precocious puberty, 62
  in prostate cancer, 62–64
Lipids, and ORT, 198
Liver, and ORT, 195–200
Luteal phase, and IVF, 145–147
Luteinizing hormone, *see* LH
Luteinizing hormone releasing hormone, *see* LHRH

Male fertility control, **113–131**
Medroxyprogesterone acetate, depot, *see* DMPA
Meiosis-inducing substance (MIS), 224, 229
Meiosis-preventing substance (MPS), 224, 229
Menopausal flushes, 64, 177–182
Menopause, and ORT, **177–206**
Menorrhagia, 58
Menstrual cycle, **133–152**
  artificial, 148
  follicular phase of, 136–144
  luteal phase of, 145–146
  physiology of, 133–136
Menstruation, 30–31
  disorders of, 58
Mifepristone, *see* RU-486
Mullerian inhibitory substance (MIS), 89, 103

Naltrexone, 163

19-Nandrolonehexyoxyphenylpropionate,
    see Anadur
Neuropeptide Y, 10–11
19-Nortestosterone, 119–121
19-Nortestosterone decanoate, *see* Deca-
    Durabolin

Oestradiol, and IVF, 136–139
Oestrogen replacement therapy (ORT),
    177–206
    in breast cancer, 194–195
    complications of, 191–200
    in endometrial cancer, 191–194
    hot flushes and, 177–182
    hypertension, 195–196
    lipid metabolism and, 198
    liver, 195–200
    osteoporosis and, 182–187
    psychological disturbances, 189–191
    route of administration and, 198–200
    skin, 189
    thromboembolism, 187–188, 196–198
Oocyte maturation inhibitor (OMI), 229
Oocytes—
    aspiration, 144–145
    in IVF, 143–144
Opioids, and pulsatility, 9–10
Org-30276, 125
Osteoporosis, 51, 182–187
Ovarian cysts, 38–40
Ovary, control, 224–231
    corpus luteum and, 230–231
    folliculogenesis, 224–230
Ovulation rate, 224–230

Parathyroid hormone (PTH), 184–185
Peritubular cells, 237–238
Polycystic ovary syndrome (POC), 58
Porcine follicular fluid, inhibin in, 99–100
Premenstrual syndrome (PMS), 59–60
Progesterone—
    gap junction and, 214–218
    oocyte aspiration, 144–145
Prolactin, 11–13
    and oocyte aspiration, 145
Pro-opiomelanocortin (POMC), 233
Prostaglandins, 211, 214
Prostate cancer, 62–64
Psychological disturbance, and ORT,
    189–191
Puberty, 23–35, 171
    development, 26–29
    disorders, 31–35
    experimental (pulsatile), 25–26
    menstruation and, 30–31
    normal, 24–25
    precocious, 62
Pulsatility, **1–21, 23–41**
    abnormal reproduction, 37–40

gonadal feedback, 4–6
gonadotrophins, 1–2
    and infertility, 35–37
neural mechanisms, 6–9
neuropeptidergic involvement in, 9–11
prolactin secretion, 11–13
and puberty, 23–35

Rat interstitial cell testosterone bioassay, *see*
    RICT
RICT, 153, 154, 157, 159, 167, 171
RS-68439, 125
RU-486 (mifepristone), **207–221**
    clinical uses of, 208–209
    gap junctions and, 214–218
    mechanism of action, 209–213
    parturition induction and, 213–214
    and uterine contraction, 213–218

Seminal plasma, inhibin of, 101–102
Seminiferous tubules, 231–234
Sertoli cells, 234–238
    culture cells, rat, 91–92
    germ cells, 234–237
    peritubular cells, 237–238
Sertoli culture cells, rat, 91–92
Sex hormone binding globulin (SHBG), 74
Skin, and ORT, 189
Spermatogenesis, 231–238
    control of, **71–87, 113–131**
Substance P, 10–11

Tamoxifen, 61, 164, 216
Testes, control, 231–238
    Sertoli–germ cell interactions, 234–237
    Sertoli–peritubular cell interactions,
        237–238
    tubule–Leydig cell interactions, 231–234
Testicular function, gonadotrophin regula-
    tion, 73–75
Testosterone, 71–81
    as cream, 118
    and danazol, 119
    esters, 114, 116
    enanthate, 81, 82, 115, 127
    and gestagens, 117–118
    and LHRH agonist analogues, 121–125
    and LHRH antagonist analogues, 125
    and male fertility control, 114–117
    propionate, 114
    rat interstitial cell bioassay, *see* RICT
    undecanoate (Andriol), 116, 124
Thromboembolism, and ORT, 196–198
Thyrotrophin-releasing hormone (TRH),
    12–13
Transforming growth factor-β, 102–103

Vasoactive intestinal peptide (VIP), 10–13